T0400776

ADVANCED CANCER

MANAGING SYMPTOMS AND QUALITY OF LIFE

HEALTH AND HUMAN DEVELOPMENT

JOAV MERRICK - SERIES EDITOR

NATIONAL INSTITUTE OF CHILD HEALTH AND HUMAN DEVELOPMENT,
MINISTRY OF SOCIAL AFFAIRS, JERUSALEM, ISRAEL

HEALTH AND HUMAN DEVELOPMENT

ADVANCED CANCER

MANAGING SYMPTOMS AND QUALITY OF LIFE

NATALIE PULENZAS
BREANNE LECHNER
NEMICA THAVARAJAH
EDWARD CHOW
AND
JOAV MERRICK
EDITORS

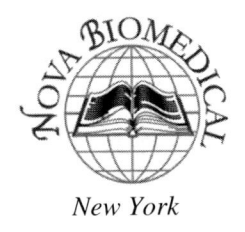

NOVA BIOMEDICAL

New York

For permission to use material from this book please contact us:
Telephone 631-231-7269; Fax 631-231-8175
Web Site: http://www.novapublishers.com

NOTICE TO THE READER

Additional color graphics may be available in the e-book version of this book.

Library of Congress Cataloging-in-Publication Data

ISBN: 978-1-62808-239-5

LCCN: 2013941187

Published by Nova Science Publishers, Inc. † New York

Contents

Introduction

Advanced cancer: Managing symptoms and quality of life in cancer

Natalie Pulenzas Pulenzas, BSc(C)[1], Breanne Lechner, BSc(C)[1]
Nemica Thavarajah, BSc(C)[1], Edward Chow, MBBS 1,
and Joav Merrick, MD, MMedSc, DMSc2,3,4,5

[1]Department of Radiation Oncology, Odette Cancer Centre,
Sunnybrook Health Sciences Centre, University of Toronto, Toronto, Ontario, Canada
[2]National Institute of Child Health and Human Development, Jerusalem, Israel
[3]Office of the Medical Director, Health Services, Division for Intellectual and
Developmental Disabilities, Ministry of Social Affairs and Social Services,
Jerusalem, Israel
[4]Division of Pediatrics, Hadassah Hebrew University Medical Center,
Mt Scopus Campus, Jerusalem, Israel
[5]Kentucky Children's Hospital, University of Kentucky, Lexington, US

Bone metastases are a common event for cancer patients. We have developed an innovative and unique clinical research program dedicated to palliative radiation oncology at the Odette Cancer Centre, Sunnybrook Health Sciences Centre and specifically a multidisciplinary clinic for bone metastases. The development of this program introduces an effective strategy to conduct research in palliative radiation oncology.

Symptom control is very important for the quality of life for bone and brain metastases patients. This is an evolving active field of research as greater emphasis is being placed into understanding the goals of improving not only a patient's survival, but the ability for therapies to improve the quality of a patient's life.

Beyond management and technical research, studies aimed at bettering our understanding of what patients in palliative care face at the end of life are important for the service we need to provide to this population. In particular, some leading research in patient and physician communication with respect to palliative patients, and models to predict survival so that we can better understand when to focus more of symptom control as opposed to cancer control. As cancer patients live longer, we foresee greater efforts in this area of cancer research to better serve our patients at the end of their life.

The concept of quality of life (QOL) is inherently complex since it purposely incorporates a multitude of factors. However, the emphasis on holistic patient care which incorporates QOL has increased. This is evident by the number of health-related QOL measures that have been published in recent times in this field and in particular in cancer related study populations, where the EORTC QLQ-C30 is the most frequently used QOL tool. This measure is a general QOL measure that uses 30 core questions in attempt to assess overall QOL.

Quality of life (QOL) is a subjective, multidimensional measurement that reflects physical symptoms, functional ability, psychosocial aspects and health perceptions of patients. In advanced cancer patients, QOL is often a more meaningful clinical endpoint for clinical trials due to shorter patient life expectancies, whereas traditional endpoints such as survival are less relevant. In most cases, QOL assessments are performed in the form of questionnaires, completed by either the patient themselves, or via proxy.

Bone metastases are a frequent complication of advanced cancer and for example breast and prostate carcinomas commonly metastasize to bone, occurring in their disease trajectory in up to 70% of patients. In addition, 15% to 30% of lung, thyroid, and renal cell carcinomas metastasize to bone. Although the exact incidence of bone metastases is unknown, it is estimated that 70-85% of cancer patients have bone metastases at the time of autopsy. Bone metastases are a common cause of intractable pain as well as skeletal related events. Traditionally, primary outcomes in clinical trials examining bone metastases have focused on objective endpoints of these skeletal related events, such as pathological fractures, spinal cord compression, analgesic use, or hypercalcemia.

Brain metastases are the most common intracranial neoplasm in adults. The majority of brain metastases originate from primary lung (40–50%), breast (15–25%) or skin (5–20%) cancer and occurs in 10–15% of patients with advanced cancer and depending on the location may cause patients to present with a wide range of neurological symptoms including headaches, focal weakness, mental disturbances, behavioural changes, seizures, speech difficulties, and ataxia. While survival and local brain tumour control are important endpoints, quality of life (QOL) is arguably the more relevant given the prognosis of this patient population. In this book we present the EORTC QLQ-C30 questionnaire, which was used in a multi-center study with patients recruited from Edmonton, Alberta, Canada; Kaohsiung, Taiwan; Kerala, India; Nicosia, Cyprus; Sao Paulo, Brazil; Taipei, Taiwan; Tanta, Egypt; and Toronto, Ontario, Canada with brain and bone metastases. It was found that the difficulties bone and brain metastases patients experience are different in several ways. Patients with bone metastases have more pain and reduced physical functioning. However, patients with brain metastases have more severe role functioning deficits. With use of the QLQ-C30, it was also found that there is ambiguity regarding the root of patient issues. Future studies that require more comprehensive disease-specific findings should include disease-specific assessment modules such as the QLQ-BM22 and QLQ-BN20. Important domains such as the minimal clinically important difference should also be established in individual subgroups of patients to assist in clinical trial design.

SECTION ONE: CASE REPORTS

In: Advanced Cancer
Editors: N. Thavarajah, N. Pulenzas, B. Lechner et al.

ISBN: 978-1-62808-239-5
© 2013 Nova Science Publishers, Inc.

Chapter 1

A unique case of long-bone disease responding to radiotherapy alone

Martin Leung, BSc, MD(C)[1], Janet Nguyen, BSc(C)[1],
Joel Rubenstein, MD[2], Edward Chow, MBBS[1],
Lori Holden, MRT(T)[1], Kristopher Dennis, MD[1]
and Florencia Jon MRT(T)[*1]

[1]Departments of Radiation Oncology
[2]Diagnostic Radiology, Odette Cancer Centre,
Sunnybrook Health Sciences Centre, University of Toronto,
Toronto, Ontario, Canada

Abstract

The femur is the most common site for long bone metastases. Complications from long-bone metastases include severe pain, compromised functionality, and most importantly, the possibility of impending pathological fractures. Although radiotherapy is an effective treatment for palliative pain control, surgery is utilized to treat metastatic lesions causing bio-mechanical instabilities. We report a unique case of a breast cancer patient with multiple bony metastases, including an impressive asymptomatic 20cm long lesion in the left femur that did not require surgical intervention. Pre and post radiation treatment was assessed by magnetic resonance imaging (MRI), showing a response to radiotherapy treatment.

---

* Correspondence: Ms Florencia Jon, BSc, MRT (T), Department of Radiation Therapy, Sunnybrook Odette Cancer Centre, 2075 Bayview Ave, Toronto, Ontario, M4N 3M5 Canada. E-mail: Florence.Jon@sunnybrook.ca.

Introduction

Bone metastases commonly occur in breast cancer patients, arising in 20-60% of patients clinically, as well as up to 70-85% at the time of autopsy (1-3). The majority of breast cancer patients with bone metastases have predominantly osteolytic lesions, while approximately 15-20% of them have predominantly osteoblastic lesions (4). Long bones are classified as being longer than they are wide, and mainly grow by elongation of the diaphysis. 3.5% of breast cancer patients develop long-bone metastases, and of those, 88% experience metastases in the femur (5). In long bone metastases, patients typically present with severe pain or biomechanical instability. In extreme cases, pathological fractures may occur, leading to a significant decrease in a patient's quality of life (QoL) and may necessitate surgical treatment (6).

We present a case of a patient with primary breast cancer with metastatic disease in the manubrium, sternum, L4 and L5, and most significantly an impressive 20cm long lesion in the left femur which was asymptomatic and required no surgical intervention.

Case report

A 62 year-old female was diagnosed with left breast cancer in March 2004 in China. Biopsy results determined it was invasive ductal carcinoma which was 3x4cm in size, along with 4/6 lymph nodes that were found to be positive. She underwent mastectomy and chemotherapy shortly afterwards. Unfortunately, she suffered a recurrence in her supraclavicular fossae and left chest wall in 2006, also in China. She was again treated with chemotherapy utilizing Xeloda and Gemcitabine, but this treatment was discontinued in February 2006. Upon discussion with the patient, it was decided she wanted to discontinue chemotherapy and was subsequently treated with Femara.

The patient was initially seen in Canada in August 2007. Her breast cancer biopsy performed in September 2007 showed recurrence of invasive ductal carcinoma, and was negative for estrogen and progesterone receptors as well as for HER2/neu. She showed an improved response to Taxotere treatment. On progression, she was switched to Gemcitabine and Platinol treatment and again showed a complete response. She recurred again on the left chest wall in November 2009 and was referred for consideration of radiotherapy.

She was planned for radical radiation treatment to the left chest wall, supraclavicular, and axillary areas, 5000cGy in 25 fractions. Metastatic work-up performed simultaneously included a bone scan (see figure 1), which showed diffuse regions of increased activity through the mid-diaphysis of the left femur, as well as increased activity in the manubrium. Magnetic resonance imaging (MRI) was recommended for the left femur. The MRI (see figure 2) performed in January 2010 showed an extensive intramedullary lesion measuring approximately 20 cm in length in the left femur. This abnormality corresponded to the area of increased activity on the patient's previous bone scan. Quite astonishing was the fact that the lesion was asymptomatic – the patient showed no pain and had no difficulty walking. The orthopedic surgeon deemed surgery not necessary as there was no impending pathological fracture and no cortical erosion. Subsequently, the patient underwent palliative radiation to the left femur, 3000cGy in 10 fractions in February 2010.

A bone scan and an MRI scan of the left femur were arranged in the following months to evaluate the status of the patient. The bone scan again showed increased activity involving the manubrium and sternum, mild increased activity in the region of L4 and L5, as well as uptake along the left femoral shaft that was not significantly changed compared to the previous scan. The MRI scan showed regression of the large femoral lesion to 17cm (Figure 3), suggesting a response to radiation. As was the case before, the metastatic lesion was asymptomatic. Unfortunately, the patient passed away several months later.

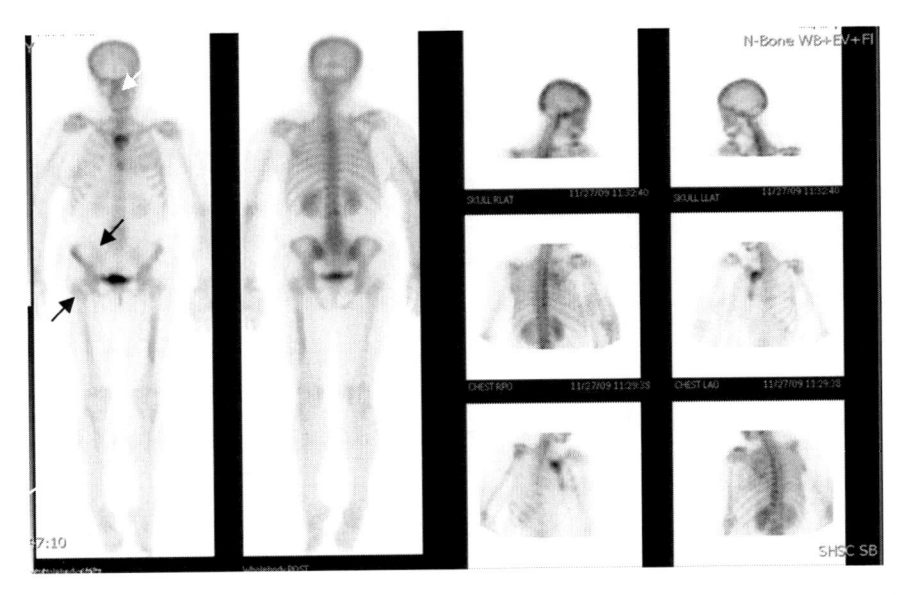

Figure 1. Bone scan (January 2010) showing diffuse regions of increased activity throughout the mid-diaphysis of the left femur (see arrows), as well as increased activity in the manubrium.

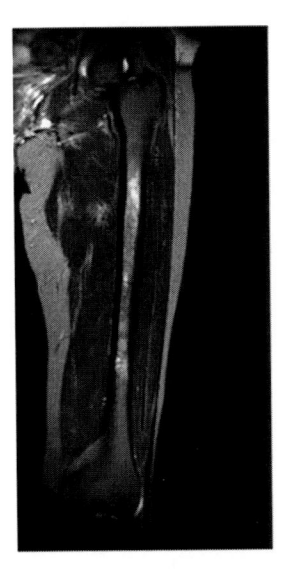

Figure 2. MRI of the left femur (January 2010), showing an extensive intramedullary lesion measuring approximately 20 cm in length extending from the subtrochanteric portion of the femur into the distal third of the femur.

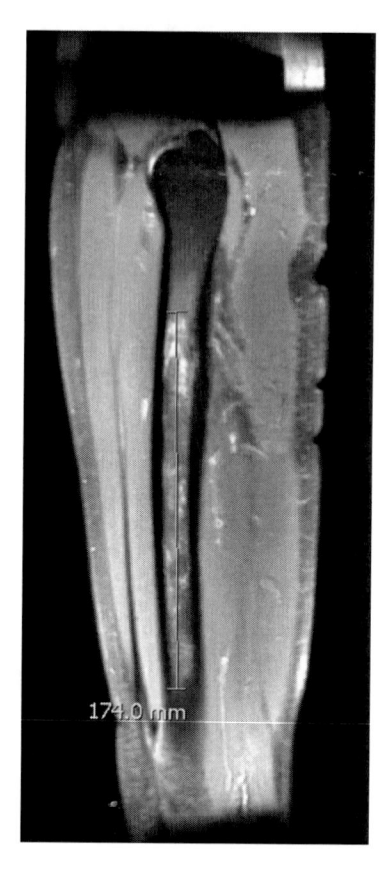

Figure 3. MRI of the left femur (April 2010), again noting an extensive 17cm intramedullary lesion with heterogeneous areas of bright signal intensity on the fluid sensitive images compatible with metastatic disease.

Discussion

Patients with long bone metastases usually present with severe pain or compromised functionality (6). However, in our unique case, there was no clinical manifestation of any symptoms, including pain or compromised functionality, impending pathological fracture, or cortical destruction, thus negating the necessity for surgical stabilization. Fibrous dysplasia can sometimes mimic bone metastases, especially in asymptomatic long length long-bone lesions. However, the presence of multiple concurrent skeletal lesions strongly suggested a diagnosis of metastatic disease in our case (7-8).

Lesions in weight-bearing bones may require prophylactic surgical stabilization. The incidence of post irradiation fracture was detailed by Keene et al (9), who studied metastatic breast carcinoma of the proximal femur. Their group found that 18% of the lesions fractured, while 26% of the lesions showed progression in size. Bunting et al (10) found that 41% of the irradiated lesions fractured. In our case, MRI results suggested improvement following the palliative radiotherapy. In a study performed by Menck et al (11), they defined metastatic measurement ranges requiring prophylactic internal fixation for pathological lesions of the femur. The criteria included ratio between width of metastasis and bone = 0.60 and/or cortical destruction in axial bone length = 13mm in the neck, and = 30mm in other parts of the femur, or involvement of the cortex circumference = 50%. Mirels (12) developed a scoring system to quantify the risk of pathological fractures from metastatic disease in long bones. It included safe irradiation without the risk of fracture for lesions with a score of 7 or lower, while lesions with a score of 8 or higher would require prophylactic internal fixation before irradiation.

Palliative radiation is usually administered for pain relief, and is not utilized for bio-mechanical fixation. Few long-bone lesions approaching the size of that presented here are treated with radiotherapy alone. This specific case demonstrated that administering palliative radiation to a weight-bearing bone can cause regression in an asymptomatic long-bone large lesion post-MRI.

Acknowledgments

We thank the Michael and Karyn Goldstein Cancer Research Fund and Mrs. Stacy Yuen for administrative support.

References

[1]   Beals RK, Lawton GD, Snell WE. Prophylactic internal fixation of the femur in metastatic breast cancer. Cancer 1971;28:1350-4.

[2]   Abrams HL, Spiro R, Goldstein N. Metastases in carcinoma; analysis of 1000 autopsied cases. Cancer 1950;3:74-85.

[3]   Habermann ET, Sachs R, Stern RE, Hirsh DM, Anderson WJ JR. The pathology and treatment of metastatic disease of the femur. Clin Orthop Relat Res 1982;169:70-82.

[4]   Roodman GD. Mechanisms of bone metastasis. N Engl J Med 2004;350:1655-64.

[5]   Knutson CO Spratt JS Jr. The natural history and management of mammary cancer metastatic to the femur. Cancer 1970;26:1199-203.

[6]   Majerovic M, Augustin G, Jelincic Z, Bukovic D, Burcar I, Smud D, et al. Endomedullary radiofrequency ablation of metastatic lesion of the right femur 5 years after primary breast carcinoma: a case report. Coll Antropol 2008;4:1267-9.

[7]   Malawer M. Treatment of metastatic bone disease. Musculoskeletal Cancer Surgery 2001;11:215-30.

[8]   De La Mota J, Bijoy Thomas M, Micaily B, Espaillat-Rijo L, Hernandez E. Polyostotic fibrous dysplasia mimicking bone metastases in a patient with advanced-stage cervical cancer. Gynecol Oncol 2010;116:584-5.

[9]   Keene JS, Sellinger DS, McBeath AA, Engber WD. Metastatic breast cancer in the femur: a search for the lesion at risk of fracture. Clin Orthop 1986;203:282-8.

[10]   Bunting R, Lamont-Havers W, Schweon D, Kliman A. Pathological fracture risk in rehabilitation of patients with bony metastases. Clin Orthop 1985;192:222-7.

[11]   Menck H, Schulze S, Larsen E. Metastasis size in pathologic femoral fractures. Acta Orthop Scand 1988;59:151-4.

[12]   Mirels H. Metastatic disease in long bones. A proposed scoring system for diagnosing impending pathologic fractures. Clin Orthop Relat Res 1989;249:256-64.

In: Advanced Cancer
Editors: N. Thavarajah, N. Pulenzas, B. Lechner et al.

ISBN: 978-1-62808-239-5
© 2013 Nova Science Publishers, Inc.

Chapter 2

Painful sacral insufficiency fracture simulating metastatic disease from primary breast cancer

Florencia Jon, MRT(T)[*,1]*, Janet Nguyen, BSc(C)*[1]*,
Joel Rubenstein, MD*[3]*, Lori Holden, MRT(T)*[1]*, Michelle Ross, RN*[1]*,
Gunita Mitera, MRT(T)*[1]*, Kristopher Dennis, MD*[1]
and Edward Chow, MBBS[1]

[1]Departments of Radiation Oncology
[2]Pathology and [3]Diagnostic Radiology, Sunnybrook Odette Cancer Centre,
University of Toronto, Toronto, Ontario, Canada

Abstract

Patients with sacral insufficiency fracture (SIF), caused by abnormally decreased bone density, often have similar symptoms to those with sacral bone metastases. SIF may often be misdiagnosed particularly in cases where there is a previous history of confirmed malignancy. We present a case of a patient with known breast cancer and persistent pain who was referred for palliative radiation for suspected painful bone metastases. Closer inspection of a previously performed bone scintigraphy revealed only an insufficiency fracture to the sacrum, characterized by its distinct H-shaped pattern. It is essential to differentiate between metastatic disease and insufficiency fractures to ensure prompt and proper treatment is administered.

[*] Correspondence: Ms Florencia Jon, BSc, MRT (T), Department of Radiation Therapy, Sunnybrook Odette Cancer Centre, 2075 Bayview Ave, Toronto, Ontario, M4N 3M5 Canada. Tel: 416-480-4998; Fax: 416-480-6002; Email: Florence.Jon@sunnybrook.ca.

Introduction

Sacral insufficiency fracture (SIF) is a type of stress fracture that occurs during normal stress on a sacrum with abnormally decreased density. It is most commonly found in women older than 60 years old with osteoporosis (1). Patients with a SIF usually complain of lower back and pelvic pain, which simulate those symptoms experienced by patients with pelvic or sacral metastatic disease. As a result of similar symptom presentation, SIF is often overlooked and misdiagnosed in patients with previously confirmed malignancy. Bone scintigraphy, Positron emission tomography-computed-tomography (PET/CT) and Magnetic resonance imaging (MRI) are all useful tools in detecting SIF. The characteristic H-shaped uptake pattern in the bone scan accompanied by no other metastases elsewhere usually represents strong evidence of SIF. This case report will demonstrate the importance of proper diagnosis and awareness of SIF to prevent patient anxiety and inappropriate referrals and treatments.

Case report

An 85 year old woman presented with a three week history of increased confusion, weakness and persistent low back pain, and was referred for consideration of radiation treatment to her lower back. She was admitted to the emergency department at her local hospital with the diagnosis of weakness "Not Yet Diagnosed" (NYD). At 75 years of age she was diagnosed with a node-negative invasive ductal carcinoma of the left breast. She underwent a lumpectomy of her left breast, and was offered no chemotherapy or radiation treatment at that time. Her past surgeries included cholecystectomy, left total knee replacement, tonsillectomy, sinus surgery and cataract removal. Her other medical conditions included osteoarthritis, hypertension, hypercholesterolemia and a lung granuloma. Upon admission, she was prescribed Meloxicam and Tylenol #3 for pain control which was ineffective. With persistent pain that was sufficient enough to limit her mobilization, a bone scan was ordered and showed increased uptake in the sacroiliac joints and sacrum region, highly suggestive of metastatic disease from breast cancer (see figure 1). An MRI was eventually planned to confirm diagnosis, but was rescheduled due to a machine impediment.

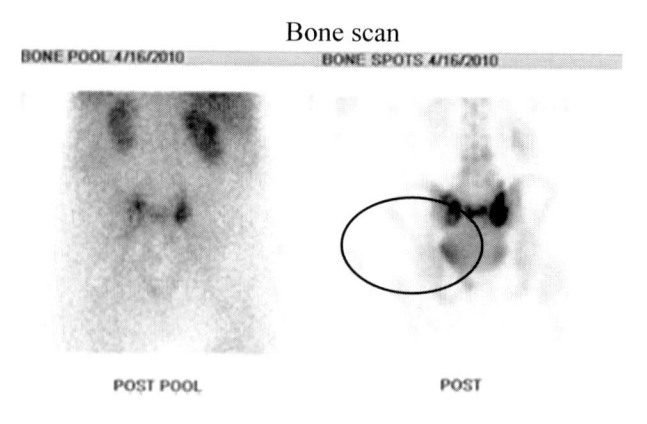

Figure. 1. Note H-shaped increased activity in the sacrum, best appreciated on the posterior scan. (Circle)

CT Lumbar-sacral spine

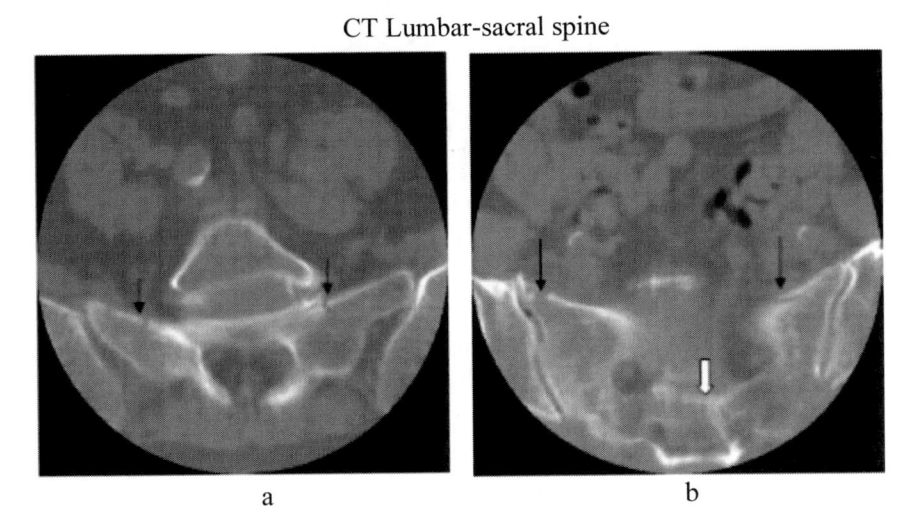

a   b

Figure 2. a) There are discontinuities in the anterior cortex of both sacral alae due to fractures (black arrows). b) Anterior cortical breaks (black arrows) are again seen with linear sclerosis and lucency in both sacral alae, plus horizontal extension across the midline (white arrow).

Other imaging modalities performed included computed tomography (CT) of the lumbar spine and sacrum (see figure 2) with contrast, which suggested advanced degenerative disc disease from L2 to L5, plain radiographs of the hips/pelvis that described early osteoarthritis, and a chest radiograph, CT of the head and a renal imaging study all showing no significant findings. Based on the report of the bone scan suggestive of metastatic disease, the patient was referred for possible pelvic radiation. The goal was for pain relief that was otherwise not controlled with pain medications. Upon arrival, the images were sent for a second opinion since no other imaging previously performed supported the conclusion of sacral metastases. The reviewing radiologist commented that the increased activity that presented in the bone scan was in fact a sacral insufficiency fracture because of the classic H-shaped pattern. The lumbar CT scan also correlated with the bone scan and showed fracture lines at these locations.

With the conclusion from the radiologist that this was not a pathological fracture, the patient was sent back to the referring hospital with the recommendations of referral for orthopedic care as well as a medical oncologist for an opinion regarding possible bone disorders i.e. multiple myeloma. Two weeks after the initial appointment to our clinic, a telephone follow-up was made with the on-call physician at the referring hospital. Due to the patient's poor performance status and general weakness to undergo further investigations, no referral was subsequently made to a medical oncologist, and the patient remained in hospital. As for orthopedic care, the patient was not offered any treatment for her SIF at the present time.

Discussion

Despite the fact that SIF is quite common in the elderly population, the diagnosis of SIF is still often confused with malignant disease in many cases. A case report documented by Lee et al (2) demonstrated the difficulty of diagnosis at early stage of SIF due to lack of trauma history and inadequate information from radiographs. The 69 year old patient underwent extensive laboratory workup as well as both bone scintigraphy and FDG-PET in order to confirm the diagnosis of SIF (2). Tsuchida et al (3) examined the effectiveness of FDG-PET in detecting SIF, in two patients with previous known malignant disease suffering from low back pain at presentation. The PET scan showed increased uptake in the distinct H-sign in the sacral area, and when correlated with CT images, a fracture line was seen under the bone window which corresponded with the FDG uptake. These two patients were diagnosed with SIF instead of metastatic disease. A study by Gotis-Graham et al (4) reviewed clinical records, radiographs, CT and bone scintigraphy to diagnose 20 cases of SIF in a five year period. This study also concluded that bone scan seemed to be the modality of choice to detect SIF, followed by a CT scan. Plain radiographs gave the least information and showed sclerosis in only four out of 20 patients (4).

Maheshwari et al (5) reported that 64% and 43% of patients with SIFs complain of low back and buttock pain, respectively, and 22% were asymptomatic at the time of diagnosis. The authors suggested that the difficulty in recognizing SIFs lays in the fact that findings on routine radiographs are often overlooked because of the overlying bowel shadow and calcification (5). Although bone scintigraphy is sensitive in detecting SIF because of the distinct H-shaped uptake, only up to 45% of sacral insufficiency fractures show this pattern. FDG-PET can be a useful diagnostic tool for bone lesion(s), especially with the classic H-shaped uptake in the sacrum, but may occasionally fail to distinguish whether the lesion is benign or malignant. This is particularly difficult to differentiate in patients with a previous history of malignancy. Fayad et al (6) and Ravenel et al (7) recorded the standardized uptake value (SUV) in their reports of SIF, but different values have been noted, hence SUV cannot be used to distinguish between benign bone lesions and metastatic bony disease. However, according to a study by Fujii at al (8), they reviewed bone scans of 26 patients with suspected SIF retrospectively and found that the H sign and its variant manifested in the scans are quite reliable in detecting SIF. The study showed the diagnostic criteria of the H sign had a 96% sensitivity and 92% positive predictive value (8).

According to Tsuchida et al (3) CT is one of the most useful modalities for the detection of SIF. The bone window of the CT can exhibit the fracture lines directly with the cross sectional images, which are sometimes uncertain on plain radiographs. CT and MRI can also help to confirm the fracture and exclude a destructive process, but a biopsy is sometimes needed to rule out the possibly of malignant tumour (9). As for the case described by Maheshwari et al (5), a biopsy was performed to rule out neoplasm, but it is generally not preferable if radiographs are sufficient to make a diagnosis.

There are some controversies as to which modality is best suited for the diagnosis of SIF. According to Fayad et al (10), MRI is most useful in the distinction of pathological fractures and stress fractures of long bones after inconclusive radiography outcomes; however the usefulness of CT scan is also well documented. Newhouse et al (1) concluded that CT is preferable if there is a need to evaluate an area of concern for osseous destruction. Other literature shows MRI as a more useful imaging technique in the diagnosis of occult insufficiency fractures in the pelvis because it can distinguish between the abnormal and normal bone marrow (9). However, literature also supports FDG-PET and bone scintigraphy to be more reliable in detecting SIF because of the increased uptake in the sacrum area that showed the characteristic H-sign pattern (8,11).

Despite the many discussions on sacral insufficiency fractures, confusion remains surrounding the proper clinical diagnosis of this medical condition. This is especially difficult with patients that have previous malignancy because the presentation of SIF mimics that of metastatic disease. Even though the bone scan showed the H-shaped pattern of SIF and CT lumbar confirmed the fracture lines, the radiologist still commented that the patient has metastatic disease secondary to breast cancer. Coincidentally, because of machine problem, the MRI was not done to confirm diagnosis. Our case study demonstrates the necessity for clinicians to familiarize themselves with the classic characteristics of SIF in order to make prompt and accurate diagnoses. Once sacral insufficiency fracture is diagnosed, conservative treatments such as bed rest along with analgesic medications are usually recommended (4). Sacroplasty is the newly accepted treatment choice, but is not suitable for all patients (2). Follow-up until the resolution of symptoms has taken place is recommended.

Conclusion

Sacral insufficiency fracture is not uncommon in the elderly, yet it is often overlooked. It is very important for clinicians to recognize the presentation of SIF in radiological imaging in order to avoid extensive workup, unnecessary delay of diagnosis and possibly improper treatment. Conservative treatments are usually sufficient to provide good relief of symptoms.

Acknowledgments

We thank the Michael and Karyn Goldstein Cancer Research Fund and Stacy Yuen.

References

[1] Newhouse KE, el-Ljpiru. Buckwalter. Occult sacral fractures in osteopenic patients. J Bone Joint Surg Am 1992;74:1472-7.

[2] Lee YJ, Bong HJ, Kim JT, Chung DS. Sacral insufficiency fracture, usually overlooked cause of lumbosacral pain. J Korean Neurosurg Soc 2008;44:166-9.

[3] Tsuchida T, Kosaka N, Sugimoto K, Itoh H. Sacral insufficiency fracture detected by FDG-PET/CT: Report of 2 cases. Ann Nuclear Med 2006;20(6):445-8.

[4] Gotis-Graham L, McGuigan T, Diamond T, Portek I, Quinn R, Sturgess A, Tulloch R. Sacral insufficiency fractures in the elderly. J Bone Joint Surg 1994;76-B:882-6.

[5] Maheshwari AV, Kounine MM, Soaita M, Kumar D, Pitcher DJ. Osteoporotic insufficiency fractures of the pelvis simulating a malignancy in an elderly man. Am J Orthop 2009;38(2):E45-8.

[6] Ravenel JG, Gordon LL, Pope TL, Reed CE. FDG-PET uptake in occult acute pelvic fracture. Skeletal Radiol 2004;33(2):99-101.

[7] Fayad LM, Cohade C, Wahl RL, Fishman EK. Sacral fractures: a potential pitfall of FDG positron emission tomography. AJR 2003;181:1239–43.

[8] Fujii M, Abe K, Hayashi K, Sosuda S, Yano F, Watanabe S, et al. Honda sign and variants in patients suspected of having a sacral insufficiency fracture. Clin Nuclear Med 2005;30(3):165-9.

[9]	Theodorou SJ, Theodorou DJ, Schweitzer ME, Kakitsubata Y, Resnick D. Magnetic resonance imaging of para-acetabular insufficiency fractures in patients with malignancy. Clin Radiol 2006;61(2):181-90.

[10]	Fayad LM, Kawamoto S, Kamel IR, Bluemke DA, Eng J, Frassica FJ, Fishman EK. Distinction of long bone stress fractures from pathologic fractures on cross-sectional imaging: How successful are we? AJR 2005;185:915-24.

[11]	Halac M, Mut SS, Sonmezoglu K, Yilmaz M, Ozer H, Uslu I. Avoidance of misinterpretation of an FDG positive sacral insufficiency fracture using PET/CT scans in a patient with endometrial cancer: A case report. Clin Nuclear Med 2007;32(10):779-81.

In: Advanced Cancer
Editors: N. Thavarajah, N. Pulenzas, B. Lechner et al.

ISBN: 978-1-62808-239-5
© 2013 Nova Science Publishers, Inc.

Chapter 3

Pathological fracture of the tibia in a patient with invasive ductal carcinoma of the breast: A case report of a rare finding

Esther Chan, MD(C), Florencia Jon, MRT(T),
Lori Holden, MRT (T), Kristopher Dennis, MD
and Edward Chow, MBBS*

Rapid Response Radiotherapy Program, Department of Radiation Oncology,
Odette Cancer Centre, Sunnybrook Health Sciences Centre,
University of Toronto, Toronto, Ontario, Canada

Abstract

While bone metastases are common among patients with cancer, metastases to the tibia are rare. The present report describes the case of a 57-year-old woman with invasive ductal carcinoma of the breast who presented with a pathological tibial fracture. She had just recently complained of bone pain and been diagnosed with diffuse metastatic disease despite a 7-year disease-free interval following her primary treatment. Bone metastases cause significant morbidity and negatively impact overall quality of life. This report highlights the importance of a thorough work-up using clinical skills which have been shown to be the most successful tools for identifying bone metastases during follow-up visits in patients with known malignancy. Early diagnosis allows physicians to employ proven prophylactic treatments which help to prevent pathological fractures and other complications of bone metastases, ultimately preventing further declines in overall quality of life.

---

* Correspondence: Edward Chow, MBBS, MSc, PhD, FRCPC, Department of Radiation Oncology, Odette Cancer Centre, Sunnybrook Health Sciences Centre, 2075 Bayview Avenue, Toronto, ON, Canada, M4N3M5, Canada, Tel: (416) 480-4998, Fax: (416) 480-6002; E-mail: Edward.Chow@sunnybrook.ca.

Introduction

Since 1991, approximately 23,000 new cases of breast cancer have been diagnosed in Canada every year (1). While the lifetime risk of developing breast cancer has been steadily decreasing, 1 in 9 Canadian women will still develop breast cancer, making it the most commonly diagnosed female cancer (1). Depending on the prognostic factors associated with a given woman's disease, 30-70% of primary breast cancer metastasize (2). Metastatic breast cancer has an affinity for spreading to the bones (3). The majority of these localize to the axial skeleton while bone metastases that occur distal to the elbows and knees are rare (4). However, as survival times of primary breast cancer patients continue to improve, the incidence of these rare metastases will increase, creating a new challenge for physicians to recognize in clinical practice. It is with this in mind that we present an uncommon case of metastatic disease to the tibia that presented in a woman seven years following her primary treatment for an invasive ductal carcinoma of the breast. From this report we hope to improve clinical awareness of below-knee metastases in patients with breast cancer.

Case report

A 57-year-old Caucasian woman with a history of breast carcinoma presented to her medical oncologist with a 6-week history of bilateral pain centred over her sacroiliac (SI) joints. The pain was new and began with the introduction of a new swimming regimen. She also related a history of left leg numbness but denied any pain, weakness or functional impairment and was otherwise healthy and active. She had a history of a left-sided, grade 3, invasive ductal carcinoma that was treated 7 years prior with lumpectomy and adjuvant breast radiotherapy, Taxol-based chemotherapy, Tamoxifen and Aromasin, and was currently enrolled in a clinical trial of extended adjuvant Letrozole vs. placebo.

Although the bilateral nature of the pain, the change in exercise patterns and her post-menopausal status suggested the cause of her symptoms could be either degenerative change or osteoarthritis, given her history of breast cancer imaging was organised. A CT scan of her pelvis unfortunately revealed bilateral bone metastases in the region of her sacroiliac joints which accounted for her symptoms. Subsequent CT scans of her hips, abdomen, chest, head and a bone scan (Figure 1) were performed. These revealed extensive visceral and bony metastatic disease, including a mixed sclerotic-lytic lesion in her right tibial diametaphysis which was entirely asymptomatic.

Despite the extensive nature of her disease, she felt well aside from the before mentioned symptoms until she sustained a pathological fracture at the site of the tibial metastasis while walking down the stairs in her home (see figure 1a). This occurred only 3 days following the bone scan that identified that asymptomatic tibial lesion. She was subsequently admitted to hospital where she was assessed by the orthopaedic surgery service and was also seen in our outpatient palliative radiotherapy clinic. She underwent open reduction and internal fixation using a proximal tibial locking plate (see figure 1b) and was scheduled to begin post-operative radiotherapy (20Gy in 5 fractions) in the hope of reducing her risk of local recurrence and promoting bone repair.

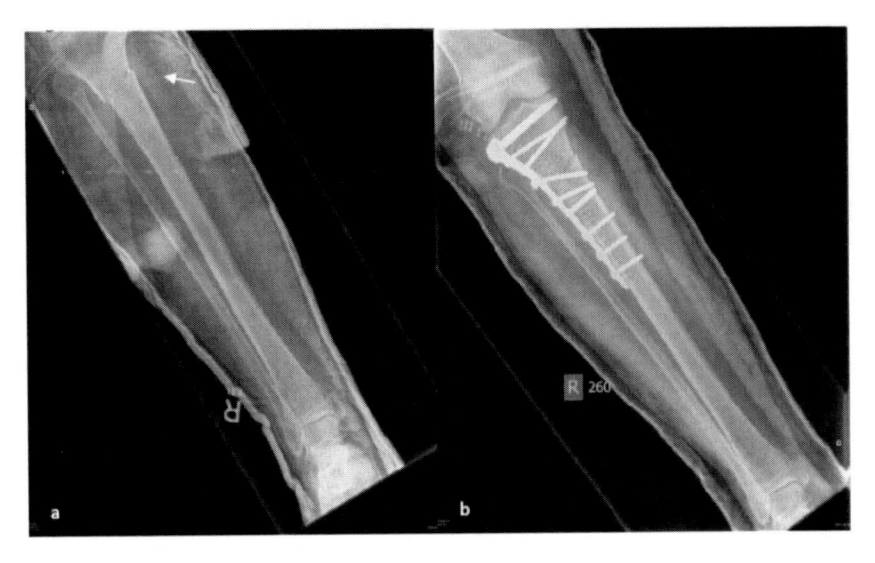

Figure 1a. Plain radiograph anteroposterior view of the right leg. There is a fracture in proximal tibia diametaphysis with slight medial displacement (see white arrow). 1b: Plain radiograph anteroposterior view of the same right leg following open reduction and internal fixation with a proximal locking plate.

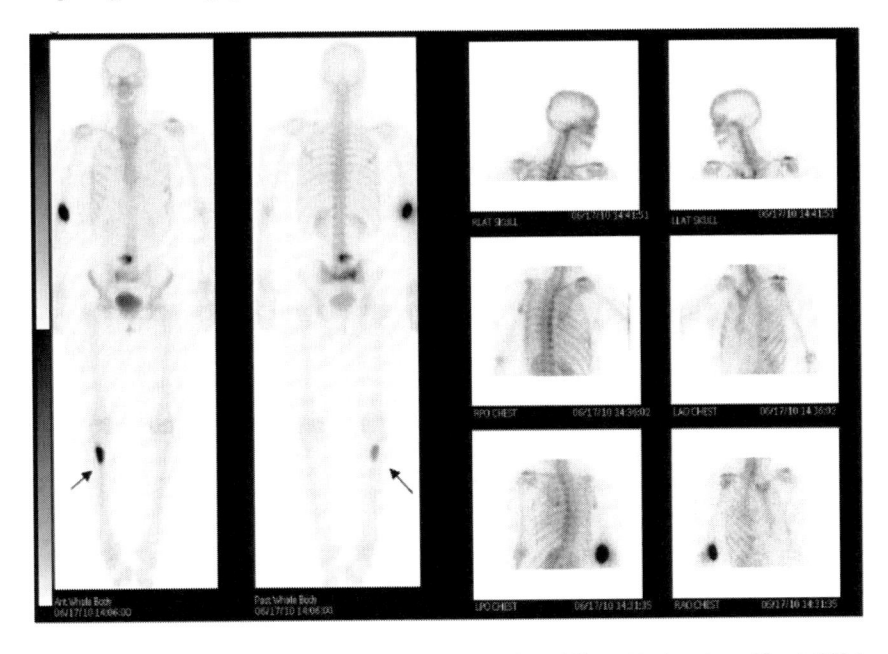

Figure 2. Whole body and right and left anterior and posterior oblique Technetium-99m-MDP bone scans views (see black arrow). In the whole body view, tracer localizes to the right proximal tibia where there is metastatic bone disease. Sacral promontory metastases are also visible.

Discussion

Metastatic breast cancer most commonly affects the skeletal system and like most bone metastases from other sites, breast cancer metastases tend to locate in the axial skeleton. In a review of seven autopsy series, approximately 71% of patients with breast carcinoma were found to have metastatic bone disease at the time of death (5). Of these, 67% and 62% of the metastases developed in the vertebrae and the pelvis compared to the only 3% that affected the tibia (5). Thus, although skeletal metastases are a fairly common finding in breast cancer patients, disease within the tibia similar to that in the present case is rare. Since 1981, breast cancer survival has been steadily increasing and age-adjusted mortality rates from breast cancer are at an all time low (1). As a result of prolonged survival following breast cancer treatment, physicians have an increasing chance of encountering tibial metastases in clinical practice. In order to decrease the morbidity associated with these dangerous bone metastases and provide appropriate care, they must also be able to recognize and diagnose these uncommon lesions in addition to the more common lesions within the vertebrae and pelvis when suspecting metastatic disease in patients with a history of breast cancer.

Detecting skeletal metastases

Although the primary disease may be treated successfully, the risk of breast cancer recurrence can continue for 15 years following initial diagnosis (6). During this time, patients are recommended to have regular follow-up visits with their oncologist or family physician who will collect a history, perform a breast examination, and order a diagnostic mammogram (6). While the majority of these clinical exams are focused on detecting local recurrences, physicians collect valuable information during the history about symptoms that may alert them to metastatic disease. While empiric bone scintigraphy and x-rays are highly sensitive tests for identifying bone metastases, studies have shown that a detailed history and physical exam are still the best tools for detecting secondary bone disease during follow-up visits (7, 8). In a retrospective study evaluating various clinical tests used to identify recurrent disease, the authors found that 66% of bone metastases from breast cancer were detected by the history and physical alone (8). Thus, clinical skills are able to identify the majority of bone metastases. This is not surprising as pain is usually the first symptom of bone disease (9). In a study examining the first signs of recurrent disease, 404 out of 425 patients with metastatic bone disease were symptomatic (7). Therefore, the majority of metastatic bone cancer recurrences should be recognizable during history taking. Moreover, these studies showed that scintigraphs performed during routine follow-ups do not contribute to identifying significantly more cases of bone metastases. Of the 238 scintigraphs performed during routine follow-up in the previous study, only an additional 6% of bone metastases were detected (8). While bone scans are very successful at confirming bony lesions in patients with a history of pain, they require long wait times to attain and may cause toxicity in patients with renal disease. Therefore, a thorough history and physical examination are still arguably the most efficient tools for identifying bone metastases during follow-up visits. Although the patient in our case did not have symptoms from her tibial metastasis prior to her fracture, her six week history of pain centered over her sacroiliac joint prompted her doctor to order a pelvic CT. Due to metastatic disease found on her pelvic CT, subsequent radiographs and bone scans were performed revealing tibial metastases. If attention were not paid to her reported lower back pain, then the bone scan would not have been ordered and her tibial metastasis would have remained undetected. Case reports such as these that emphasize the importance of clinical skills will hopefully aid physicians in the early detection of bone metastases and prevention of debilitating fractures.

Morbidity, survival, and influences on quality of life

Metastatic breast cancer (MBC) is generally considered an incurable disease (10). Metastatic bone disease results in a substantial amount of morbidity thereby negatively impacting patients' quality of life. Most skeletal morbidity result from skeletal related events and include: pain, the need for radiotherapy and/or surgery to treat the pain, hypercalcemia, pathologic fracture, and spinal cord compression (9). Symptoms of these events, such as, bone pain or fatigue, anorexia and constipation associated with hypercalcemia (11), have been identified in quality of life studies to independently and significantly impact overall quality of life; the greater symptoms these patients have, the worse their overall quality of life (12). Moreover, debilitating pathological fractures and paralysis associated with spinal cord compression reduced mobility and limit physical functionality, also affecting overall quality of life (12). Yet, while their skeletal morbidity greatly impairs their quality of life, patients with metastatic bone disease have been observed to have longer survival times following diagnosis of metastatic disease (10,13, 14) compared to those with visceral metastases. Studies examining survival of metastatic breast cancer patients also show an increasing trend in overall survival time that has changed from a median of 18 months to 23.6 months between 1983-2001 (10) and studies of treated patients with hormone-receptor positive breast cancer report survival times as high as 45 months (14). Thus, patients with metastatic breast cancer affecting the bones are living for longer periods of time with symptomatic skeletal morbidities. Detecting these skeletal metastases is essential for providing appropriate palliative care. Early clinical studies have shown that treatments with bisphosphonates, Taxol-based chemotherapy, hematopoietic colony-stimulating factors, and antibiotics are successful for improving pain and managing drug toxicities (9-11, 14). Moreover, early recognition and diagnosis is imperative for the use of non-systemic treatments like prophylactic radiation treatment (9) or surgery (11) in order to prevent high-risk lesions from progressing to pathological fractures. Because breast cancer is highly associated with pathological fractures (11) and long bones and weight bearing bones are at greatest risk of fracturing (11), early recognition of tibial metastases is necessary in order to provide pre-emptive care and maintain these patients' quality of life.

Conclusion

Although distal skeletal metastases to sites such as the tibia are rare, the high prevalence of breast cancer and prolonged survival following diagnosis of primary and secondary disease means that oncologists and family physicians will increasingly encounter patients with these lesions in practice. Attention and awareness to the possibility of distal skeletal metastases is necessary in order to utilize the most successful tools for initially detecting this type of bone disease: clinical history and physical examination. From these exams a history of skeletal related pain can be identified and the possibility of metastases may be confirmed with x-rays and bone scans. There is a need for early identification of bone metastases to make use of prophylactic treatments and deliver appropriate palliative care. By providing appropriate treatment, physicians can prevent complications due to skeletal related events and help patients with metastatic breast cancer preserve their overall quality of life. We hope we may increase awareness of uncommon tibial metastases.

Acknowledgments

We thank the Michael and Karyn Goldstein Cancer Research Fund and Mrs. Stacy Yuen for administrative support.

References

[1]   Canadian Cancer Society's Steering Committee: Canadian Cancer Statistics 2010. Toronto: Canadian Cancer Society, 2010.

[2]   Cardoso F, Castiglione M. Clinical recommendations for diagnosis, treatment, and follow-up. Ann Oncol 2009;20:15-8.

[3]   Coleman RE, Rubens RD. The clinical course of bone metastases from breast cancer. Br J Cancer 1987;55:61-6.

[4]   Leeson MC, Makley JT, Carter JR. Metastatic skeletal disease distal to the elbow and knee. Clin Orthopaedics Relat Res 1986;206:94-9.

[5]   Lee Y-TN. Breast carcinoma: Pattern of metastasis at autopsy. J Surg Oncol 1983;23:175-80.

[6]   Khatcheressian JL, Wolff AC, Smith TJ, Grunfeld E, Muss HB, Vogel VG, et al. American Society of Clinical Oncology 2006 update of breast cancer follow-up and management guidelines in the adjuvant setting. J Clin Oncol 2006;24:5091-7.

[7]   Pivot X, Asmar L, Hortobagyi GN, Theriault R, Pastorini F, Buzdar A. A retrosepctive study of first indicators of breast cancer recurrence. Oncology 2000;58:185-90.

[8]   Cowan JD, and Kies MS. Detection of recurrent breast cancer. South Med J 1981;74:910-12.

[9]   Chow E, Finkelstein JA, Coleman RE. Metastatic cancer to the bone. In: Devita V, Hellman S, Rosenberg S, eds. Cancer: Principals and practice of oncology. Philadelphia, PA: Lippincott Williams Wilkins, 2009:2510-22.

[10]   Gennari A, Conte P, Rosso R, Orlandini C, Bruzzi P. Survival of metastatic breast carcinoma patients over a 20-year period. Cancer 2005;104:1742-50.

[11]   Coleman RE. Clinical features of metastatic bone disease and risk of skeletal morbidity. Clin Cancer Res 2006;12:6243-9.

[12]   Cassie A, Culleton S, Nguyen J, Zhang L, Zeng L, Holden L, et al. What QLQ-C15-PAL symptoms matter most for overall quality of life in patients with advanced cancer? Manuscript in print. Toronto:ON: Sunnybrook Hosp, Univ Toronto, 2010.

[13]   Plunkett T, Smith P, Rubens R. Risk of complications from bone metastases in breast cancer: implications for management. Eur J Cancer 2000;36:476-82.

[14]   Andre F, Slimane K, Bachelot T, Dunant A, Namer M, Barrelier A, et al. Breast cancer with synchronous metastases: Trends in survival during a 14-year period. J Clin Oncol 2004;22:3302-8.

In: Advanced Cancer
ISBN: 978-1-62808-239-5
Editors: N. Thavarajah, N. Pulenzas, B. Lechner et al.   © 2013 Nova Science Publishers, Inc.

Chapter 4

Renal mass – primary or metastatic? The search for a definitive diagnosis

Justin Kwong, BSc(C)[1], Florencia Jon, MRT(T)[*,1],
Linda Sugar, MD[2], Bonnie O'Hayon, MD[3], Lori Holden, MRT(T)[1],
Janet Nguyen, BSc(C)[1], Michelle Ross, RN[1], Cassandra Uy,
MD(C)[1], Luluel Khan, MD[1], Kristopher Dennis, MD[1]
and Edward Chow, MBBS[1]

[1]Departments of Radiation Oncology,
[2]Pathology and [3]Diagnostic Radiology, Sunnybrook Odette Cancer Centre,
University of Toronto, Toronto, Ontario, Canada

Abstract

Although renal cell carcinoma and renal metastases usually have unique characteristics on CT imaging, without documented evidence of primary disease progression and/or widespread metastases elsewhere in the body, it is impossible to differentiate the two with certainty without biopsy as renal metastases in a patient with a known history of cancer can easily mimic renal cell carcinomas on imaging. Here, we report a case of a patient with known adenocarcinoma of the lung who presented with a large renal mass radiologically compatible with a new primary renal cell carcinoma. Interestingly, however, a fine needle aspiration of the renal mass showed features compatible with metastases from lung adenocarcinoma. This case demonstrates the necessity of a biopsy to definitively differentiate renal cell carcinoma from metastases to ensure that appropriate therapeutic management is conducted.

[*] Correspondence: Ms Florencia Jon, BSc, MRT (T), Department of Radiation Therapy, Sunnybrook Odette Cancer Centre, 2075 Bayview Ave, Toronto, Ontario, M4N 3M5 Canada. Tel: 416-480-4998; Fax: 416-480-6002; Email: Florence.Jon@sunnybrook.ca.

Introduction

Two percent of all cancer patients are diagnosed with renal cell carcinoma (1). With the widespread use of imaging modalities, most renal masses are incidentally discovered in asymptomatic patients. Most patients with renal masses do not present with any kidney-related symptoms, including hematuria and pain. Definitive diagnosis of a renal mass as a primary tumor or metastatic lesion is required in order to deliver optimal therapeutic management. Without radiographic evidence of primary disease progression over time or pre-existing extra-renal metastases, it is difficult to differentiate between primary and secondary renal lesions unless histopathological confirmation is obtained. Although highly sensitive, computed tomography (CT) does not suffice as a tool for definitive diagnosis of disease. Herein we present the case of a patient with radiological evidence of a new primary renal cell carcinoma that was later found to be a renal metastasis from a primary lung adenocarcinoma following biopsy of the lesion.

Case report

A 64 year old female was diagnosed with lung adenocarcinoma in 2008 and subsequently underwent left pneumonectomy. After surgery, the patient was given adjuvant Cisplatin and Vinorelbine which ended in April 2009, and Pemetrexed which ended in March 2010. The patient had not received any previous radiation. Towards the end of April, 2010, she was referred to the Rapid Response Radiotherapy Program (RRRP) of Sunnybrook Odette Cancer Centre due to hematuria and pain along the right flank with a worst pain score of 7/10 in the previous 24 hours. The patient previously required blood transfusion on two occasions to compensate for blood loss. Ultrasound of the abdomen, performed February 2010, revealed that gall bladder, bile ducts, left kidney, spleen, aorta and inferior vena cava (IVC) were unremarkable. CT scan of Chest/Abdomen/Pelvis, performed March 2010, revealed a large right renal mass measuring 6.65x8.14cm (Figure 1). The appearance of a liver mass, measuring 4.4x3.8cm, in the posterior segment of the liver was compatible with residual disease from a previous fungal infection of the liver. There was no bony destruction and the spleen, pancreas, left kidney and left adrenal appeared grossly normal. There were three small nodules in the right lower lobe, measuring approximately 3mm, 3mm and 5mm.

On the CT scan, it appeared that the renal mass was a new primary for which palliative radiotherapy (RT) would not have been the preferred treatment. Further opinion was sought from two Radiation Oncologists, specializing in both lung and genitourinary tract cancers, who thought that the kidney mass might in fact be a new primary, so the patient was referred to the Urology service for consideration of surgical resection. The patient was then referred for an assessment by Urology in Sunnybrook for a second opinion and consideration of surgical resection.

Further inquiry revealed she had undergone fine needle aspiration of the renal mass in October 2009. The diagnosis was adenocarcinoma, consistent with a metastasis from a lung primary. By immunohistochemistry, the tumour was CK7 positive, focally CEA positive, CD10 negative and TTF-1 negative. The morphology was very similar to that previously seen in the patient's primary lung tumour (Figure 2 and 3).

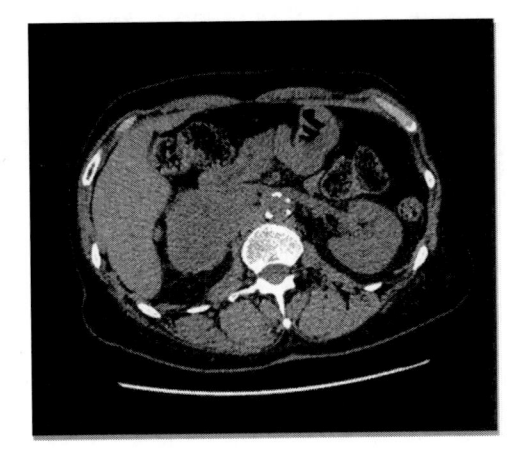

Figure 1. Unenhanced axial CT suggesting gross infiltration of right kidney and renal hilum.

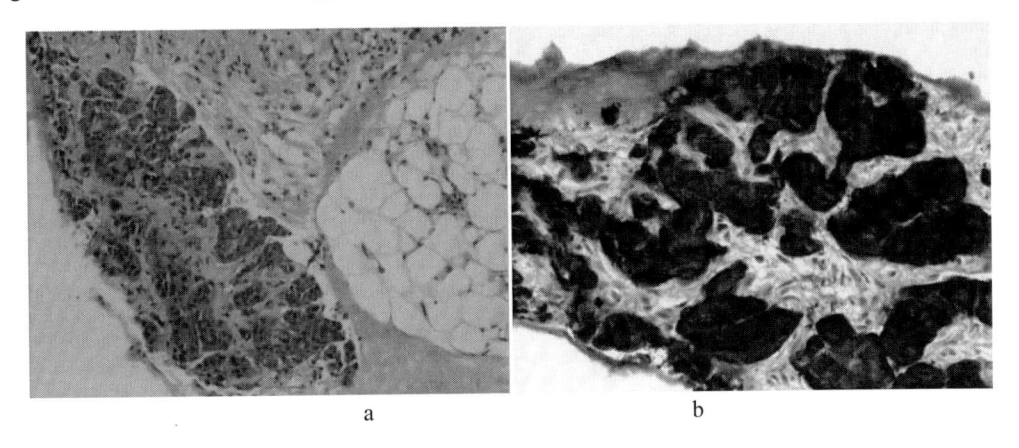

a   b

Figure 2. Renal tumour biopsy: a) There are nests and cords of cells with round to oval nuclei, prominent nucleoli and abundant amphophilic cytoplasm. b) CK7 shows diffuse strong cytoplasmic staining.

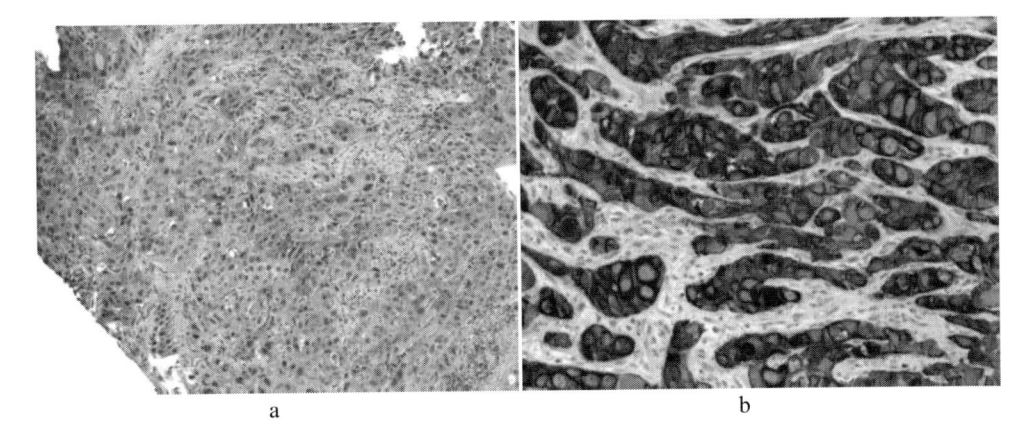

a   b

Figure 3. Lung biopsy: a) There are nests and cords of cells with round to oval nuclei, prominent single or multiple nucleoli, and abundant amphophilic cytoplasm. Focally there is gland formation. b) CK7 shows strong diffuse cytoplasmic staining.

The Urology service deemed the patient a poor surgical candidate due to the large size of the kidney mass. The next day, the patient was started on palliative RT with 2000cGy in five fractions directed to the right renal mass. She was premedicated with Ondansetron 8mg PO BID to prevent nausea and vomiting. At 3-weeks post-radiation during a telephone follow-up interview, the patient reported that her hematuria had ceased and she had but mild fatigue as a result of radiotherapy.

Discussion

The occurrence of renal carcinoma as a second primary is 4.5 times more common than the occurrence of a renal metastasis (2). When renal metastases occur, they most commonly originate from primary tumours in the lung followed by breast, stomach, melanoma and contralateral kidney. Other origins include carcinomas of the colon, ovaria, uterus and prostate (3). The symptoms of renal metastases, which include hematuria and pain, are often clinically silent and arise in only 20% of patients (4,5). For this reason, clinical identification of symptoms of renal metastases from lung carcinoma is rare (6). In contrast, renal metastases are frequently discovered post-mortem, during autopsy (7). As well, small renal masses are often reported incidentally due to the widespread use of imaging modalities (3).

Although rare, some patients may present with hematuria and pain corresponding to an enlarged renal mass on a CT scan. At this point, physicians are faced with the task of determining radiologically if the renal mass is a new primary or metastases.

Our patient presented with the appearance of another primary renal cell carcinoma while it was in fact biopsy proven renal metastases. According to features of renal cell carcinoma found in the relevant literature, the patient's images did indeed suggest that the renal mass was a new primary.

Firstly, our patient's renal mass was 6.65x8.14cm which is characteristic in size of a new primary. Most metastases are <3cm while primary renal masses are typically >6cm (8). The size of metastatic masses typically ranges from microscopic to several millimeters and only rarely are they larger than 3cm (9-11).

Secondly, renal metastases typically occur in patients with widespread metastatic disease and not in those with controlled or limited metastases, as present in our patient (4,12,13). Renal metastases are typically diffuse and bilateral (14). As well, among patients with cancer metastatic to the kidney, only 10% have isolated renal metastases (13). In our patient, the only other lesion suspicious for metastases was within the liver which also appeared compatible with a residual fungal infection.

A study by Prkacin et al (3) established criteria to differentiate renal cell carcinomas from metastases. After retrospectively reviewing 25 cases of kidney neoplasms, fourteen CT characteristics were chosen to characterize renal masses: bilateralism, number, location, size, shape, margin, calcification, involvement of the renal vein, involvement of collecting system, hydronephrosis, perirenal extension, attenuation, thickening of Gerota's fascia and lymphadenopathy. The characteristics of our patient's renal mass included: unilateral, one mass, 6.1-9cm, and round; all of which according to Prkacin et al's criteria indicate renal cell carcinoma. Renal metastases are typically small, multicentric and bilateral although less than 2% of renal cell carcinomas may have these characteristics (13).

With technological advancement, the increased use of computed tomography may lead to an increased frequency of radiological detection of renal masses. Although renal cell carcinomas and metastases usually display unique radiological features, metastases may mimic renal cell carcinomas. Angiomyolipoma, lymphoma, renal anomalies and other pseudotumors can also mimic renal cell carcinoma (15). As confirmed by this case report, however, one cannot always rely on a CT scan to provide the definitive diagnosis for a renal mass. For this, a biopsy is required. This is affirmed by Choyke et al (13) who claimed that without evidence of primary disease progression and/or widespread metastases elsewhere in the body, it is impossible to differentiate renal metastases from renal cell carcinoma without histopathological evidence. Although radiological images may indicate a probable diagnosis, biopsy is required for definitive diagnosis (8).

Accuracy of diagnosis is essential for the arrangement of optimal therapeutic management and to avoid needless surgery. Uzal et al (6) indicated that patients with renal metastases could expect better treatment response and survival so long as optimal treatment was administered. Randomised trials showed that cisplatin-based chemotherapy may improve short-term survival in patients with renal metastases, especially in patients with limited sites of distant metastases (16). In patients with renal carcinoma, nephrectomy was indicated, while this was not the case for patients with renal metastases (3). In contrast, radiotherapy and chemotherapy are not appropriate for first-line management of early-stage localized renal cell carcinoma, but can often be useful for disseminated metastatic disease.

Due to its high sensitivity, CT imaging is considered the most precise imaging modality to identify renal masses. To ensure optimal treatment for patients with secondary renal cell carcinoma or metastases, the only method to achieve definitive diagnosis is via biopsy (13).

Acknowledgments

We thank the Michael and Karyn Goldstein Cancer Research Fund and Stacy Yuen.

References

[1] Paglino C, Imarisio I, Rovereto B. Epidemiology, molecular epidemiology, and risk factors for renal cell carcinoma. Oncol Rev 2007;1:120-7.

[2] Pagani JJ, Bernardino ME. Incidence and significance of serendipitous CT findings in the oncologic patient. J Comput Assist Tomogr 1982;6:268-75.

[3] Prkacin I, Naumovski-Mihalic S, Dabo N, Palcic I, Vujanic S, Babic Z. Comparison of CT analyses of primary renal cell carcinoma and of metastatic neoplasms fo the kidney. Radiol Oncol 2001;35(2):105-10.

[4] Mitnick JS, Bosniak MA, Rotherberg B, Megibow AJ, Raghavendra BN, Subramanyam BR. Metastatic neoplasm to the kidney studied by computed tomography and sonography. J Comput Assist Tomogr 1985;9:43-9.

[5] Honda H, Coffman CE, Berbaum KS, Barloon TJ, Masuda K. CT analysis of metastatic neoplasms of the kidney. Acta Radiol 1992;33:29-44.

[6] Uzal MC, Kocak Z, Uygun K, Altaner S, Gozen S, Unlu E. A case of isolated bilateral renal metastases from carcinoma of the lung. Turk J Cancer 2004;34(2):81-4.

[7]   Becker WE, Schellhammer PF. Renal metastases from carcinoma of the lung. Br J Urol 1986;58:
        494-8.
[8]   Pagani JJ. Solid renal mass in the cancer patient: second primary renal cell carcinoma versus renal
        metastasis. J Comput Assist Tomogr 1983;7(3):444-8.
[9]   Klinger ME. Secondary tumors of the genitourinary tract. J Urol 1951;65:144-53.
[10]   Newsam JE, Tulloch WS. Metastatic tumors in the kidney. Br J Urol 1966;38:1-6.
[11]   Bosniak MA, Stern W, Lopez F, Tehranian N, O'Connor SJ. Metastatic neoplasm to the kidney.
        Radiology 1969;92:989-93.
[12]   Pickhardt PJ, Lonergan GJ, Davis CJ, Kashitani N, Wagner BJ. From the archives of the AFIP:
        infiltrative renal lesions – radiologic-pathologic correlation. RadioGraphics 2000; 20:215-43.
[13]   Choyke PL, White EM, Zeman RK, Jaffe MH, Clark LR. Renal metastases: clinicopathologic and
        radiologic correlation. Radiology 1987;162:359-63.
[14]   Richmond J, Sherman RS, Diamond HD, Craver LF. Renal lesions associated with malignant
        lymphomas. Am J Med 1962;32:184-97.
[15]   Israel GM, Bosniak MA. How I do it: evaluating renal masses. Radiology 2005;236:441-50.
[16]   Weick JK, Crowley J, Natale RB, Hom BL, Rivkin S, Coltman CA, Taylor SA, Livingston RB. A
        Randomized trial of five cisplatin-containing treatments in patients with metastatic non-small-cell lung
        cancer: a southwest oncology group study. J Clin Oncol 1991;9:1157-62.

In: Advanced Cancer
Editors: N. Thavarajah, N. Pulenzas, B. Lechner et al.

ISBN: 978-1-62808-239-5
© 2013 Nova Science Publishers, Inc.

Chapter 5

Suspicious perianal lesion in a patient with renal cell carcinoma

Cassandra Uy, MD(C)[1], Florencia Jon, MRT(T)[*1],*
Corwyn Rowsell, MD[2], Bonnie O'Hayon, MD[3], Sherif Hanna, MD[4],
Georg Bjarnason, MD[5], Lori Holden, MRT(T)[1],
Janet Nguyen, BSc(C)[1], Michelle Ross, RN[1],
Justin Kwong, BSc(C)[1], Arjun Sahgal, MD[1], Luluel Khan, MD[1],
Kristopher Dennis, MD[1] and Edward Chow, MBBS[1]

[1]Departments of Radiation Oncology
[2]Pathology, [3]Diagnostic Radiology, [4]Surgical Oncology and [5]Medical Oncology,
Odette Cancer Centre, Sunnybrook Health Sciences Centre,
University of Toronto, Toronto, Ontario, Canada

Abstract

The appearance of a new cutaneous lesion can lead to a variety of conclusions based upon examination by individual physicians. We present the case of a 65-year-old man with renal cell carcinoma, who presented two years following diagnosis with complaints of a suspicious perianal lesion. Cutaneous metastasis of renal cell carcinoma is a relatively rare occurrence and signifies a late stage of the disease. Diagnosis of this metastatic spread can be difficult, due to morphological similarities with other cutaneous lesions. The unique location of the lesion reported herein also brings forth differential diagnosis of squamous cell carcinoma of the anal region. Following a near-complete excisional biopsy of the lesion, the conclusion was made that no cancerous tissue was present in the lesion, thereby stressing the importance of correct diagnosis prior to treatment.

* Correspondence: Ms Florencia Jon, BSc, MRT (T), Department of Radiation Therapy, Sunnybrook Odette Cancer Centre, 2075 Bayview Ave, Toronto, Ontario, M4N 3M5 Canada. Tel: 416-480-4998; Fax: 416-480-6002; Email: Florence.Jon@sunnybrook.ca.

Introduction

The past few decades have seen an increase in the incidence of renal cell carcinoma (RCC), largely due to more technologically advanced imaging practices and an aging population (1). When compared with other cancers, RCC occurrence remains relatively rare, accounting for approximately 3% of all adult neoplasms; however, worldwide incidence and mortality rates have been rising at a rate of 2-3% every decade (2). At initial presentation of RCC, approximately 25-30% of all patients have metastatic deposits, and unusual sites of metastases are not uncommon (3). The appearance of cutaneous metastases of RCC generally denotes a late stage and widespread disease (4), making prompt diagnosis and treatment imperative. Unfortunately, the diagnosis of cutaneous metastases of RCC can be difficult, due to its infrequent presentation and likeness to other lesions (4). Ultimately, while there is a sense of urgency in identifying the cause of a cutaneous lesion so as to expedite treatment, the necessary precautions must still be taken to ensure that proper treatment is administered.

We present a case of a 65-year-old man to emphasize the importance of proper diagnosis prior to treatment.

Case report

A 65-year-old man presented with a round, indurated lesion located in the perianal region just to the left of the anus. The lesion was 3-4 cm in diameter, with evidence of ulceration. Additionally, it was bleeding profusely and caused him a great deal of discomfort.

He was initially diagnosed with renal cell carcinoma (RCC) two years prior. On presentation of bilateral leg swelling, an ultrasound was performed, revealing a large (9.5×7.0×6.5cm) right-sided renal mass. The mass extended into both the proximal and distal inferior vena cava (IVC) and external iliac veins; there was also some invasion of the perinephric fat. A right nephrectomy was performed (preserving the adrenal gland) as well as thrombectomies in the IVC and external iliac veins to remove the tumour thrombi. A non-removable IVC filter was also placed in order to discourage future occurrence of pulmonary emboli. He was also prescribed Fragmin.

Post-operatively, a pathological investigation of the resected tumour confirmed the presence of clear cell renal carcinoma, stage III (see figure 1). A CT scan also demonstrated the possibility of a thrombus within the intrahepatic vena cava.

About a year following the surgical resection of the mass, an MRI scan of the head demonstrated a 1cm nodule anterior to the pineal gland in the brain. The nodule was treated with stereotactic radiosurgery (single 21Gy).

A month following this event, an MRI of the abdomen suggested that the intrahepatic lesion was most likely a tumour rather than thrombus. The patient began sunitinib (Sutent) for tumour control. Surgical resection was not possible due to the intrahepatic location of the mass.

Two years following his nephrectomy, the patient complained of pain and bleeding caused by the perianal lesion. The lesion was suspected to be a subcutaneous metastasis of the patient's RCC with an overlying hematoma caused by his Fragmin therapy. He was referred to a radiation oncologist due to profuse bleeding of the lesion. However, the radiation oncologist suspected that this might be a squamous cell carcinoma (SCC) of the anal canal. No radiation treatment was given, as there had yet to be confirmation of this lesion as metastatic RCC or an alternate primary SCC. A CT scan of the pelvis confirmed the presence of the lesion (see figure 2).

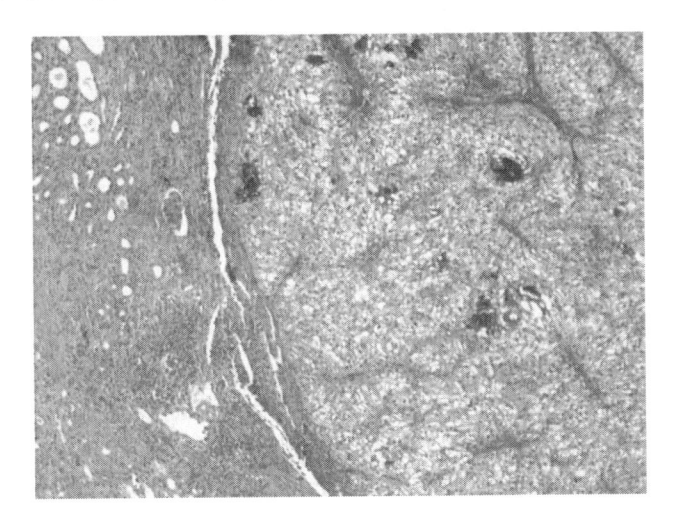

Figure 1. Primary renal cell carcinoma – clear cell type, with adjacent renal parenchyma.

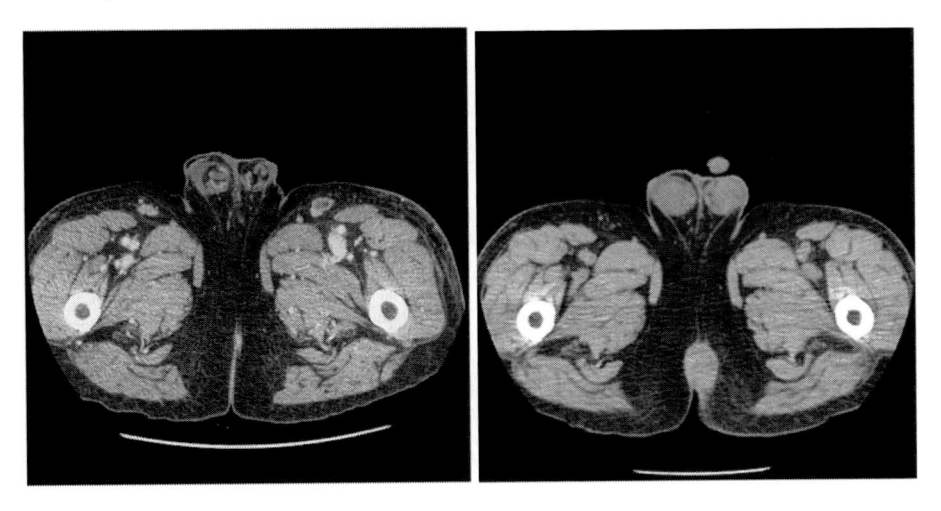

Figure 2. Left: Previous axial CT image showing unremarkable left perianal region. Right: CT performed 3 months later shows interval development of a left perianal soft tissue lesion.

The patient was seen by a gastrointestinal surgical oncologist, who drained the hematoma and excised a large portion of the lesion, which was sent for a pathology examination. A small portion of the mass was left intact due to its close proximity to the anal sphincter.

The pathology revealed the specimen was non-cancerous, presenting only inflamed squamous epithelium with condylomatous changes and hyperplasia (Figure 3). Histological features of the perianal lesion were completely different when compared with the primary RCC (see figure 1). There was a decision not to perform an additional biopsy, as the first had been quite generous. The patient continues to be followed for any signs of progression in his disease and at last follow-up there was no evidence of local progression of his disease.

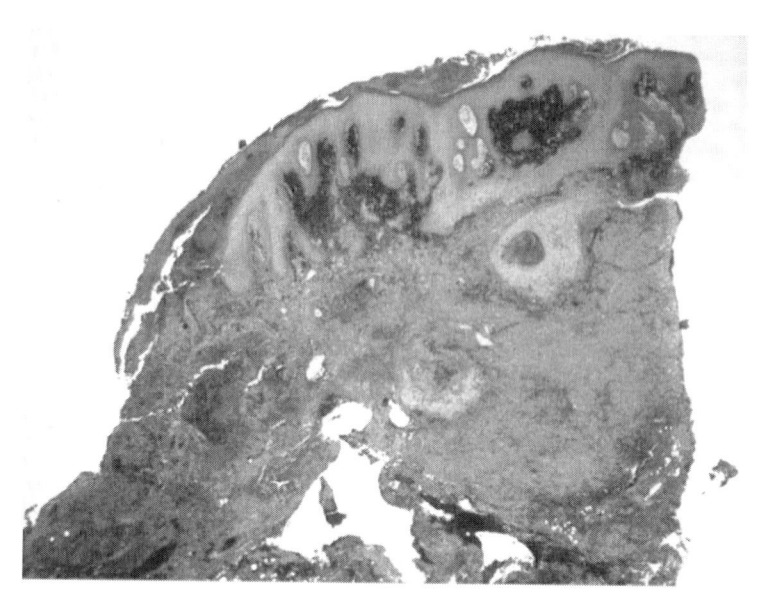

Figure 3. Perianal lesion – inflamed squamous epithelium with hyperplasia and some condylomatous changes. Extensive haemorrhage and inflammation in underlying soft tissue.

Discussion

Despite first appearing localized, the presentation of RCC metastases following nephrectomy remains possible (5), as was seen with this patient and his brain metastasis. Suspicion of further metastatic spread, therefore, was not completely unwarranted. While a subcutaneous metastasis that had gone on to ulcerate through skin was initially suspected, a brief literature search revealed no prior examples of subcutaneous metastasis of RCC. Furthermore, categorization of a lesion as cutaneous versus subcutaneous depends upon the component of skin primarily affected by pathological change, but both are considered lesions of the skin (6). As such, further discussion is carried out with cutaneous metastases in mind.

The diagnosis as a non-cancerous lesion was surprising, but cutaneous metastasis of RCC is rather rare (4,7,8). In patients with RCC, cutaneous metastasis has been reported in only 2.8% to 6.8% of cases; it is the 7th most common site of involvement (7). More frequent sites of metastases include the lung parenchyma (50-60% of patients with metastases), the bone (30-40%), and the brain (5%) (3). Cutaneous metastases are more common with other cancers, such as breast cancer in women and lung cancer in men (4,9).

Features of cutaneous metastases of RCC are varied. Lesions may present as a solitary metastasis or as multiple metastases, with either a localized or diffuse spread (8). Size of the metastatic lesions also tends to vary widely, ranging from several millimetres to a few centimetres in diameter (8). The metastatic lesion may be flesh-coloured, but can range from red hues to purple, brown, or black (4,8). In our patient's case, the presenting colour and overlying hematoma of the lesion was suspected to be secondary to his Fragmin therapy. Cutaneous spread of metastatic RCC also tends to manifest itself upon the face and scalp, although presentation upon the chest and abdominal region is also commonplace (4,8). Appearance of cutaneous metastasis in more distant regions is attributed to haematogenous spread following tumour infiltration of the renal vein (7); this also takes into account the highly vascularised nature of RCC (8). Often, metastatic lesions will demonstrate the same histologic properties as the primary cancer (8). When comparing Figures 1 and 3 for this patient, it is clear there was no evidence of metastatic spread to the perianal region.

The appearance of cutaneous lesions generally carries with it a poor prognosis (8,9). Therefore, treatment is limited and tends toward symptom palliation. Chosen treatments depend upon the degree of spread to other organs (7,8); surgical excision and radiotherapy, or a combination of the two, can be beneficial (8).

A brief review of the literature reveals no case of metastatic RCC which had presented itself as a single lesion in the perianal region. An alternate primary cancer located in the anal region would have been justly suspected.

Similar to the rarity of cutaneous metastatic RCC, SCC of the anal canal represents only 1.5% of all gastrointestinal tract malignancies (10). Furthermore, SCC of the anal margin is very rare, being tenfold less common than anal canal carcinomas (11). As noted by Jensen et al (12), lesions can present with bleeding, pain, and a palpable mass – all of which were demonstrated in this patient. Further symptoms can include change in bowel habits, discharge and pruritis ani (12). Lesions are usually ulcerated (13), which was demonstrated in this case; however, lesions also rarely invade the sphincter muscle (13), which was a concern in this patient. Due to the slow progression of anal cancers, they are often mistaken for benign conditions, making definitive diagnosis through incisional or excisional biopsy a necessity (14). Following confirmation of the cancer, common methods of treating SCC of the anal region can include surgical excision or a chemoradiotherapeutic approach (15). Surgical excision is generally reserved for well-defined tumours which are capable of being excised with wide margins (13). More advanced cancers are treated with a combination of chemotherapy (5-fluorouracil and mitomycin) and concurrent radiation, although Chapet et al (11) did present evidence that in treating SCC of the anal margin, radiotherapy alone was as effective.

As there had not yet been confirmation of cutaneous metastasis in the patient, there was a decision to withhold radiation treatment, but to proceed with surgical excision and histological examination. The decision proved wise, following the negative pathology report. As reported by Mueller et al. (8), differential diagnoses can include an opportunistic infection or a cutaneous drug reaction (a possibility due to the patient being administered sunitinib). It is interesting to note that Michalaki et al (16) recently reported a similar patient who possessed a non-cancerous abscess that mimicked progression of his metastatic RCC. They suggested that the abdominal abscess could be a side-effect of the sunitinib due to its effects on normal vasculature. Due to the possible differential diagnoses, it is generally suggested that a biopsy is performed on the lesion prior to administration of additional treatment (3), as was the case here.

Treatment of this patient would have been drastically altered based on a different conclusion from the pathology report. Had there been evidence for cancerous cells, further action would be warranted for the portion of the mass that was not resected due to its proximity to the anal sphincter. As it stands, because a conclusion of non-cancerous tissue was drawn upon pathological examination and re-examination, the patient received no further treatment for the lesion and continues to be monitored for signs of disease progression.

Acknowledgments

We thank the Michael and Karyn Goldstein Cancer Research Fund and Mrs. Stacy Yuen for administrative support.

References

[1]   Wotkowicz C, Wszolek MF, Libertino JA. Resection of renal tumors invading the vena cava. Urol Clin North Am 2008; 35:657-71.

[2]   Gupta K, Miller JD, Li JZ, Russell MW, Charboneau C. Epidemiologic and socioeconomic burden of metastatic renal cell carcinoma (mRCC): A literature review. Cancer Treat Rev 2008;34:193-205.

[3]   Motzer RJ, Bander NH, Nanus DM. Renal-cell carcinoma. N Engl J Med 1996;335(12):865-75.

[4]   Lim C, Chan R, Regan W. Case report: Renal cell carcinoma with cutaneous metastases. Australas J Dermatol 2005;46:158-60.

[5]   Nelson EC, Evans CP, Lara Jr PN. Renal cell carcinoma: Current status and emerging therapies. Cancer Treat Rev 2007;33:299-313.

[6]   Lee EH, Nehal KS, Disa JJ. Benign and premalignant skin lesions. Plast Reconstr Surg 2010;125(5):188e-98.

[7]   Kouroupakis D, Patsea E, Sofras F, Apostolika N. Renal cell carcinoma metastases to the skin: a not so rare case? Br J Urol 1995; 75:583-5.

[8]   Mueller TJ, Wu H, Greenberg RE, Hudes G, Topham N, Lessin SR, et al. Cutaneous metastases from genitourinary malignancies. Urology 2004; 63:1021-6.

[9]   Gurer CK, Karaduman A, Bukulmez G, Sahin S, Ozkaya O, Erkan I. Renal cell carcinoma with skin metastasis. J Eur Acad Dermatol Venereol 2004;18(3):386-7.

[10]   Martin FT, Kavanagh D, Waldron R. Squamous cell carcinoma of the anal canal. Surgeon 2009;7(4):232-7.

[11]   Chapet O, Gerard JP, Mornex F, Goncalves-Tavan S, Ardiet JM, D'hombres A, et al. Prognostic factors of squamous cell carcinoma of the anal margin treated by radiotherapy: the Lyon experience. Int J Colorectal Dis 2007;22:191-9.

[12]   Jensen SL, Hagen K, Shokouh-Amiri MH, Nielsen OV. Does an erroneous diagnosis of squamous cell carcinoma of the anal canal and anal margin at first physician visit influence prognosis. Dis Colon Rectum 1987;30:345-51.

[13]   Mendenhall WM, Zlotecki RA, Vauthey JN, Copelan EM. Squamous cell carcinoma of the anal margin treated with radiotherapy. Surg Oncol 1996;5:29-35.

[14]   Newlin HE, Zlotecki RA, Morris CG, Hochwald SN, Riggs CE, Mendenhall WM. Squamous cell carcinoma of the anal margin. Surg Oncol 2004;86:55-62.

[15]   Garrett K, Kalady MF. Anal neoplasms. Surg Clin North Am 2010; 90:147-61.

[16]   Michalaki V, Arkadopoulos N, Kondi-Pafiti A, Gennatas C. Abscess formation mimicking disease progression, in a patient with metastatic renal cell carcinoma during sunitinib treatment. World J Surg Oncol 2010;8(1):45.

In: Advanced Cancer
Editors: N. Thavarajah, N. Pulenzas, B. Lechner et al.

ISBN: 978-1-62808-239-5
© 2013 Nova Science Publishers, Inc.

Chapter 6

Osteonecrosis of the jaw appearing as bone metastases in a bone scan in a patient with breast cancer

Gillian Bedard, BSc(C), Liang Zeng, MD(C), Sunil Verma, MD, Natalie Lauzon, MRT(T), Lori Holden, BSc, MRT(T), Kristopher Dennis, MD, Michael Poon, MD(C) and Edward Chow*, MBBS

Rapid Response Radiotherapy Program, Department of Radiation Oncology, Odette Cancer Centre, Sunnybrook Health Sciences Centre, University of Toronto, Toronto, Ontario, Canada

Bisphosphonate therapy has increased in popularity since the late 20th century for its use in treatment of bone metastases. Osteonecrosis has been linked to the use of bisphosphonate treatment and osteonecrosis of the jaw is seen in about 1% of patients who are taking oral bisphosphonates. Those who have osteonecrosis of the jaw (ONJ) have exposed bone in the maxillofacial region for at least eight weeks without a history of radiotherapy to the jaw. This report presents the case of a patient who was found to have ONJ. This patient was kept on her bisphosphonate treatment even with the ONJ diagnosis. In the most recent bone scan, uptake was shown in the maxillofacial region and was characterized as either bone metastases or ONJ by the radiologist. Uptake in the mouth and facial region in patients who are taking oral bisphosphonates should be clinically examined by a dentist to rule out ONJ.

* Correspondence: Professor Edward Chow MBBS, MSc, PhD, FRCPCDepartment of Radiation Oncology, Odette Cancer Centre, Sunnybrook Health Sciences Centre, 2075 Bayview Avenue, Toronto, ON Canada. E-mail:Edward.Chow@sunnybrook.ca.

Introduction

Osteonecrosis of the jaw (ONJ) is defined as a condition in which there is necrotic exposed bone in the maxillofacial region for greater than eight weeks duration (1). ONJ is typically seen in 0.94% to 10% of patients who are taking bisphosphonates, and was first seen in the 19th century in workers exposed to white phosphorous (2). The mortality rate of ONJ or "phossy jaw" as it was called at the time was very high as there were no antibiotics (2). It took many years for ONJ to be linked to the use of bisphosphonates; however, today there is a confirmed link and increasing awareness (3). Although there is no well established time frame for development of ONJ, one study found that patients were more likely to develop ONJ with at least 4 years of bisphosphonate use (4).

Although they have their side effects, bisphosphonates have been effective in improving the quality of life in patients with bone metastases, osteoporosis or Paget's disease. Bisphosphonates are inhibitors of osteoclast function and are able to reduce bone pain, hypercalcemia and skeletal related events in the bone metastases population as they aid in strengthening the bone (3).

Here we present the case of a young woman who was found to have osteonecrosis of the jaw after the extended use of bisphosphonates yet the bone scan feature mimics that of bone metastases.

Case report

A 39 year old female presented to clinic with extensive bony metastases from primary breast cancer. Two and a half years after starting pamidronate, the patient developed dental pain and her medical oncologist referred her to the dentist on site. After seeing the dentist, the patient was diagnosed with osteonecrosis of the jaw. In response, her medical oncologist took her off pamidronate for a few weeks. During this time, the patient complained of generalized bony pain and aches, and her ONJ seemed to heal. It was determined that some of her bony pain may be secondary to the fact that she had not had her dose of pamidronate. Since it was determined that receiving the pamidronate would not likely worsen her ONJ condition, the patient was given the pamidronate dose due to the increase in bony pain. After receiving her scheduled doses of pamidronate, the bony pain the patient was experiencing seemed to be somewhat alleviated.

The most recent bone scan displayed widespread metastases. There was uptake in the lumbar spine, sacrum, pelvis, proximal femurs, sternum, scapulae, all ribs, both humeri and activity in the left hemimandible. The radiologist determined that the uptake in the hemimandible may be metastatic or dental (see figure 1).

This uptake was in fact dental, and determined by the dentist to be osteonecrosis of the jaw. The dentist prescribed the patient antibiotics to clear up the ONJ, and it was determined that there would be no role for surgical intervention at that time.

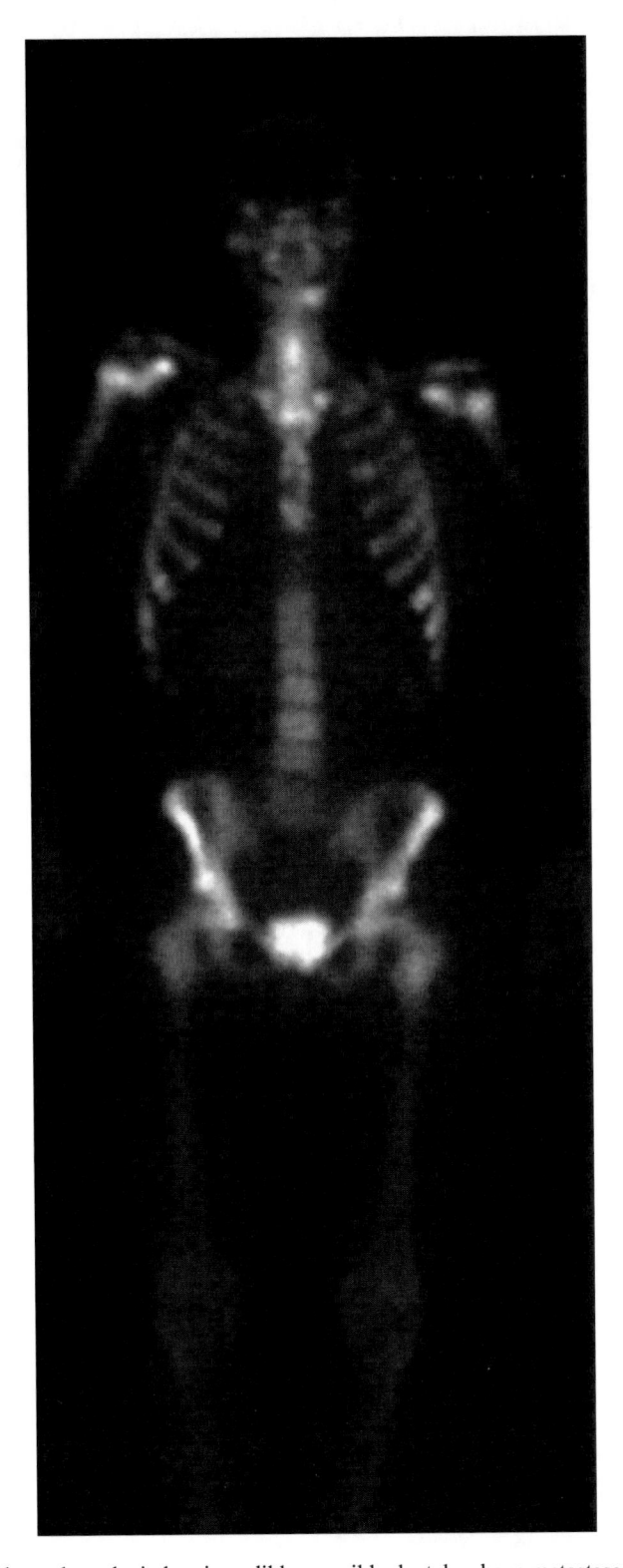

Figure 1. Bone scan showed uptake in hemimandible; possible dental or bone metastases.

Discussion

Osteonecrosis of the jaw is diagnosed clinically by dentists or oral surgeons. Patient history and clinical examination are combined to reach an accurate diagnosis for this disease (3). ONJ becomes symptomatic upon infection, and symptoms include pain, tooth mobility, mucosal swelling, erythema, and ulceration (3). Microscopic examination of the exposed bone often reveals necrotic bone with associated bacterial debris, although there are no features specifically unique to ONJ (3).

Imaging of ONJ is often difficult as it can appear to be bone metastases of the jaw. The jaw uptake is not a reliable predictor of ONJ development as demonstrated through a study by O'Connor et al. In this study, uptake on the bone scan was seen in 92% of patients with ONJ and 70% of patients without ONJ (5). Lamonica et al (6) also did a study to confirm that uptake as seen on a bone scan is not predictive of ONJ.

In this particular case, the bone scan displayed results possible for either bone metastases or ONJ from uptake shown in the jaw. This can be problematic for diagnosis if there is no clinical history norclinical diagnosis available. In this case, the importance of diagnosis of ONJ by a dentist is crucial.

Treatment for ONJ that has become infected and painful for the patient can include antibiotics, surgery and use of antibacterial mouth wash(3). Although bisphosphonate treatment can cause ONJ, it may be recommended that this treatment continue despite this, especially in the case of those with bone metastases. A multidisciplinary team should make this decision on a case-by-case basis (1). In the case of our current patient, it was determined by the dental and medical oncology teams that the bisphosphonate treatment should continue as it would be more burdensome on the patient if treatment was stopped.

This case demonstrates the importance of clinical and imaging diagnosis of ONJ, as a bone scan can show uptake in the jaw that can be attributed to ONJ or bone metastases. This case also outlines the necessity for a multidisciplinary team to be involved in the dental care of patients on bisphosphonate treatment. Treatment decisions pertaining to bisphosphonates once a patient has been diagnosed with ONJ should be made together by the oncology and dental teams involved in the patient's care.

Acknowledgments

We thank the generous support of Bratty Family Fund, Michael and Karyn Goldstein Cancer Research Fund, Joseph and SilvanaMelara Cancer Research Fund, and Ofelia Cancer Research Fund.

References

[1]   Silverman SL, Landesberg R. Osteonecrosis of the jaw and the role of bisphosphonates: a critical review. Am J Med 2009;122:33-45.

[2]   McLeod NM, Brennan PA, Ruggiero SL. Bisphosphonate osteonecrosis of the jaw: a historical and contemporary review. Surgeon 2012;10:36-42.

[3]   Ruggiero SL, Mehrotra B. Bisphosphonate-related osteonecrosis of the jaw: diagnosis, prevention, and management. Annu Rev Med 2009;60:85-96.

[4]   Lo JC, O'Ryan FS, Gordon NP, Yang J, Hui RL, Martin D, et al. Prevalence of osteonecrosis of the jaw in patients with oral bisphosphonate exposure. J Oral Maxillofac Surg 2010;68:243-53.

[5]   Bisphosphonate-induced osteonecrosis of the jaw: Risk factors and diagnostic utility of bone scans. 2007 ASCO Annual Meeting Proceedings Part I.; 2007.

[6]   Lamonica D, Li l, Padmanabhan A, O'Connor T. Diagnostic utility of bone scans for bisphosphonate-induced osteonecrosis of the jaw. J Nuclear Med 2007;48:143.

In: Advanced Cancer

Editors: N. Thavarajah, N. Pulenzas, B. Lechner et al.

ISBN: 978-1-62808-239-5

© 2013 Nova Science Publishers, Inc.

Chapter 7

Unusual presentation of osteolytic bone metastases in prostate adenocarcinoma

Michelle Zhou, BSc(C), Liang Zeng, BSc(C),
Monique Christakis, MD, Michael Poon, BSc(C),
Emily Chen, BSc(C), Natalie Lauzon, MRTT,
Nemica Thavarajah, BSc(C), Julia DiGiovanni, BSc(C)
and Edward Chow[*], MBBS

Rapid Response Radiotherapy Program, Department of Radiation Oncology, Odette Cancer Centre, Sunnybrook Health Sciences Centre, University of Toronto, Toronto, Ontario, Canada

Prostate adenocarcinoma is one of the leading causes of death in men. Bone metastases are common in patients with prostate cancer, typically being characterized as osteoblastic. Evidence shows that although osteoblastic activity is dominant, osteolytic activity is also present. Treatment for bone metastases is often multi-disciplinary and palliative, targeting pain management as well as preventing deteriorating quality of life. This report presents the case of a patient who was found to have rare osteolytic lesions rather than the typical osteoblastic lesions. The patient received radiation treatment to the lesions of the spine, right hemipelvis including the hip to mid-femur and left mid femur. In the most recent CT scan, the radiated sites showed increased sclerosis within the osteolysis and periosteal new bone formation. Radiotherapy helped alleviate the pain and promote healing in the affected bones.

[*] Correspondence: Professor Edward Chow MBBS, MSc, PhD, FRCPC, Department of Radiation Oncology, Odette Cancer Centre, Sunnybrook Health Sciences Centre, 2075 Bayview Avenue, Toronto, ON Canada M4N 3M5. E-mail: Edward.Chow@sunnybrook.ca.

Introduction

Prostate cancer is one of the prevalent causes of death from cancer in men (1). Prostate cancer often metastasizes in the bone leading to bone pain, impaired mobility and pathological fractures (2). The amount of osteoblastic and osteolytic activity determines the type of metastatic bone lesion (1). Bone metastases formed from prostate cancer are often characterized as osteoblastic due to the significant amount of osteoblasts in close proximity to prostate cancer cells. Despite the prevalence of osteoblastic metastases, there is also evidence of underlying osteolytic activity (1, 3). Evidence suggests that prostate cancer causes increased bone production due to osteoclast resorption of bone and then osteoblast mediated replacement of resorbed bone, with osteoblast eventually outweighing the osteoclast resorption. Prostate cancer metastatic to bones remains incurable and current treatments are mostly palliative, including radiotherapy for pain and pharmacological management of bone pain (2). Here we present the case of a man who was found to have prostate cancer metastatic to bones, leading to diffuse osteolytic lesions.

Case report

A 76 year old male was referred to clinic in May 2011 for consideration of radiation therapy (RT) for painful left pelvic and also thoracic vertebrae bone metastases. A CT scan of the spine revealed diffuse osteolytic lesions throughout the spine. The differential diagnosis was multiple myeloma but his PSA level was abnormally high. Due to presence of abnormal PSA level, the patient then underwent a biopsy of the bone metastases, which confirmed the origin of prostate cancer. The biopsy, although not always performed, was important as it helped with the diagnosis of prostate cancer.

The lesions at the cervical vertebrae were most prominent at C3 and C7 (Figure 1). There were pathological fractures at T1, T2 and T3, with the T1 vertebral approximately 30% compromised with soft tissue extending into the spinal canal. There were also mild retropulsion of the bone from the posterior cortex at T3 and disruption of the posterior cortex at T6 with minimal soft tissue encroachment on the spinal cord. Bony destruction of the posterior vertebral body at L1 and L3 was also present (Figure 2). The upper regions of both thoracic and lumbar vertebrae, cervical vertebrae and the lesion at T6 were treated with 20 Gy in 5 fractions.

A CT scan of the pelvis and hips revealed extensive lytic destruction in the left hemi pelvis, left sacrum and coccyx with slight expansion plus extraosseous extension into the iliac fossae and posterior gluteal area (Figure 3). Lytic destruction was also present in the right femoral neck extending to the femoral head, right hemi pelvis and lower lumbar spine. The patient was referred to an orthopedic surgeon however; prophylactic surgery was not suitable because the risk of fracture of the right proximal femur was not exceedingly high. The patient underwent palliative radiation treatment in August 2011 to the right hemi pelvis including the hip to mid-femur and left mid femur of 30 Gy in 10 fractions and received morphine for pain control.

After the treatment, there was progressive improvement leading to the eventual absence of pain. CT scans showed increased sclerosis within the osteolysis and periosteal new bone formation about the left ilium suggestive of response to treatment (Figure 4). The radiation provided increased healing and the patient was referred for physiotherapy.

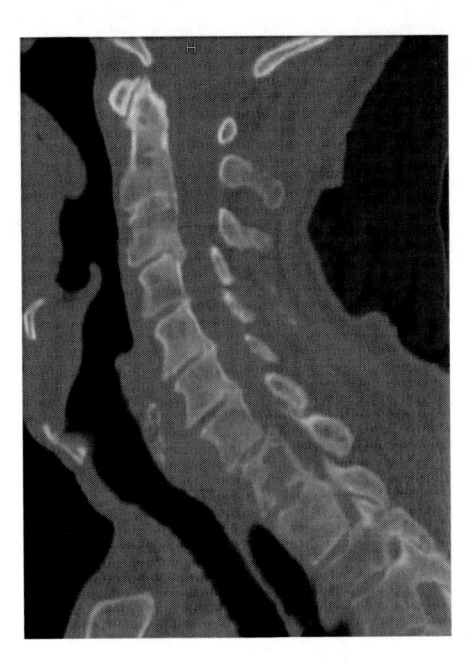

Figure 1. CT scan (May 2011) of the cervical vertebrae showing the osteolytic lesions.

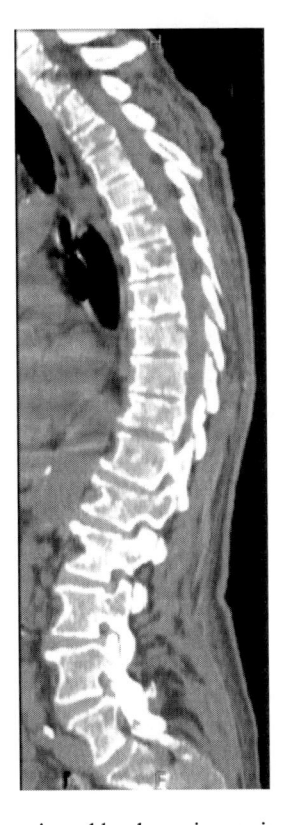

Figure 2. CT scan (May 2011) of the thoracic and lumbar spine again with extensive osteolysis.

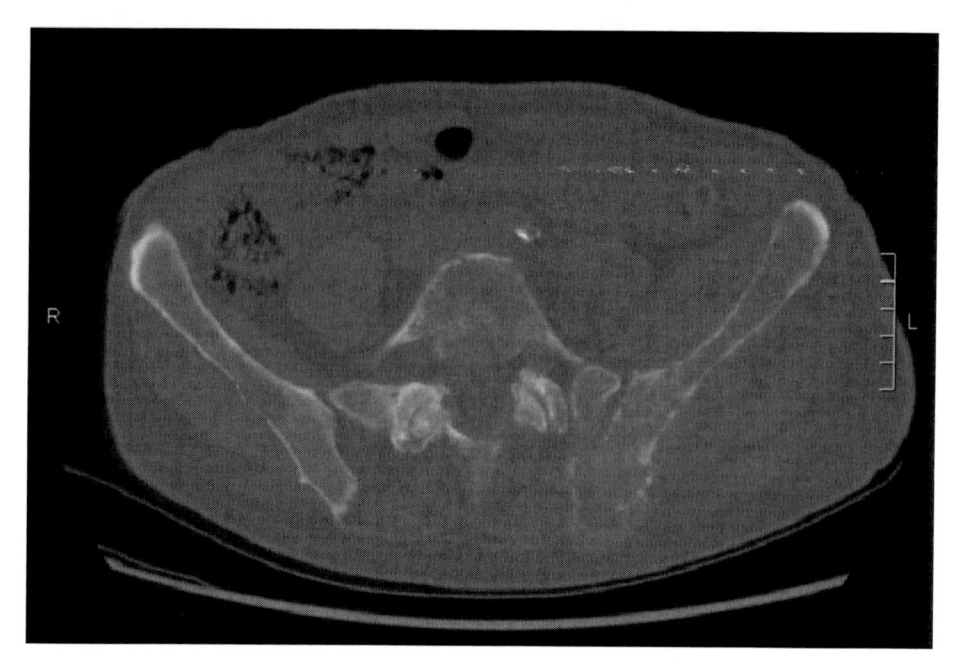

Figure 3. Axial CT images (May 2011) showing lytic destruction in left and right hemipelvis.

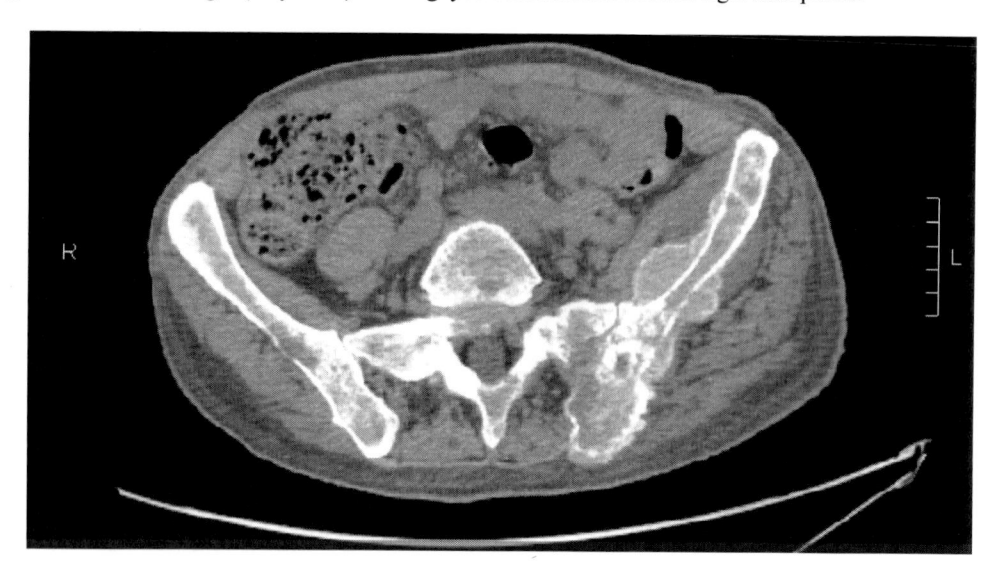

Figure 4. CT scan (June 2011) post radiation treatment showing osteolytic lesions in both the left and right hemipelvis. Increased density of extraosseous soft tissue and sclerosis within osteolysis and development of new bone suggestive of response to treatment.

Discussion

Bone, specifically the axial skeletal, is frequently the site of metastatic disease in prostate cancer patients (4, 5). Metastases formed from prostate cancer are predominantly osteoblastic although both osteolytic and osteoblastic activities are activated (2, 5). Development of bone metastases requires the activation of not only osteoblastic activity but also osteoclastic activity (2). Clinical trials report bone metastases being asymptomatic during the early stages of the disease, but can lead to 35 - 45% of the patients experiencing bone pain, 14 – 22% experience pathological fracture and 3 – 7% experiencing spinal cord compression (4). Due to the effects of bone metastases, treatment aims at reducing the existing bone-related symptoms and prolonging deterioration of a patient's quality of life or survival (4).

Acetaminophen and non-steroidal anti-inflammatory drugs are typically the first pharmaceutical drug administered for pain control. As the disease progresses, opioids may also be given to the patient in a step-wise fashion (5). Palliative treatment options are often multi-disciplinary, including chemotherapy, osteoclast-inhibitory agents, corticosteroids, external-beam radiotherapy or surgery (2,5). External beam radiation therapy has been proven to provide pain relief in up to 80% of patients with bone metastases (5). Standard pharmaceutical treatments include androgen ablation to increase osteoclastic bone resorption and bone loss, while treatment with zoledronic acid prevents bone loss from androgen deprivation and reduces bone metastases. Bisphosphonates, a class of bone resorption inhibitors prevent bone loss in advanced prostate adenocarcinoma (3).

In this particular case, the patient referred to clinic presented bone metastasis with high osteoclast resorption, leading to osteolytic rather than osteoblastic lesions. The patients received radiation to the affected areas. Subsequent CT scan administered after radiation presented indication of response to treatment.

Conclusion

Prostate cancer resulting in osteolytic bone metastases is a rare occurrence. Typically, prostate cancer leads to osteoblastic lesions. This case study shows that radiation is an effective treatment for osteolytic bone metastases as the CT scans showed response to treatment.

Acknowledgments

We thank the generous support of Bratty Family Fund, Michael and Karyn Goldstein Cancer Research Fund, Joseph and Silvana Melara Cancer Research Fund, and Ofelia Cancer Research Fund. We thank Stacy Yuen for the secretarial assistance. The authors have no conflicts of interest to disclose.

References

[1]   Logothetis CJ, Lin SH. Osteoblasts in prostate cancer metastasis to bone. Nat Rev Cancer 2005;5:21-8.

[2]   Keller ET, Brown J. Prostate cancer bone metastases promote both osteolytic and osteoblastic activity. J Cell Biochem 2004;91:718-29.

[3]   Guise TA, Mohammad KS, Clines G, Stebbins EG, Wong DH, Higgins LS, et al. Basic mechanisms responsible for osteolytic and osteoblastic bone metastases. Clin Cancer Res 2006;12:6213-16.

[4]   Autio KA, Scher HI, Morris MJ. Therapeutic strategies for bone metastases and their clinical sequelae in prostate cancer. Curr Treat Options Oncol 2012 [Epub ahead of print].

[5]   Goyal J, Antonarakis ES. Bone-targeting radiopharmaceuticals for the treatment of prostate cancer with bone metastases. Cancer Lett 2012 [Epub ahead of print]

In: Advanced Cancer
Editors: N. Thavarajah, N. Pulenzas, B. Lechner et al.

ISBN: 978-1-62808-239-5
© 2013 Nova Science Publishers, Inc.

Chapter 8

Asymptomatic presentation of lung and bone metastases in a patient with breast cancer

Michael Poon, BSc(C), Emily Chen, BSc(C), Linda Probyn, MD, Liang Zeng, BSc(C), Natalie Lauzon, MRTT, Lori Holden, MRTT and Edward Chow, MBBS*

Rapid Response Radiotherapy Program, Department of Radiation Oncology, Odette Cancer Centre, Sunnybrook Health Sciences Centre, University of Toronto, Toronto, Ontario, Canada

Bone metastases are often one of the first signs of disseminated disease, especially in patients with breast cancer. It has been found that up to 79% of patients experience severe pain in the period before palliative therapy. This case describes a fifty year old female, who clinically presents with numerous pulmonary nodules yet remains asymptomatic. Despite multiple pelvic osteolytic lesions and progressive deterioration, the patient reports no pain, can bear weight, has good exercise tolerance and is not short of breath. This report highlights that clinical symptoms do not always reflect computer tomography imaging features or the extent of disease and metastases. Imaging features seen do not necessarily equate to the amount of pain experienced by patients.

Introduction

Metastases are typically associated with clinical manifestations indicative of patients' health. Bone metastases are often one of the first signs of disseminated disease, especially in patients

* Correspondence: Professor Edward Chow MBBS, MSc, PhD, FRCPC Department of Radiation Oncology, Odette Cancer Centre, Sunnybrook Health Sciences Centre, 2075 Bayview Avenue, Toronto, ON Canada. E-mail: Edward.Chow@sunnybrook.ca.

with breast cancer (1). In these patients, treatment intent is typically palliative aimed towards reducing pain, preventing fractures, maintaining activity and possibility prolonging survival.

In this report, we present the case of a middle aged woman whose radiological imaging reveal multiple pelvic and lung metastases associated with breast cancer, yet remains asymptomatic and painless.

Case report

A 50 year old female patient breast cancer patient was seen in Rapid Response Radiotherapy Program at the Odette Cancer Centre, Sunnybrook Hospital on September 29, 2011, presenting with multiple pulmonary nodules (see figure 1). In spite of these numerous pulmonary nodules, the patient was asymptomatic. The patient was noted to have been in Hong Kong for two weeks with her mother, whom was recently diagnosed with tuberculosis. Queries were raised as to whether pulmonary nodules were from infectious origins or were suspected lung metastases consistent with breast cancer. As such, a CAT scan guided biopsy of one of the pulmonary lesions was ordered. A whole body bone scan was ordered in search of possible bony lesion as well.

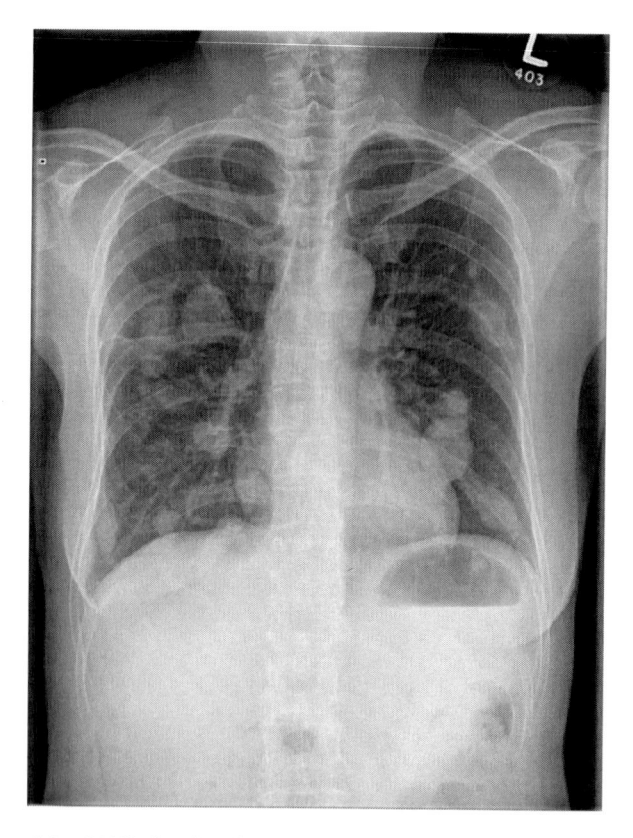

Figure 1. X-ray of chest (May 2012) showing the multiple pulmonary nodules.

The whole body bone scan completed October 18, 2011 showed bilateral ischial uptake (increased ischial tuberosity) and a subsequent follow-up CT identified multiple lytic lesions in her pelvis. This included a permeative destructive lesion in the right ischial tuberosity with mixed lytic and sclerotic components and bony expansion with a small amount of extraosseous soft tissue. A prominent lytic lesion involving the left ischial tuberosity extending into the posterior acetabular column with patchy areas of sclerosis was also found. This was consistent with metastases given the clinical history of breast cancer. Further deterioration was seen with a cortical breech at the inferior margin compatible with pathologic fracture and degenerative changes to the lower lumbar spine and sacroiliac joints. The core biopsy from the right lower lobe lung nodules was positive for breast malignancy, and was both estrogen and progesterone positive indicating possible response to hormone therapy.

Yet again, the patient remained totally asymptomatic, denying any pain, even when ambulating or bearing weight. She had good exercise tolerance and was not short of breath either. While X-ray scans did not portray a need for prophylactic surgery, the patient proceeded with prophylactic radiation treatment as the lesion was in a weight bearing area. The patient received a prescribed dose of 30 Gy in 10 fractions and tolerated the treatment very well. There were no reports of episodes of pain flares, nausea or vomiting. The patient was restarted on Tamoxifen as of November 2011 and was tolerating it well. Previously, she stated she had only taken Tamoxifen for a short period of time due to liver discomfort. Clodronate was started December 2011.

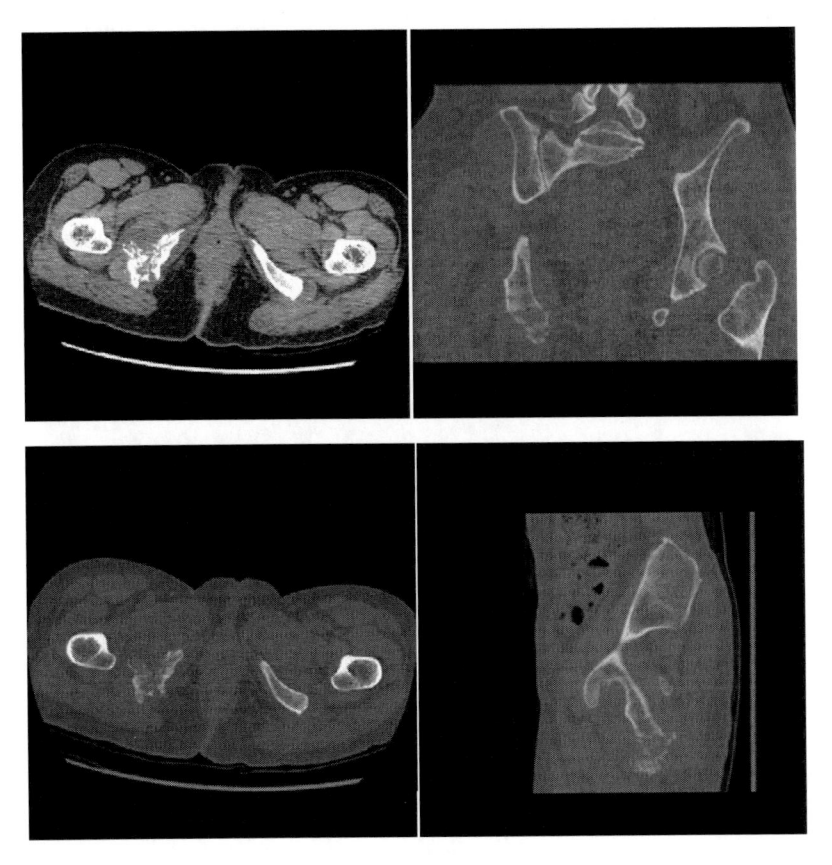

Figure 2. Multiple views of pelvic CT scan (April 2012) illustrating a permeative destructive lesion in the right ischial tuberosity with mixed lytic and sclerotic components.

Despite treatment, progressive osteolysis of the bone metastasis in the pelvis was shown on the repeat CAT scan April 2012 (Figure 2). Even with the deterioration shown on the scans, she remained completely asymptomatic and was feeling better than she had been in a long time. Unfortunately, the tumour was progressing with increased size of lung lesions in conjunction with some new lytic bony lesions.

Discussion

In the progression of metastatic disease, symptoms indicating deterioration of health are expected as part of a patient's normal disease trajectory. Diagnosis of bone metastases in breast cancer patients is typically associated with increased morbidity (2). These bone metastases clinically manifest as pain and can lead to many issues including skeletal related events such as spinal cord compression and use of radiation (2). It has been found that up to 79% of patients experience severe pain in the period before palliative therapy (3). However, despite progressive deterioration and a worsening of her condition seen in imaging, this patient remained asymptomatic. She denied experiencing pain or discomfort, uncharacteristic of her physical state.

The imaging of this patient revealed extensive metastases. Multiple pulmonary nodules and lytic lesions were discovered without the expected clinical symptoms of coughing, dyspnea, or fatigue. For this reason, diagnostically, it is important to recognize clinical symptoms do not always reflect computer tomography imaging features or extent of disease. Imaging features seen do not necessarily equate to if pain is experienced or the severity of pain experienced by patients. A comprehensive assessment of patient symptoms is required.

There is a lack of consensus regarding the optimal treatment of asymptomatic patients with bone metastases. This contention arises from how treatment of bone metastases is primarily palliative in nature. Among others, the aims of treatment are to relieve pain, improve function, and better quality of life (4). Therefore without clinical signs of distress, an optimal course of action requires careful consideration of a patient's immediate and future prognosis. Whether to actively observe or to opt to treat requires relative risk to benefit assessment and forethought towards potential treatment side effects. Some investigators have recommended a no-treatment policy for asymptomatic patients (5). In this case, radiotherapy was ordered prophylactically as lesions were located in a weight bearing area of the pelvis. This was performed in the hopes of delaying the osteolytic progression of bone metastasis. Because of the primary being breast cancer, the patient was put on the respective systemic therapy.

Conclusion

Use of diagnostic imaging is extremely important, but is not always reflective of patients' clinical symptoms. Imaging features do not necessarily equate to pain response. Bone and lung metastases can sometimes present atypically as asymptomatic.

Acknowledgments

We thank the generous support of Bratty Family Fund, Michael and Karyn Goldstein Cancer Research Fund, Joseph and Silvana Melara Cancer Research Fund, and Ofelia Cancer Research Fund.

References

[1] Nielsen OS. Palliative treatment of bone metastases. Acta Oncol 1996;35 Suppl 5:58-60.

[2] Roodman GD. Mechanisms of bone metastasis. N Engl J Med 2004;350(16):1655-64.

[3] Janjan N. Bone metastases: approaches to management. Semin Oncol 2001;28(4 Suppl 11):28-34.

[4] Nielsen OS. Palliative radiotherapy of bone metastases: there is now evidence for the use of single fractions. Radiother Oncol 1999;52(2):95-6.

[5] Nielsen OS, Munro AJ, Tannock IF. Bone metastases: pathophysiology and management policy. J Clin Oncol 1991;9(3):509-24.

In: Advanced Cancer
Editors: N. Thavarajah, N. Pulenzas, B. Lechner et al.

ISBN: 978-1-62808-239-5
© 2013 Nova Science Publishers, Inc.

Chapter 9

Prophylaxis with radiation treatment after surgery to the cervical spine for established heterotopic ossification

Gemma Cramarossa, BHSc (C), Emily Chen, BSc (C),
Liang Zeng, BSc (C), Cyril Danjoux, MD, Kevin Higgins, MD,
Nicholas Phan, MD, Richard Aviv, MD, Natalie Lauzon, MRTT,
Kristopher Dennis, MD and Edward Chow[*], MBBS

Odette Cancer Centre, Sunnybrook Health Sciences Centre, University of Toronto,
Toronto, Ontario, Canada

Radiation treatment for prophylaxis of heterotopic ossification following surgery has not been comprehensively described in sites other than the pelvis. The present case describes a 54 year old male with previous spinal cord injury at the C5-C6 level who was experiencing dysphagia caused by the presence of osteophytes from heterotopic ossification. The osteophytes in that area of previous trauma were indenting the posterior pharyngeal wall at the C3-C4 and C4-C5 spinal levels, as evidenced by a CT scan. They were resected, followed by a single radiation dose of 8 Gy the following day. Since then, the patient has been feeling well with no difficulty in swallowing. Further studies are necessary to confirm that radiation is effective at preventing or at least decreasing the risk for heterotopic ossification after surgery to remove osteophytes in sites outside the pelvis.

Introduction

Heterotopic ossification (HO) is the abnormal formation of bone in soft tissue outside the skeleton (1,2). It may be caused by a number of factors including central nervous system

[*] Correspondence: Professor Edward Chow MBBS, MSc, PhD, FRCPC, Department of Radiation Oncology, Odette Cancer Centre, Sunnybrook Health Sciences Centre, 2075 Bayview Avenue, Toronto, ON, Canada M4N 3M5. E-mail: Edward.Chow@sunnybrook.ca.

disorders, injury, bone or joint surgery or hereditary causes (1-3). Radiation treatment is often prophylactic in nature and there are few reports on successful irradiation for established HO outside the pelvis. Of these reports, all cases were established HO in the pelvis which were treated with single or multiple fractions (4,5). Although radiation treatment for prophylaxis of HO has been reported to be successful in many studies after bone and joint surgery to the pelvis, little is known about whether it is effective in the cervical spine and what the optimal dose of radiation would be. A single case report by Lo et al. in 1996 reported excision of an osteophyte in the C3-C4 region of the spine and administration of a single radiation dose of 6 Gy the following day (6). Recurrence of the osteophyte was reported, however noted to be less prominent.

The present case is a middle-aged quadriplegic who underwent surgery after the presence of osteophytes were discovered in his C spine and he subsequently received radiation treatment to the area to prevent the reformation of HO.

Case report

A 54 year old male was injured in a car accident 20 years ago which required a C5-C6 decompression and fusion as a consequence of a cervical spine fracture, resulting in quadriplegia. The patient has ankylosing spondylitis. He began to experience worsening dysphagia over a few months, beginning around May 2011. Initially he began to find it difficult to swallow pills, however he could still eat solid foods including meat and vegetables. By August 2011, he required a liquefied diet. He had been referred to the Rapid Response Radiotherapy Program (RRRP) at the Odette Cancer Centre, Sunnybrook Hospital for a consultation regarding lower back pain in May of 2011, but this treatment was put on hold as dysphagia became a more pressing concern.

In June of 2011, flexible nasopharyngoscopy was performed which confirmed the effects of osteophytes at the C3-C4 and C4-C5 spinal levels. The osteophyte around C3-C4 was quite large and was evidently causing an indentation in the patient's posterior pharyngeal wall, pushing the epiglottis anteriorly. A CT scan of the neck was ordered at the end of June which clearly displayed the prominent osseous overgrowths in the area. Overgrowth of the anterior longitudinal ligament was seen at inferior C3 and superior C4, with osteophytes extending 1 cm anterior to the C4 body proper. The displacement of the posterior pharyngeal mucosa was notable (Figure 1). The osteophyte at the level below, C4-C5, was smaller. A CT scan of the thoracic and lumbar spine revealed osteophytes in these areas as well, however they were not causing any pressing issues.

Those involved in the patient's care reasoned that the osteophyte slowly progressed over the years and was presenting a concern now because of the size it had reached and the area it was infringing upon. Surgical resection involving anterior cervical decompression and drilling of C3-C4 and C4-C5 osteophytes was performed on August 30, 2011 with no complications. An awake-tracheotomy was required because of the airway narrowing. The following day, he received a single radiation treatment of 8 Gy post-surgery to prevent osseous regrowth in that cervical spine region.

A plain X-ray in October did not show any abnormal osseous growth and alignment of the cervical spine was normal. The patient was seen again at the RRRP in May 2012 and reported that he was no longer having problems with dysphagia. A CT scan in May showed minor C3-C4 and C4-C5 marginal osteophytes that appear stable (Figure 2). This imaging confirms that the difference between pre- and post-treatment is evident. Further follow-up imaging should continue to monitor whether the osteophytes remain stable and if heterotopic ossification reoccurs.

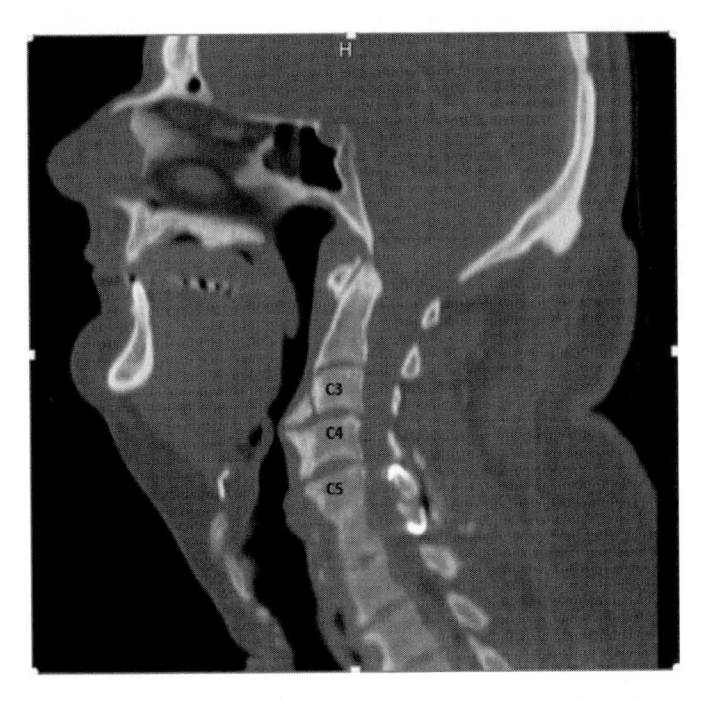

Figure 1. CT scan prior to resection of osteophytes. Narrowing of the pharynx is evident.

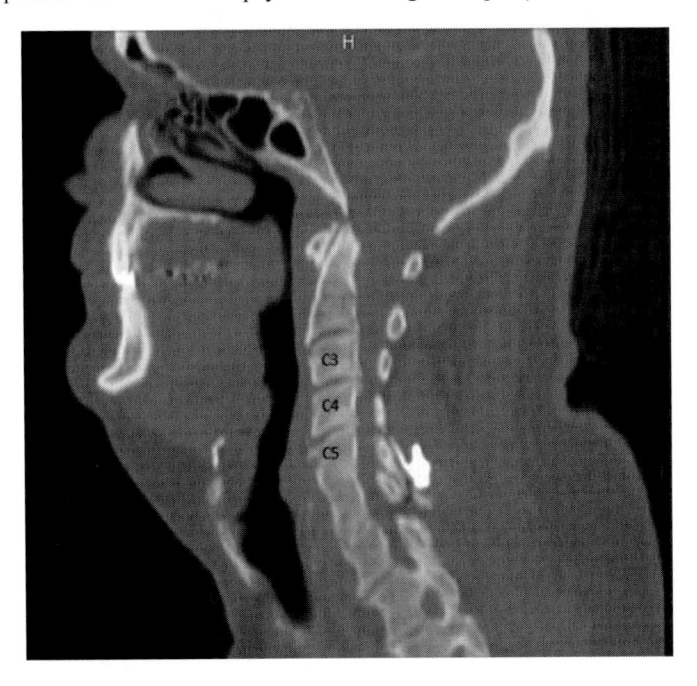

Figure 2. CT scan approximately 8 months after treatment. Minor osteophytes visible at C3-C4 and C4-C5.

Discussion

Heterotopic ossification may present following bone or joint surgery or as a consequence of central nervous system (CNS) injury (1-3). In patients undergoing surgery due to HO, as in this case report, there may be an increased risk of HO following surgery. Other risk factors include ankylosing spondylitis and osteoarthritis, as reported in studies involving surgery to the hip (7-10). The incidence of HO in patients with spinal cord injuries is between 20% and 25%, likely a result of immobilization (3). The incidence of clinically significant HO is low following hip surgery, however radiographic evidence is present in approximately 56% of patients (11). Since the patient presented with HO and ankylosing spondylitis as well as a history of spinal cord injury, he was at high risk for recurrence of HO.

Due to the limited literature on radiation treatment for established HO as well as irradiation for HO in non-pelvic regions of the body, the patient's physicians discussed whether radiation treatment would be appropriate as well as what dose they deemed to be safe and effective. It was agreed given this patient's likelihood of developing post-surgery HO that radiation would be offered. The single case report by Lo et al. stated that a single dose of 6 Gy was given to their patient, who was also experiencing dysphagia, the day after C3-C4 osteophytes were removed (6). Follow-up studies revealed recurrence of the osteophyte. Taking this case into consideration, as well as other studies which reported a single dose of 8 Gy as effective for prophylaxis of HO in the hip, the decision to give a higher dose of 8 Gy was made in the hopes of preventing reoccurrence (12-13).

Further studies on radiation treatment for established HO and for the prophylaxis of HO in non-pelvis areas must be conducted to collect data on success rates as well as conclusively determine the optimal dose fractionation. Current literature may be lacking not only due to the low incidence of this phenomenon, but also may be due to unsuccessful radiation treatment which is not reported as often as successful results. Another reason for the limited literature may be due to lack of follow-up as these patients are rarely followed long term by radiation oncologists and surgical follow-up is variable. The patient in this report is not currently experiencing dysphagia or other related symptoms, however this finding is reported less than a year after treatment. Further studies should be conducted to assess if and how long after resection and radiation treatment clinically significant osteophytes may reappear in the cervical spine.

Conclusion

Radiation treatment may be effective for preventing reccurrence of heterotopic ossification in the cervical spine. The potential benefit of irradiation must be weighed against the potential risk of creating a radiotherapy-induced malignancy. Radiation should be considered for patients at high risk of HO and the literature on the subject must be expanded in order for physicians to be informed when making radiation treatment decisions following surgery for established HO.

Acknowledgments

We thank the generous support of Bratty Family Fund, Michael and Karyn Goldstein Cancer Research Fund, Joseph and Silvana Melara Cancer Research Fund, and Ofelia Cancer Research Fund.

References

[1]   McCarthy EF, Sundaram M. Heterotopic ossification: a review. Skeletal Radiol 2005;34:609-19.

[2]   Vanden Bossche L, Vanderstraeten G. Heterotopic ossification: a review. J Rehabil Med 2005;37:129-36.

[3]   Garland DE. A clinical perspective on common forms of acquired heterotopic ossification. Clin Orthop Relat Res 1991;13-29.

[4]   Schaeffer MA, Sosner J. Heterotopic ossification: treatment of established bone with radiation therapy. Arch Phys Med Rehabil 1995;76:284-6.

[5]   Jang SH, Shin SW, Ahn SH, Cho IH, Kim SH. Radiation therapy for heterotopic ossification in a patient with traumatic brain injury. Yonsei Med J 2000;41:536-9.

[6]   Lo TCM, Pfeifer BA, Smiley PM, Gumley GJ. Case report: radiation prevention of heterotopic ossification after bone and joint surgery in sites other than hips. Br J Radiol 1996;69:673-7.

[7]   De Lee J, Ferrari A, Charnley J. Ectopic bone formation following low friction arthroplasty of the hip. Clin Orthop 1976;121:53–9.

[8]   Michelsson JE, Rauschning W. Pathogenesis of experimental heterotopic bone formation following temporary forcible exercising of immobilized limbs. Clin Orthop 1983;176:265–72.

[9]   Ekelund A, Brosjo O, Nilsson OS. Experimental induction of heterotopic bone. Clin Orthop 1991;263:102–12.

[10]   Kjaersgaard-Andersen P, Ritter MA. Prevention of formation of heterotopic bone after total hip arthroplasty. J Bone Joint Surg Am 1991;73:942–7.

[11]   Thomas BJ. Heterotopic bone formation after total hip arthroplasty. Orthop Clin North Am 1992;23:347–58.

[12]   Board TN, Karva A, Board RE, Gambhir AK, Porter ML. The prophylaxis and treatment of heterotopic ossification following lower limb arthroplasty. J Bone Joint Surg Br 2007;89:434-40.

[13]   Pellegrini VD Jr, Konski AA, Gastel JA, Rubin P, Evarts CM. Prevention of heterotopic ossification with irradiation after total hip arthroplasty: radiation therapy with a single dose of eight hundred centigray administered to a limited field. J Bone Joint Surg Am 1992;74:186-200.

In: Advanced Cancer
Editors: N. Thavarajah, N. Pulenzas, B. Lechner et al.

ISBN: 978-1-62808-239-5
© 2013 Nova Science Publishers, Inc.

Chapter 10

Good surgical outcome and long survival in a patient with occipitocervical instability requiring occiput to C3 fixation

Michael Poon, BSc(C), Michael Ford, FRCSC, Liang Zeng, MD(C), Monique Christakis, FRCPC, Emily Sinclair, MRTT, Natalie Lauzon, MRTT, Marko Popovic, BHSc(C) and Edward Chow*, MBBS

Rapid Response Radiotherapy Program, Department of Radiation Oncology, Odette Cancer Centre, Sunnybrook Health Sciences Centre, University of Toronto, Toronto, Ontario, Canada

Spinal metastases in the occipitocervical junction typically present with pain secondary to neck instability. Non-traumatic upper cervical instabilities are quite rare and are usually connected to C1 or C2 metastasis, rheumatoid polyarthritis, infection or congenital malformations. In many cases, these instabilities are symptomatic and can cause bilateral or quadrilateral limb paresthesias, sharp neck pain or upper back pain. Occipitocervical fixation is typically required for the treatment of these conditions. Commonly, rigid constructs are employed where plates are typically fixed into place with screws or wires. This report presents the case of a breast cancer patient who had neck instability and extensive left C1 destruction. Surgical stabilization from the patient's posterior occiput to C3 was performed with excellent results. The patient regained ambulatory function, with no intra-operative or post-operative complications. Exceptional survival was observed as well, with an improvement in quality of life, for 47 months to date.

* Correspondence: Professor Edward Chow MBBS, MSc, PhD, FRCPC Department of Radiation Oncology, Odette Cancer Centre, Sunnybrook Health Sciences Centre, 2075 Bayview Avenue, Toronto, ON Canada. Email:Edward.Chow@sunnybrook.ca.

Introduction

The third most common site of metastasis is the skeletal system, following lung and liver (1). It has been found that upon autopsy, vertebral body metastases have been found in over one third of all cancer patients (1). Metastases to this region may cause the loss of vertebral body structural integrity due to metastatic destruction and produce instability (1). For this reason, treatment of spinal metastases around the atlanto-axial region is required. However,flexion, extension, lateral bending, and rotation must be limited while accounting for poor bone quality and possible pannus (2). In many cases, these unique biomechanical and anatomical characteristics complicate occipitocervical stabilization procedures (3).

Patients with spinal metastases in the occipitocervical junction typically present with pain secondary to neck instability. Occipitocervical fixation is required for the treatment of upper cervical instabilities not related to trauma. Plates are typically fixed into place with screws or wires. However, this type of fixation is counter-indicated in the treatment of patients with osteoporosis or significant thinning of the occipital bone (4). Non-traumatic upper cervical instabilities are quite rare and are usually connected to C1 or C2 metastasis (as was the case with this patient), rheumatoid polyarthritis, infection or congenital malformations (4,5). We document the case of a woman with breast cancer who presents with cervical instability in her neck, whom by employing a rigid fixation construct has regained ambulatory function and has exceeded survival expectations.

Case report

A 70 year old female patient with breast cancer presented in the Rapid Response Radiotherapy Program (RRRP) at the Odette Cancer Centre, Toronto, Canadaon May 16, 2008 with severe neck pain for consideration of radiation treatment. Pathology revealed that the tumor was an invasive ductal carcinoma, both estrogen and progesterone positive but negative for HER2/NEU. The sentinel lymph node biopsy at that time showed 1 of the 2 intramammary lymph nodes was positive for metastatic cancer. By recommendation of the surgeon, since one of the two sentinel lymph nodes was positive for tumor cells, a complete axillary lymph node dissection was planned. However, because of a complicating infection, the procedure was postponed. Upon the patient's full recovery, the possibility of carrying out the initial surgery with subsequent palliative radiotherapy was revisited.

An x-ray taken subsequent to her visit to RRRP indicated that the patient had an unstable neck. Review of the x-ray showed occipitocervical instability secondary to left C1 lateral mass destruction, causing the loss of ambulatory ability. An orthopedic surgeon was consulted with regard to how to treat the patient as well as viability of surgical intervention. The patient was promptly scheduled for an occipital cervical fusion up to C3 on the posterior aspect of her cervical spine.

The patient underwent surgery to stabilize from her posterior occiput to C3 in June 2008. The right lateral mass of C1 and the right pars of C2 were noted to be destroyed by tumour on the computer tomography (CT) scan (see figure 1). No attempt was made to place instrumentation into those sites. Lateral mass screws were inserted into the left lateral mass of C1 and at C3; a pars screw was inserted at C2. The occipital plate was applied and a rod was appropriately contoured and fixed to the screws. Excellent purchase was obtained in C3 secondary to fairly large osteophytes with good quality sclerotic bone. Additional adjuvant fixation was carried out using an interspinous cable through the spinous processes of C2 and C3 around the rods of the construct. Polymethyl methacrylate (PMMA) bone cement was laid onto the posterior cervical spine and up onto the skull to further reinforce the construct. Intraoperative x-rays demonstrated the implants were in good position (see figure 2). There were no intraoperative complications and the patient was transported to the recovery room in good condition. Neural monitoring signals were intact throughout the procedure.

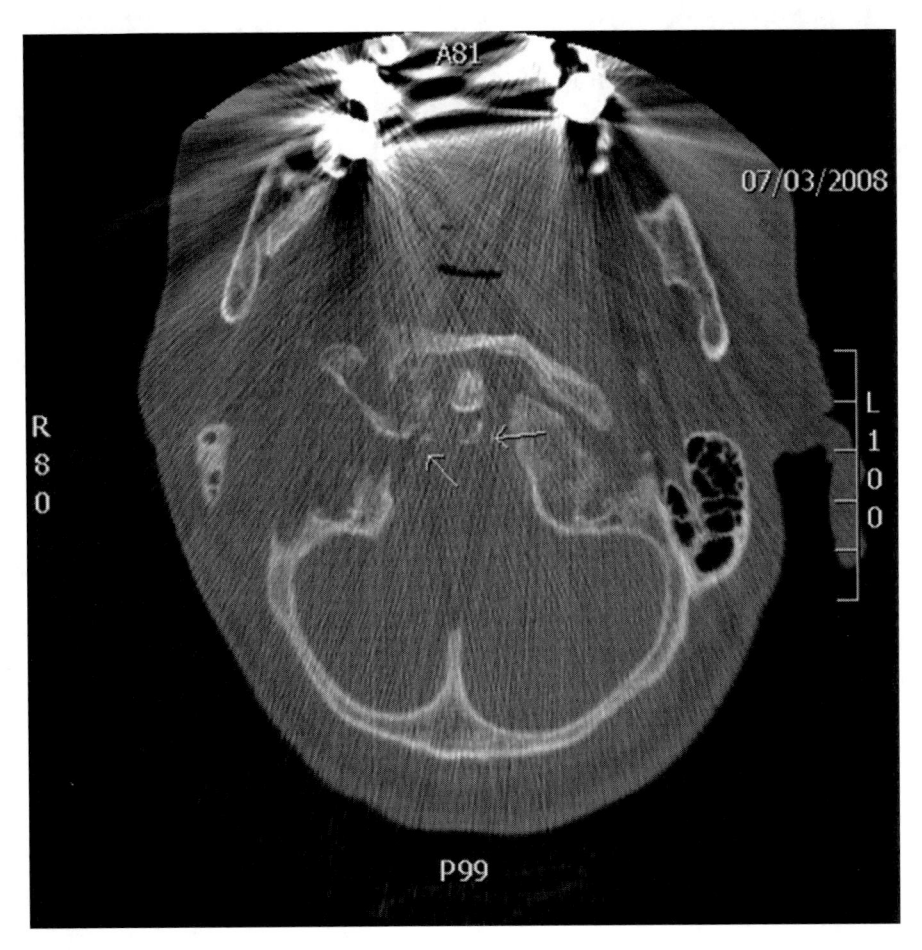

Figure 1. Cervical spine CT (July 2008) before surgeryshowingthe destruction of the right lateral mass of C1 and the right pars of C2.

The patient returned to the RRRP on July 31, 2008. The results of her surgical stabilization were excellent; she reported that she was able to walk again. Post-operative radiation of 2000 cGy in 5 fractions was delivered to her neck and it was suggested that she should discuss the possibility of systemic treatment. For the last two years, she had been ontamoxifen. Since she had her stabilization, she has experienced mild stiffness in her neck but there is no pain in her neck nor radiating down her arms. She denies any paresthesias or weakness in the arm.

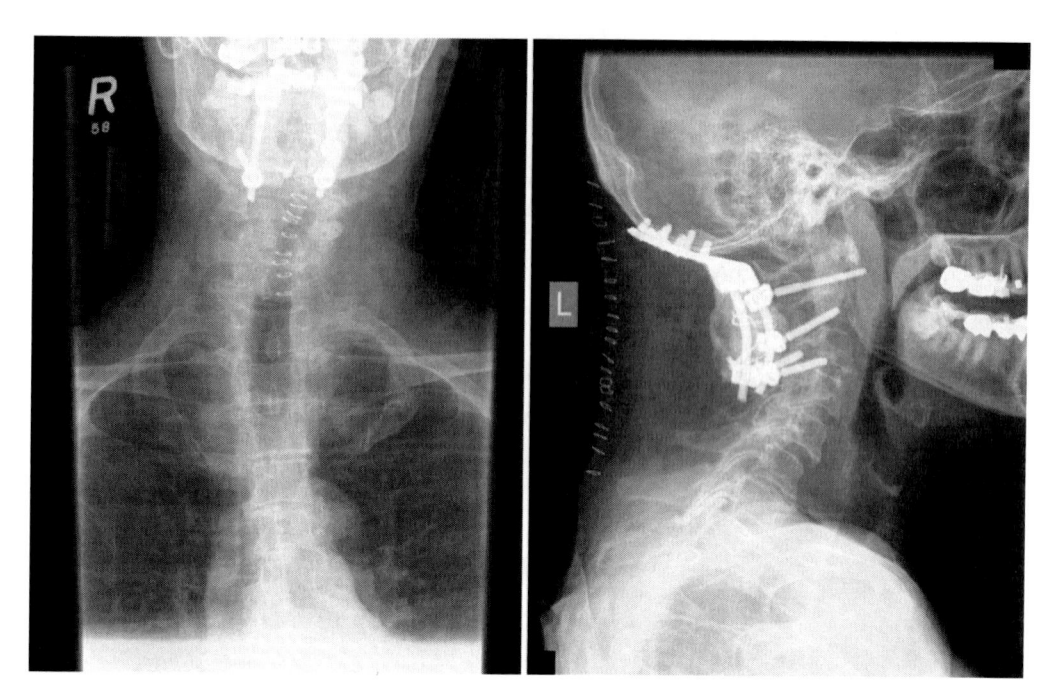

Figure 2. Intra-operative x-ray of cervical spine and occipitocervical(July 2008) demonstrating the implants to be in good position.

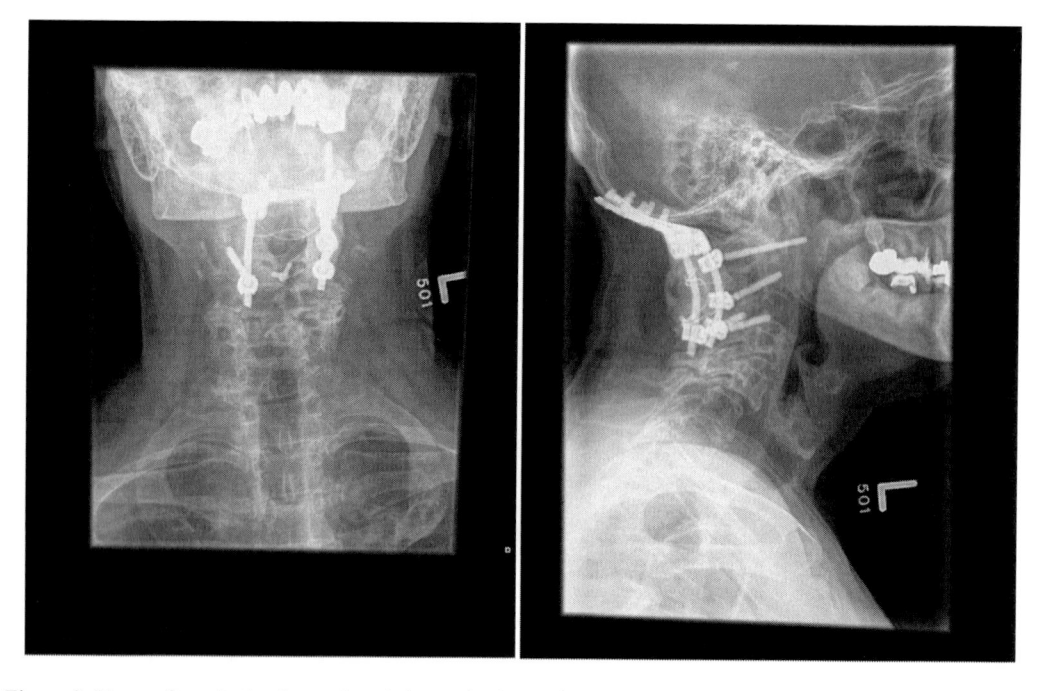

Figure 3. X-ray of cervical spine and occipitocervical construct (May 2012) 4 years post occipitocervical stabilization showingstable, minor degenerative listhesis below her construct with no other significant changes.

The patient is now 3-4 years post-occiput to C3 fusion for metastatic disease. The patient is doing extremely well. She is no longer taking pain medications and has managed to gain weight. She has developed some stiffness but still reports no pain or neurological symptoms.

X-ray shows minor degenerative listhesis that is stable below her construct with no other significant change (see figure 3). There is no evidence of any recurrence of tumor.

Discussion

Non-traumatic upper cervical instabilities are quite rare and are commonly connected to C1 or C2 metastasis. In many cases, these instabilities are symptomatic and can cause bilateral or quadrilateral limb paresthesias, sharp neck pain or upper back pain (6).This need for arthrodesis has buoyed various methods for occipitocervical fixation. As Garrido et al (5) found, clinical complications rates are significantly lower in patients treated with rigid occipitocervical fixation methods (10%) compared to non-rigid (48%). In this case, a rigid internal fixation construct was used as it provides immediate stability and eliminates the need for poorly tolerated external fixators. The results were very positive; the patient regained ambulatory function with no intraoperative or post-operative complications to report.

In a retrospective study by Fourney et al (3) of patients with C-1 or C-2 metastases that underwent surgery at the University of Texas MD Anderson Cancer Center between 1994 and 2001, the mean follow-up period was found to be 8 months. This study sought to review surgical strategies to stabilize the spine and advocated the use of posterior stabilization of the spine, citing the durable pain relief and preservation of ambulatory status (3). This result acquiesces with the similar outcome the patient presented experienced. However, through Kaplan-Meier analysis, the median survival was only reported to be 6.1 months (3). In the patient presented, not only was a good surgical outcome seen but much longer survival as well. This exceptional survival was observed, with an improvement in quality of life, for 47 months to date. This far surpasses the median survival of 6.1 months previously expected from literature.

This case adds to the literature advocating the use of posterior stabilization of the spine and avoidance of poorly tolerated external fixators. In the 4 years post-occiput to C3 fusion, occipitocervical stabilization has provided pain relief and preservation of the patient's ambulatory status, improving the quality of her life.

Acknowledgment

We thank the generous support of Bratty Family Fund, Michael and Karyn Goldstein Cancer Research Fund, Joseph and Silvana Melara Cancer Research Fund, and Ofelia Cancer Research Fund. We thank Ms Stacy Yuen for the secretarial support.

References

[1]   Ratliff JK, Cooper PR. Metastatic spine tumors. South Med J 2004;97(3):246-53.
[2]   Bongartz EB. Two asymmetric contoured plate-rods for occipitocervical fusion. Eur Spine J 2004;13(3):266-73.

[3]   Fourney DR, York JE, Cohen ZR, Suki D, Rhines LD, Gokaslan ZL. Management of atlantoaxial metastases with posterior occipito cervical stabilization. J Neurosurg 2003;98(Suppl 2):165-70.

[4]   Paquis P, Breuil V, Lonjon M, Euller-Ziegler L, Grellier P. Occipitocervical fixation using hooks and screws for upper cervical instability. Neurosurgery 1999;44(2):324-31.

[5]   Garrido BJ, Myo GK, Sasso RC. Rigid versus non rigid occipitocervical fusion: a clinical comparison of short-term outcomes. J Spinal Disord Tech 2011;24(1):20-3.

[6]   Cook C, Brismee JM, Fleming R, Sizer PS,Jr. Identifiers suggestive of clinical cervical spine instability: a Delphi study of physical therapists. PhysTher 2005;85(9):895-906.

In: Advanced Cancer   ISBN: 978-1-62808-239-5
Editors: N. Thavarajah, N. Pulenzas, B. Lechner et al.   © 2013 Nova Science Publishers, Inc.

Chapter 11

Pain relief through palliative radiation therapy in a patient with cervical spine bone metastases

*Rehana Jamani, BSc(C)[1], Liang Zeng, MD(C)[1],
Linda Probyn, MD[2], Natalie Lauzon, MRTT[1], Lori Holden, MRTT[1],
Nemica Thavarajah, BSc(C)[1], Erin Wong, BSc(C)[1]
and Edward Chow, MBBS[1]**

[1]Rapid Response Radiotherapy Program, Department of Radiation Oncology,
[2]Department of Medical Imaging, Sunnybrook Health Sciences Centre,
University of Toronto, Toronto, Ontario, Canada

Abstract

In up to 75% of cases, prostate cancer metastasizes to the bone, often to the spine. Metastatic destruction often leads to a loss of vertebral body structural integrity, thus leading to instability. As a result of instability, patients often experience intense pain. Radiation therapy is generally known to provide pain relief and tumour control for patients with bone metastases; however, it does not improve bone stability. We present with a prostate cancer patient with bone metastases to the cervical spine (C-spine) leading to basilar invagination. The result of this was limited neck motion and severe pain. The metastases were treated with external beam radiation. At the most recent follow-up, the patient had regained neck movement and had experienced significant pain relief.

* Correspondence: Professor Edward Chow MBBS, MSc, PhD, FRCPC, Department of Radiation Oncology, Odette Cancer Centre, Sunnybrook Health Sciences Centre, 2075 Bayview Avenue, Toronto, ON Canada. E-mail: Edward.Chow@sunnybrook.ca.

Introduction

Metastasis to the bone is common in patients with advanced prostate cancer, occurring in up to 75% of patients (1). In particular, vertebral body metastases are generally found in more than one third of autopsied cancer patients (2). The median survival of patients with prostate cancer metastatic to the bone is 12-53 months (1).

There are multiple treatment options for spinal metastases including surgery and radiotherapy. Indications for surgery include spinal instability from pathological fracture, neurological compression, and disease or pain unresponsive to radiotherapy, chemotherapy, or hormone therapy. In cases where a patient is unable to undergo an open surgical procedure (for example due to co-morbidities), minimally invasive approaches are available. Vertebroplasty and kyphoplasty are two such options for the treatment of spinal instability. By improving a patient's spinal instability, the goal is to reduce their pain level (1).

Radiation therapy is known to be effective in providing pain relief, and in most cases of vertebral body metastases, is the first therapy considered (3). Metastatic destruction often leads to a loss of vertebral body structural integrity, thus leading to instability (2). Pain is often the first symptom that presents in patients with spinal metastases, often as a result of instability (4). Radiation therapy is generally known to provide pain relief and tumour control for patients with bone metastases; however, it does not improve bone stability (3). Previous research has shown that as many as one-third of patients treated with radiotherapy experience total pain relief, independent of primary cancer or lesion type, and a further one-third experience some level of pain relief (1). The following case demonstrates the effectiveness of radiation therapy as a method of pain relief for a patient with spinal metastases.

Case report

A sixty-seven year old male patient with prostatic adenocarcinoma and painful bone metastases was seen in the Rapid Response Radiotherapy Program (RRRP) at the Odette Cancer Centre (OCC), Toronto, Canada. The patient presented with limited neck rotation, difficulty with lateral flexion, and pain in the bilateral hip area. Previous scans showed multiple spots of metastatic disease including the skull base involving the clivus, the cervical spine (C1), and the bilateral femora. A single 8 Gy fraction of radiation was given to the area after plain films showed no risk of fracture in the femora. The patient was referred to be seen in the orthopedic clinic regarding the disease in the skull base and cervical spine and was prescribed a soft collar.

CT scans completed after the patient's appointment in the RRRP showed basilar invagination (figures 1 and 3). As such, the orthopedic surgeon recommended posterior occipitocervical instrumented fusion followed by post-operative radiotherapy to stabilize the patient. The patient declined the surgical approach and chose instead to begin with radiation treatment.

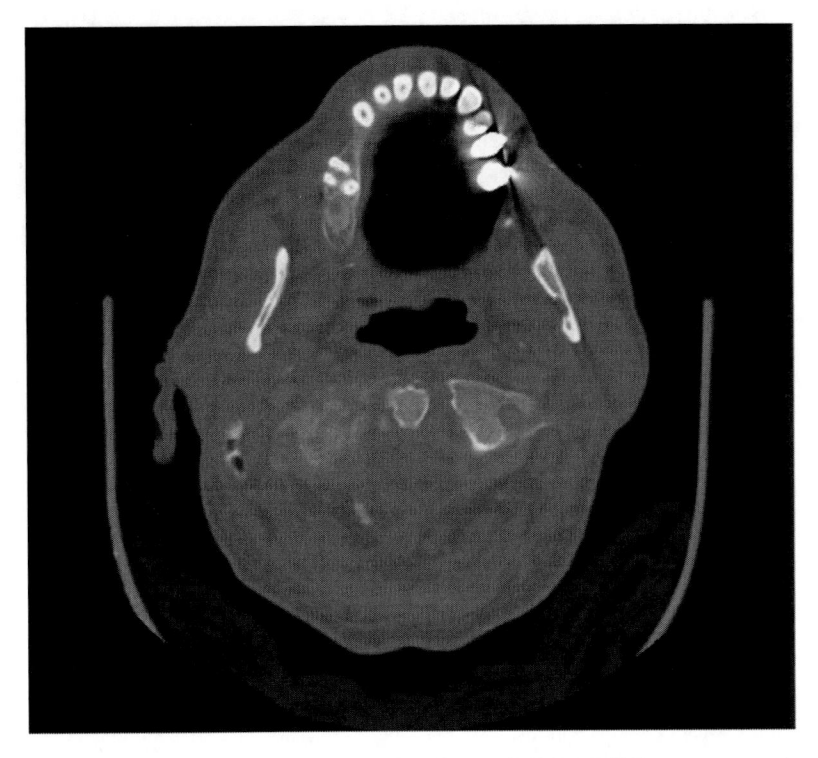

Figure 1. Axial CT image through the C1 level on bone window (W3000, L600) pretreatment demonstrating a predominately lytic lesion in the right C1 lateral mass.

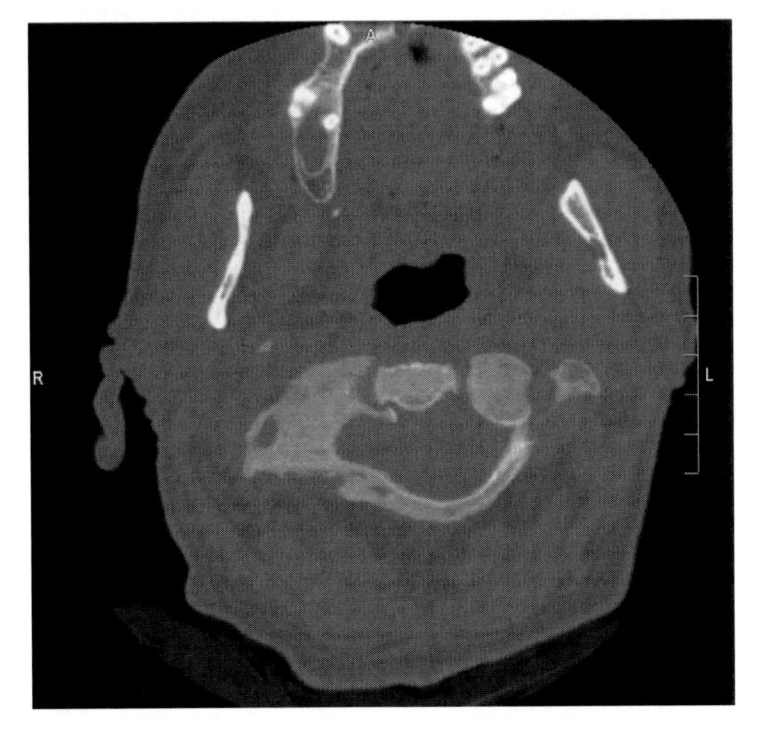

Figure 2. Axial CT image through the C1 vertebra on bone window (W3000, L600) post-treatment demonstrating increased sclerosis of the lesion involving the C1 lateral mass.

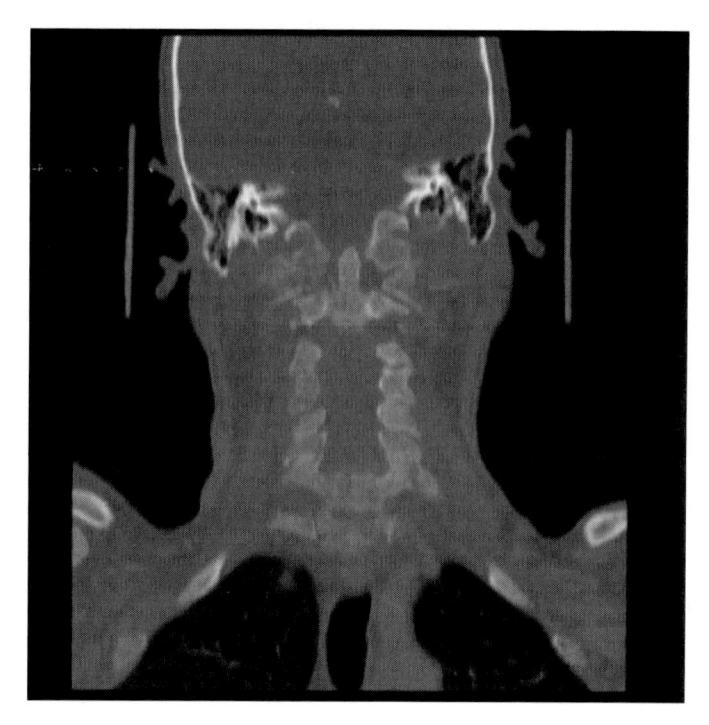

Figure 3. Coronal CT image on bone window (W3000, L600) pretreatment demonstrating a predominantly lytic lesion with the right C1 lateral mass with lateral displacement and mal-alignment between the C1 and C2 lateral masses.

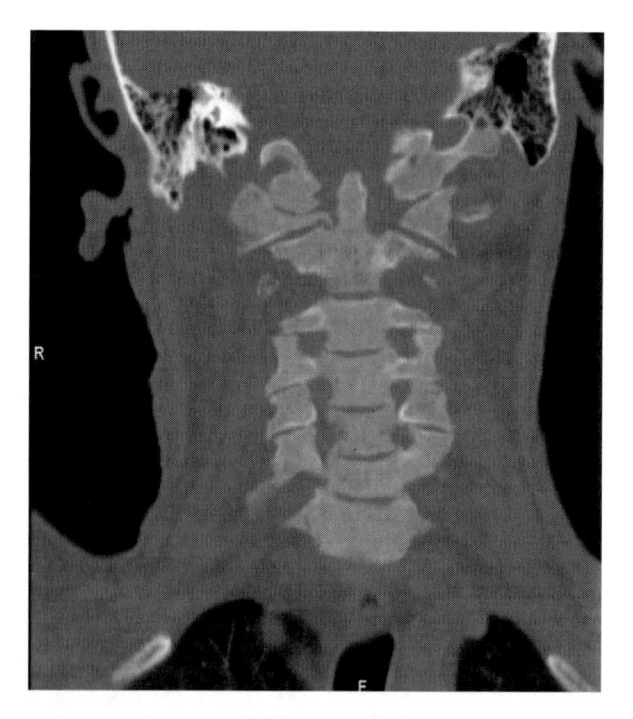

Figure 4. Coronal CT image on bone window (W3000, L600) post-treatment demonstrating increased sclerosis of the C1 lateral mass laterally displacing and mal-alignment between the C1 and C2 lateral masses is unchanged.

The patient received 20 Gy in 5 fractions to the cervical spine in May 2012 and was seen post-treatment in the Fracture Clinic. Surgery was once again offered as an option to address stability. Due to the decrease in pain from the radiation treatment and the higher risks associated with surgery post-radiation, the patient opted to remain with the nonsurgical approach.

The patient was last seen on July 13, 2012 in the Bone Metastases Clinic (BMC) at the OCC with the repeat imaging (Figures 2 and 4). He no longer had pain associated with neck movement and as such, no longer required the use of a collar. It was decided that due to the positive response to radiation, no further treatment was needed for the neck at present. The patient will continue to be followed closely.

Discussion

Non-traumatic upper cervical instabilities are uncommon. They generally occur as a result of rheumatoid poly-arthritis, complex congenital malformations, or C1 or C2 metastasis, as seen in this patient (5). Cervical instabilities often cause symptoms such as bilateral or quadrilateral limb paresthesias, upper back pain, or sharp neck pain (6). Uncontrolled cancer-related pain occurs in over 70% of patients with metastases (7).

The need to treat bone metastases with radiotherapy is indicated by pain, risk for pathological fracture, or spinal cord compression. Due to the lower tolerance to radiation of the spinal cord, radiotherapy doses administered to spinal metastases are often palliative. The treatment is intended to cause tumour regression and ideally alleviate symptoms for the long term (7). Localized external beam radiotherapy aims to relieve symptoms, restore function, and stop disease progression. This has shown to be an effective treatment modality for patients with bone metastases. Previous studies have shown that 80-90% of such patients treated with various fractionations of radiotherapy have experienced pain relief (3). In addition, it has been shown that prostate cancer patients are likely to experience a decrease in pain early post-treatment. Radiation is an effective option for patients with metastases to the cervical spine as studies have shown that the location of vertebral metastases (cervical, lumbar, or thoracic) does not impact patient response to the treatment (8).

This case demonstrates the effectiveness of radiotherapy as a method of relieving pain and restoring mobility. In the two months since radiation treatment to the cervical spine, the patient has experienced substantial pain relief and has regained the function of his neck, significantly improving his overall quality of life.

Acknowledgments

We thank the generous support of Bratty Family Fund, Michael and Karyn Goldstein Cancer Research Fund, Joseph and Silvana Melara Cancer Research Fund, and Ofelia Cancer Research Fund. We thank Ms Stacy Yuen for secretarial assistance.

References

[1]   Nguyen J, Chow E, Cramarossa G, Finkelstein J, Goh P. Handbook of Bone Metastases for healthcare professionals. Toronto: Odette Cancer Centre, Sunnybrook Health Sciences Centre, 2011.

[2]   Ratliff JK, Cooper PR. Metastatic spine tumors. South Med J 2004;97(3):246-53.

[3]   Chow E, Wu J, Barnes ET. Cancer drug discovery and development. Bone metastases: Experimental and clinical therapeutics. Totowa: Humana Press, 2005:323-36.

[4]   Katagiri H, Takahashi M, Inagaki J, Kobayashi H, Sugiura H, Yamamura S, Iwata H. Clinical results of nonsurgical treatment for spinal metastases. Int J Radiat Oncol Biol Phys 1998;42(5);1127-32.

[5]   Paquis P, Breuil V, Lonjon M, Euller-Ziegler L, Grellier P. Occipitocervical fixation using hooks and screws for upper cervical instability. Neurosurgery 1999;44(2):324-31.

[6]   Cook C, Brismee JM, Fleming R, Sizer PS Jr. Identifiers suggestive of clinical cervical spine instability: a Delphi study of physical therapists. Phys Ther 2005;85(9):895-906.

[7]   Janjan NA. Radiation for bone metastases. Cancer 1997;80:1628-45.

[8]   Nguyen J, Chow E, Zeng L, Zhang L, Culleton S, Holden L, Mitera G, Tsao M, Barnes E, Danjoux C, Sahgal A. Palliative response and functional interference outcomes using the brief pain inventory for spinal bony metastases treated with conventional radiotherapy. Clin Oncol (R Coll Radiol) 2011;23(7):485-91.

In: Advanced Cancer
Editors: N. Thavarajah, N. Pulenzas, B. Lechner et al.

ISBN: 978-1-62808-239-5
© 2013 Nova Science Publishers, Inc.

Chapter 12

Single fraction palliative radiation treatment in the treatment of bone metastases with soft tissue mass

Nicholas Lao, Michael Poon, BSc(C), Linda Probyn, MD, Marko Popovic, BHSc(C), Ronald Chow, Natalie Lauzon, MRTT and Edward Chow, MBBS[*]

Rapid Response Radiotherapy Program, Department of Radiation Oncology, Odette Cancer Centre, Sunnybrook Health Sciences Centre, University of Toronto, Toronto, Ontario, Canada

Abstract

Pain associated with bone metastases can substantially decrease the quality of life (QOL) in cancer patients; single or multiple fraction radiation treatment is commonly used to treat uncomplicated bone metastases. However when the bone metastasis is associated with soft tissue mass, we tend to deliver multiple radiation treatments. We present a case report involving a 56-year old female breast cancer patient presenting with a right femur bone metastasis with soft tissue mass. The patient was treated with a single 8 Gy fraction of radiation and responded well to the treatment with good pain relief and shrinkage of the soft tissue mass.

[*] Correspondence: Professor Edward Chow MBBS, MSc, PhD, FRCPC Department of Radiation Oncology, Odette Cancer Centre, Sunnybrook Health Sciences Centre, 2075 Bayview Avenue, Toronto, ON Canada. E-mail: Edward.Chow@sunnybrook.ca.

Introduction

Bone metastases occur in up to 85% of breast cancer patients [1]. For these patients, pain is a common symptom [2]. Palliative treatments for bone metastases are aimed at reducing pain experienced by the patient and improving their overall quality of life (QOL) [3]. Treatment options include single or multiple fraction radiotherapy for pain. Debate exists in the literature on which one is optimal for palliative cancer patients [2]. When the bone metastasis is associated with soft tissue mass, we tend to deliver multiple radiation treatments.

In this report, we present the case of a middle-aged woman with primary breast cancer who developed a right femur bone metastasis with soft tissue mass lesion and was treated with a single 8 Gy of radiation.

Case report

In November of 2008, a 56-year old female with a right breast carcinoma was referred to the Odette Cancer Centre, Sunnybrook Hospital. Breast lumpectomy and sentinel node biopsy were performed and positively identified the cancer as an invasive ductal carcinoma. The lesion was of high-grade and measured 2.3 cm. It was also found to be ER/PR negative and HER-2 negative. One sentinel lymph node was removed and found to be negative for metastatic disease. The biopsy also revealed perineural invasion without invasive tumor necrosis. An abdominal ultrasound performed showed no evidence of metastatic disease within the liver. She began four cycles of chemotherapy with good tolerance. Radiotherapy of 5000 cGy was delivered in 25 fractions to the right breast and completed in March of 2009. Afterwards, the patient developed shingles for which she received Calamine Lotion and antiviral medications.

In April 2012, the patient developed local recurrence and was treated with mastectomy and lymph node dissection. There were at least seven lymph nodes found involved with extranodal extension. The tumor itself measured 0.6 x 0.1 cm. The patient was at a very high risk of distant metastases.

In June 2012, the patient was referred to the Bone Metastases Clinic after a painful lesion of 4-5 cm developed in her right distal femur. A computed tomography (CT) scan showed that the lesion was both intramedullary and extramedullary and primarily soft tissue without definite evidence of cortical breach (Figure 1). No prophylactic fixation was needed as there was no significant loss of structural bone. She received a single 8 Gy.

A post-radiation CT scan was performed on the right femur. The soft tissue mass had substantially decreased in size, and new endosteal and periosteal bone had formed in the femur (Figure 2). The patient also reported substantial pain relief.

Discussion

Radiation is a common treatment for pain in patients with bone metastases. Treatments in Canada usually consist of multiple fractions or a single fraction [4]. In this case, the patient received a single 8 Gy radiation to her right femur and experienced good pain relief as well as a good response in the post-radiation CT scan. These responses indicate the efficacy of single fraction radiation to bone for the palliative treatment of bone metastases in both reducing pain and shrinking the soft tissue mass.

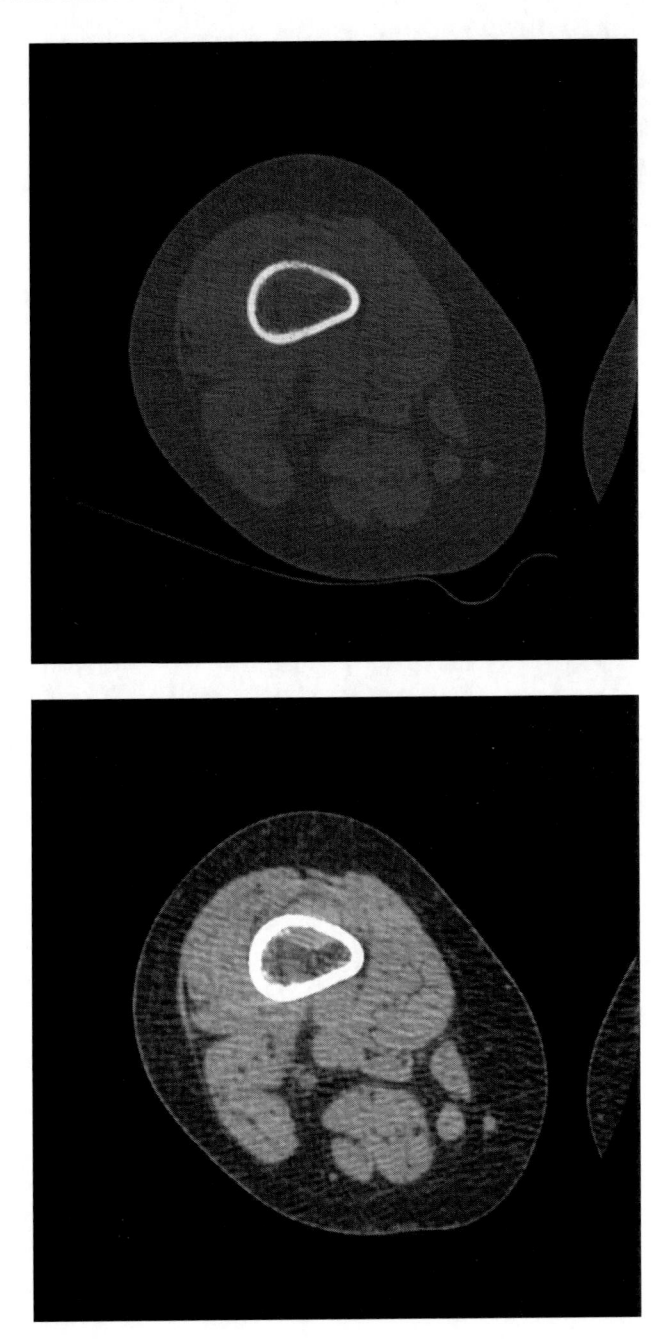

Figure 1. Axial CT images through the right femur pre-radiation treatment on soft tissue and bone windows demonstrating a cortical-based soft tissue mass at the anterior femur with endosteal, intramedullary and extraosseous components compatible with metastases from breast carcinoma with permeative change of the cortex.

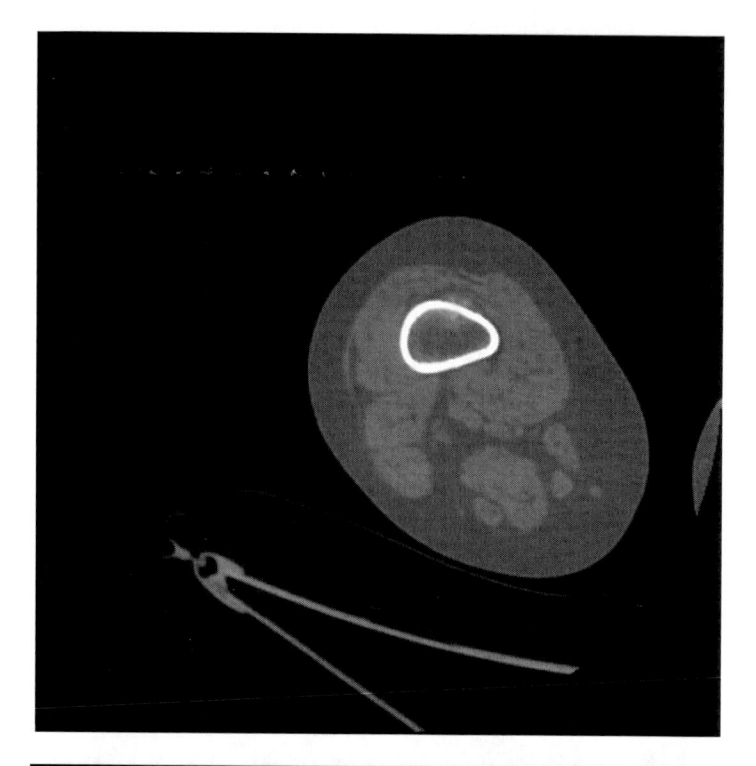

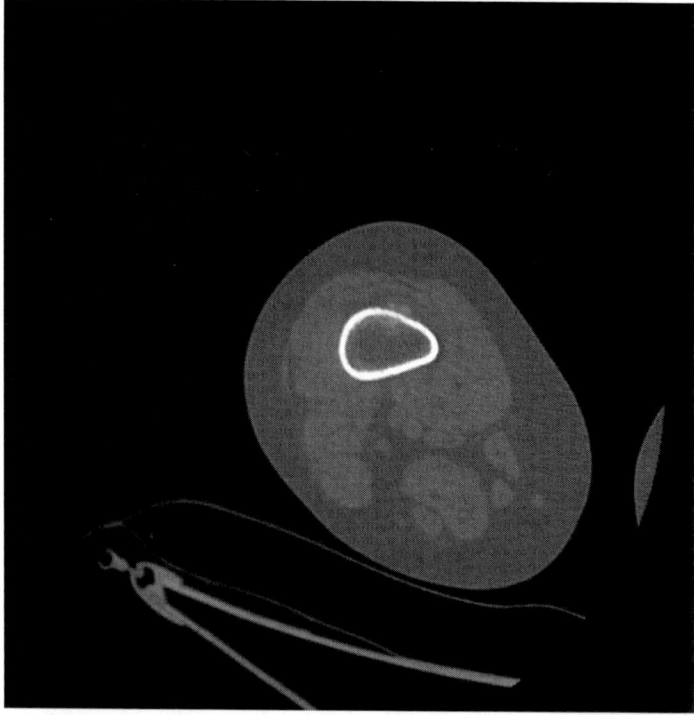

Figure 2. Axial CT images through the right femur post-radiation treatment on soft tissue and bone windows and sagittal reformatted image on bone windows demonstrating a decrease in size of the soft tissue mass in the intramedullary and extraosseous components with residual permeative change of the cortex and periosteal reaction related to a treatment response.

Acknowledgments

We thank the generous support of Bratty Family Fund, Michael and Karyn Goldstein Cancer Research Fund, Joseph and Silvana Melara Cancer Research Fund, and Ofelia Cancer Research Fund. We thank Stacy Yuen for secretarial assistance.

References

[1]   Verbeeck A. Bone metastases from breast cancer: Guidelines for diagnosis. A case report from the chiropractic office. J Manipulat Physiol Ther 2004; 27(3): 211-5.

[2]   Badzio A, Senkus-Konefka E, Jereczek-Fossa B, Adamska K, Fajndt S, et al. 20 Gy in five fractions versus 8 Gy in one fraction in palliative radiotherapy of bone metastases. A multicenter randomized study. NOWOTWORY J Oncol 2003;53(3):261-4.

[3]   Hartsell W, Scott C, Bruner D, Scarantino C, Ivker R, et al. Randomized trial for short-versus long course radiotherapy for palliation of painful bone metastases. J Natl Cancer Institute 2005;97(11):798-804.

[4]   Kachnic L, Berk L. Palliative single-fraction radiation therapy: How Much more evidence is needed? J Natl Cancer Institute 2005;97(11):786-8.

In: Advanced Cancer
ISBN: 978-1-62808-239-5
Editors: N. Thavarajah, N. Pulenzas, B. Lechner et al.   © 2013 Nova Science Publishers, Inc.

Chapter 13

Radiation therapy alone for established heterotopic ossification

Erin Wong, BSc (C)[1], Gemma Cramarossa, BHSc (C)[1], Gillian Bedard, BSc(C)[1], Linda Probyn, MD[2], Lori Holden, MRTT[1], Edward Chow, MBBS[1] and Natalie Lauzon, MRTT[1]*

[1]Rapid Response Radiotherapy Program, Department of Radiation Oncology, Odette Cancer Centre, Sunnybrook Health Sciences Centre,, [2]Department of Medical Imaging, Sunnybrook Health Sciences Centre, University of Toronto, Toronto, Ontario, Canada

Abstract

There are limited therapeutic treatment options for established heterotopic ossification. The most common treatment option is surgical resection of the bone formed followed with prophylactic radiation treatment to prevent reoccurrence. However, this presents an issue when a patient is not a surgical candidate: how is established heterotopic ossification treated then? Here, we present the case of a 55-year-old male with extensive heterotopic ossification in the pelvis area causing significant pain. Since this patient was not a surgical candidate, his options were limited. A single dose of 8 Gy radiation was prescribed to the painful area and this patient experienced significant pain relief despite no interval radiological change in the established heterotopic ossification. Further studies should be conducted to assess and understand the efficacy of radiation to palliate pain caused by heterotopic ossification.

* Correspondence: Ms. Natalie Lauzon BSc, MRTT Department of Radiation Therapy, Odette Cancer Centre, Sunnybrook Health Sciences Centre, 2075 Bayview Avenue, Toronto, ON Canada. Email: Natalie. Lauzon @ Sunnybrook.ca.

Introduction

Heterotopic ossification, or heterotopic bone formation, is a complication that can be brought about by trauma, central nervous system injuries, operations, fractures or can also occur as a result of a genetic disorder (1-3). It is a condition characterized by the formation of bone outside of the skeleton, occupying space in soft tissue (4). This bone formation can occur in areas such as the skin, muscles, and walls of vessels (5). Although the initial establishment of heterotopic ossification can be asymptomatic, with progression of this bone formation, there are instances in which it can lead to severe pain (2,6).

There are certain risk factors for the development of heterotopic ossification such as gender and past medical history. Those particularly at risk are males, patients that have had a previous history of heterotopic ossification and patients that suffer from paraplegia due to a spinal cord injury (1,6).

In terms of heterotopic ossification prevention, radiation has been recognized as a useful prophylactic treatment after hip surgery (7). There has also been evidence for its role as a prophylactic treatment in other joints such as knee and elbow or the spine (6,8). In general, this is a clinically accepted prophylactic treatment after resection of heterotopic ossification (9).

It has also been suggested through a few case reports that radiation alone may have a role as a therapeutic treatment for established heterotopic ossification, hence, not only as a prophylactic treatment. In two case reports, Schaeffer et al. and Jang et al., both reported an increase in mobility and a reduction of pain in patients with established heterotopic ossification treated with therapeutic radiation (10,11).

In the following case, a 55-year-old quadriplegic male experienced significant pain, which corresponded to areas of heterotopic ossification. Radiation treatment alone was given to the area of pain in hopes of palliation.

Case report

A 55-year-old male has been a C5 quadriplegic secondary to a motor vehicle accident in 1994. Due to the accident, he underwent an anterior cervical spine decompression and fusion at C5-6 because of a cervical spine fracture. He was referred to the Rapid Response Radiotherapy Program (RRRP) at Sunnybrook Odette Cancer Centre in 2011 due to dysphagia caused by heterotopic ossification at the C3-4 and C4-5 level. Of concern were the osteophytes at the C3-4 level, which the orthopedic surgeons felt was operable. Thus in August 2011, the patient proceeded with a C3-4 anterior cervical decompression and drilling followed by a prophylactic radiation treatment of 8 Gy in one fraction post-surgery.

This patient was then seen again in the RRRP in May of 2012 and reported no pain at the C3-5 area and no dysphagia. However, at this time, this patient had pain in the pelvic region, which corresponded with heterotopic ossification imaged on a recent CT scan. This heterotopic ossification was deemed inoperable by two different orthopedic surgeons. Since there was previous evidence from literature that radiation may be used as a therapeutic option for pain caused by heterotopic ossification, we offered this patient a single 8 Gy of radiation to the pelvic region extending to the proximal bilateral femurs to palliate the pain.

From May 11, 2012, the pre-radiation CT scan of the spine, abdomen and pelvis showed extensive bilateral heterotopic ossification in the hip regions, sacroiliac joints and anterior and medial portion of the proximal femurs (Figures 1 and 2). An aspect of ossification was seen in both the left and right iliac wing measuring 20cm and 15cm respectively. On the left, there was a bulk of ossification anterior to the hip extending from the iliac ossification (Figure 1). Treatment to the pelvic region and bilateral femurs was delivered on May 24, 2012 (Figure 3).

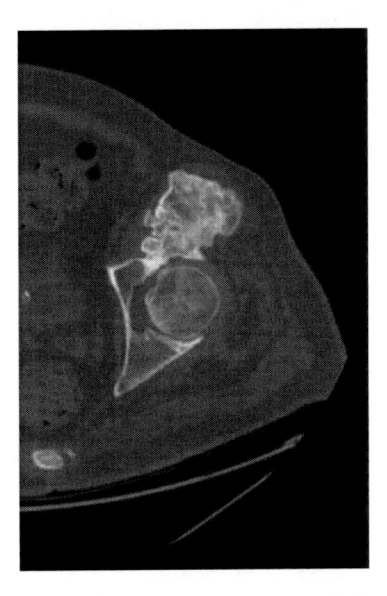

Figure 1. Axial CT scan through the pelvis prior to the therapeutic radiation treatment showing extensive heterotopic ossification anterior to the left hip.

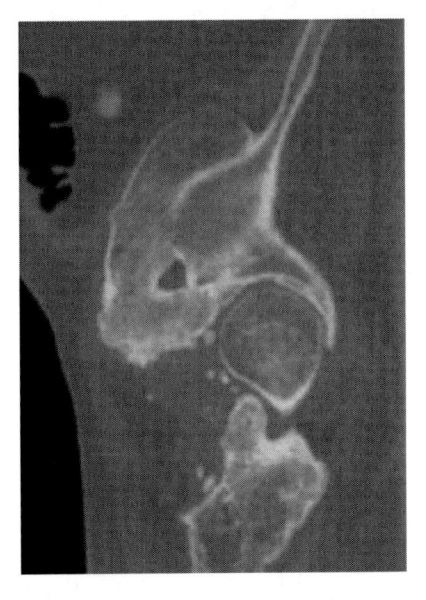

Figure 2. Sagittal reformatted CT scan through the left hip prior to the therapeutic radiation treatment showing prominent heterotopic ossification extending from the left ilium and proximal femur anterior to the hip.

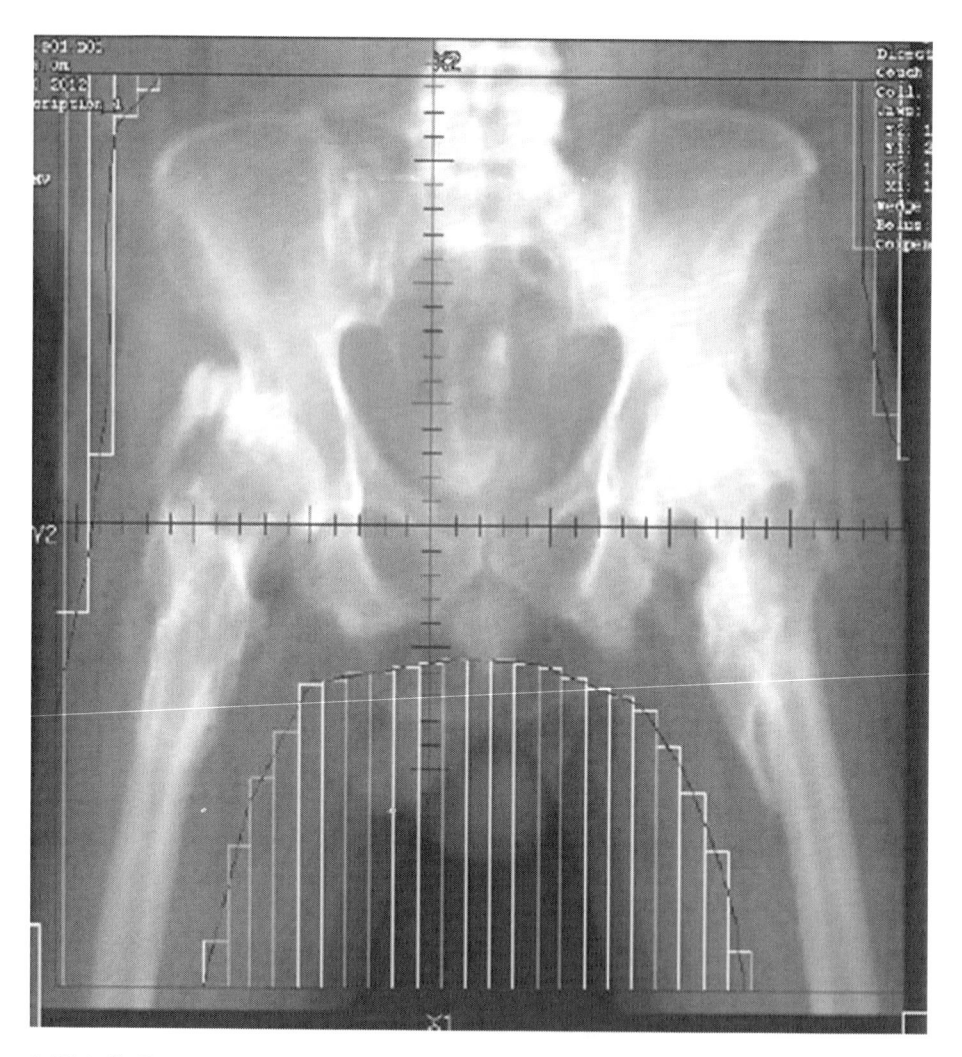

Figure 3. Digitally Reconstructed Image (DRR) representing radiation treatment volume, treated anteriorly and posteriorly for 800 cGy in 1 fraction, delivered on May 24th, 2012.

On September 12, 2012, post-radiation CT scans from the head and neck to bilateral femurs were ordered for comparison. These CT scans showed similar extensive heterotopic ossification along the same regions as noted in May of 2012 (Figures 4 and 5) with no interval change in comparison to the scans from May 11, 2012.

The patient completed a pain diary, daily at the end of each day, to track his pain post-radiation for twenty days. This diary tracked the patient's pain score out of 10, whether the pain was better, worse or the same in comparison to before radiation and the pain medications the patient took that day. As recorded in the pain diary, the patient experienced an increase in pain from the first day after radiation to the seventh day after radiation. At the eighth day after treatment, the patient began noticing some pain relief, with a decrease in pain score from 7/10 to 4/10 with no change in regular pain medication. From the eighth day and onwards, the patient's pain relief fluctuated with some days better than others, but towards the fifteenth day after treatment, pain relief occurred more consistently and at the twentieth day post-radiation, the patient recorded a pain score of 2-3/10 for most of the day. The patient was seen 4 months post-treatment on September 20, 2012. At this follow-up, the patient reported that this pain relief has been consistent and he expressed that he believes the radiation has provided palliation of pain for his extensive heterotopic ossification.

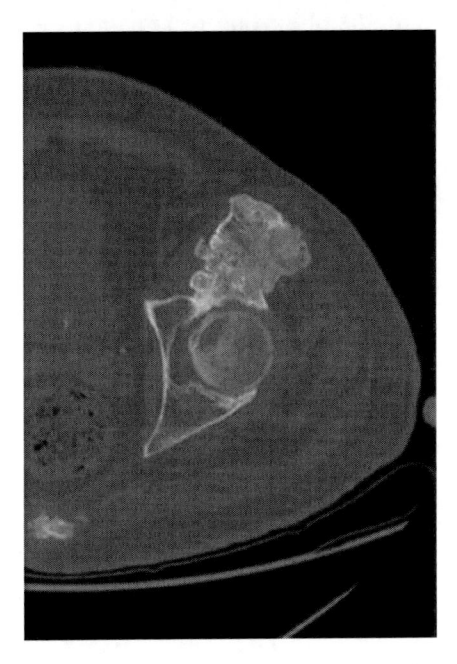

Figure 4. Axial CT scan through the pelvis post-therapeutic radiation treatment showing extensive heterotopic ossification anterior to the left hip as seen previously.

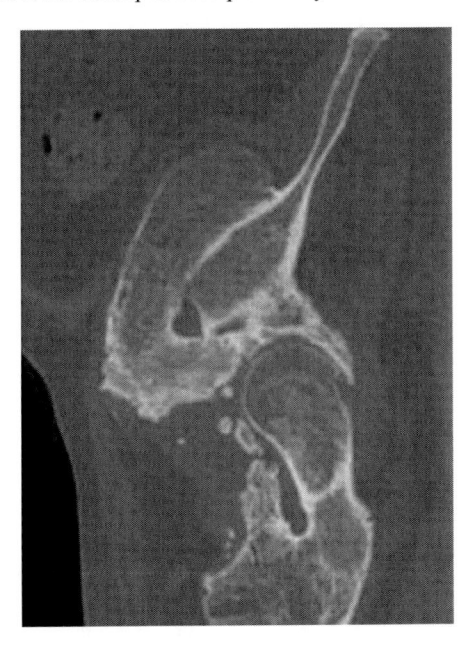

Figure 5. Sagittal reformatted CT scan through the left hip post-therapeutic radiation treatment showing prominent heterotopic ossification extending from the left ilium and proximal femur anterior to the hip as seen previously.

Discussion

In the current body of literature, the utilization of radiation for heterotopic ossification has only been established as a prophylactic treatment, mainly after bone surgery. While the available therapeutic treatment for established heterotopic ossification is severely limited, surgical resection is traditionally the only option (2,3,6,7). This leaves few options for patients that are not surgical candidates. There exists a few cases as reported by Schaeffer et al (10) and Jang et al (11) on the usage of radiation as a therapeutic treatment, giving hope to those with established heterotopic ossification.

Schaeffer et al reported two cases in which patients experienced decrease range of motion and significant pain in the hip and elbow due to the formation of heterotopic ossification in these joints. This pain was palliated and greater range of motion was seen post-radiation treatment in both patients (11). It should be noted that for the aforementioned patients, a dose fractionation schedule of 20 Gy in 10 fractions was used. Similarly, Jang et al. reported on the usage of the 20 Gy in 10 fractions on a patient that developed heterotopic ossification in both hips post-brain trauma. This patient also reported decreased pain and increased activity after the therapeutic radiation treatment (10).

In the current case, this patient suffered from quadriplegia secondary to a motor vehicle accident. It has been suggested that paraplegia is a risk factor for the development of heterotopic ossification, which may explain the extensive formation of heterotopic ossification in this patient that lead to significant pain (1). Based upon the evidence from Schaeffer et al (10) and Jang et al (11), we recommended a single dose of radiation as a therapeutic treatment for heterotopic ossification for the palliation of the pain. Despite having no interval radiological change in the heterotopic ossification formed, the patient experienced significant pain relief after radiation. During the twenty days post-treatment, the patient may have experienced a pain flare due to the radiation, as seen in the initial seven days in which he experienced increased pain. Once this increased pain subsided, pain relief was experienced, similar to other radiation-induced pain flare process. The efficacy and mechanism by which radiation acts as a therapeutic treatment for the abnormal formation of bone is still an area of uncertainty. The mechanism for the therapeutic usage of radiation for heterotopic ossification is hypothesized to be due to the stopping of osteoblastic stem cell formation thus preventing continuous bone formation which may be the cause of pain (11).

This case study and the two others that preceded it reveals an area of study that requires further investigation, however this does add to the body of literature supporting the use of radiation alone as a therapeutic treatment for heterotopic ossification. Therefore, radiation may be a possible treatment option to palliate the pain in patients with heterotopic ossification who are experiencing significant pain yet are not surgical candidates. It can be further suggested that a single dose of 8 Gy radiation may be effective in this usage. Further research should be conducted to establish the efficacy of radiation as a therapeutic treatment for heterotopic ossification as well as determining the most effective dose fractionation schedule.

Acknowledgments

We thank the generous support of Bratty Family Fund, Michael and Karyn Goldstein Cancer Research Fund, Joseph and Silvana Melara Cancer Research Fund, and Ofelia Cancer Research Fund.

References

[1] Shehab D, Elgazzar AH, Collier BD. Heterotopic ossification. J Nucl Med 2002;43(3):346-53.

[2] Pakos EE, Ioannidis JP. Radiotherapy vs. nonsteroidal anti-inflammatory drugs for the prevention of heterotopic ossification after major hip procedures: a meta- analysis of randomized trials. Int J Radiat Oncol Biol Phys 2004;60(3):888-95.

[3] Balboni TA, Gobezie R, Mamon HJ. Heterotopic ossification: Pathophysiology, clinical features, and the role of radiotherapy for prophylaxis. Int J Radiat Oncol Biol Phys 2006;65(5):1289-99.

[4] Baird EO, Kang QK. Prophylaxis of heterotopic ossification - an updated review. J Orthop Surg Res 2009;4:12.

[5] McCarthy EF, Sundaram M. Heterotopic ossification: a review. Skeletal Radiol 2005;34(10):609-19.

[6] Lo TC. Radiation therapy for heterotopic ossification. Semin Radiat Oncol 1999;9(2):163-70.

[7] Vavken P, Castellani L, Sculco TP. Prophylaxis of heterotopic ossification of the hip: systematic review and meta-analysis. Clin Orthop Relat Res 2009;467(12):3283-9.

[8] Mishra MV, Austin L, Parvizi J, Ramsey M, Showalter TN. Safety and efficacy of radiation therapy as secondary prophylaxis for heterotopic ossification of non-hip joints. J Med Imaging Radiat Oncol 2011;55(3):333-6.

[9] Vanden Bossche L, Vanderstraeten G. Heterotopic ossification: a review. J Rehabil Med 2005;37(3):129-36.

[10] Jang SH, Shin SW, Ahn SH, Cho IH, Kim SH. Radiation therapy for heterotopic ossification in a patient with traumatic brain injury. Yonsei Med J 2000;41(4):536-9.

[11] Schaeffer MA, Sosner J. Heterotopic ossification: treatment of established bone with radiation therapy. Arch Phys Med Rehabil 1995;76(3):284-6.

In: Advanced Cancer ISBN: 978-1-62808-239-5
Editors: N. Thavarajah, N. Pulenzas, B. Lechner et al.   © 2013 Nova Science Publishers, Inc.

Chapter 14

Focal myositis as a presentation of paraneoplastic syndrome in pancreatic cancer

Erin Wong, BSc (C)[1], Gillian Bedard, BSc(C)[1], Linda Probyn, MD[2],
Natalie Pulenzas, BSc(C)[1], Breanne Lechner, BSc(C)[1],
Lori Holden, MRTT[1], Edward Chow, MBBS[1]
and Natalie Lauzon, MRTT[1]*

[1]Rapid Response Radiotherapy Program, Department of Radiation Oncology, Odette Cancer Centre, Sunnybrook Health Sciences Centre, University of Toronto, Toronto, Ontario, Canada, [2]Department of Medical Imaging, Sunnybrook Health Sciences Centre, University of Toronto, Toronto, Ontario, Canada

Abstract

Paraneoplastic syndrome is rare in the field of oncology, with approximately 8 out of 100 patients displaying some manifestation of this syndrome. In terms of dermatological and rheumatological manifestations of paraneoplastic syndromes, dermatomyositis and polymyositis are common presentations. In the same family of inflammatory muscle disease as polymyositis, focal myositis occurs infrequently and its presentation as a paraneoplastic syndrome has only been suggested in a few cases. Here we present the case of a 42-year-old female with focal myositis of the right quadriceps muscles, who also has known primary pancreatic cancer, suggesting its presentation as a paraneoplastic syndrome.

* Correspondence: Ms. Natalie Lauzon BSc, MRTT Department of Radiation Therapy, Odette Cancer Centre, Sunnybrook Health Sciences Centre, 2075 Bayview Avenue, Toronto, ON Canada. Email: Natalie.Lauzon@ Sunnybrook.ca.

Introduction

Paraneoplastic syndrome is uncommon, correlating clinical features or symptoms that occur as a result of an underlying malignancy (1-3). What characterizes this syndrome is that it is not due to the infiltration of the primary tumor, compression caused by the primary tumor or the metastasized spread of the tumor (4,5). Conversely, paraneoplastic syndrome is hypothesized to be the result of tumor biological mediators produced by the primary tumor such as hormones, peptides, autocrine and paracrine mediators or immune-mediated response such as cytotoxic lymphocytes and antibodies (3,4). As there are a wide variety of causes, intuitively, there are multiple manifestations of paraneoplastic syndromes such as neurological (motor/autonomic neuropathy or Lambert-Eaton myaesthenic syndrome), endocrine (hypercalcemia or cushing syndrome), hematological (eosinophilia or granulocytosis), and dermatological and rheumatological (dermatomyositis and polymyositis) (5,6).

Dermatomyositis (DM) and polymyositis (PM) are a group of autoimmune inflammatory disorders. PM is characterized by proximal muscle weakness, while DM is characterized by both skin involvement as well as proximal muscle weakness (3,5,6). Focal myositis, which is similar to DM and PM, is the painful enlargement of muscle mass which is localized to one area of the body (7). However, unlike DM and PM, its association with a primary malignancy is very rare and has not been thoroughly studied with only a few reported cases in literature (8-12).

In this report, we present the case of a young female with metastatic pancreatic cancer experiencing significant right knee pain. Radiological imaging of this region demonstrated findings suggestive of focal myositis, as a presentation of the rheumatological manifestation of paraneoplastic syndrome.

Case report

A 42 year old female was diagnosed with pancreatic cancer in November 2011. Initially, lymphadenopathy was found in the retroperitoneal region which was subsequently biopsied. Pathology of the specimen was consistent with metastatic adenocarcinoma with the differential diagnosis of upper gastrointestinal or pancreaticobiliary tract primary. Later in July 2012, a CT scan of the chest, abdomen and pelvis revealed a multicystic mass in the pancreatic tail (see figure 1). Therefore a diagnosis of metastatic pancreatic cancer was made due to subsequent findings of enhancement in the bone of the pelvis and spine seen in the staging scans.

This patient was initially referred to the Rapid Response Radiotherapy Program (RRRP) for radiotherapy treatment to palliate bone pain in August 2012. At that time, she had pain in the pelvis and lumbar spine region radiating down the right leg which was treated with a single dose of 800 cGy. This patient also had bony metastases in the cervical spine, specifically C2, with soft tissue mass on the thecal sac which was radiated with 2000 cGy in five fractions.

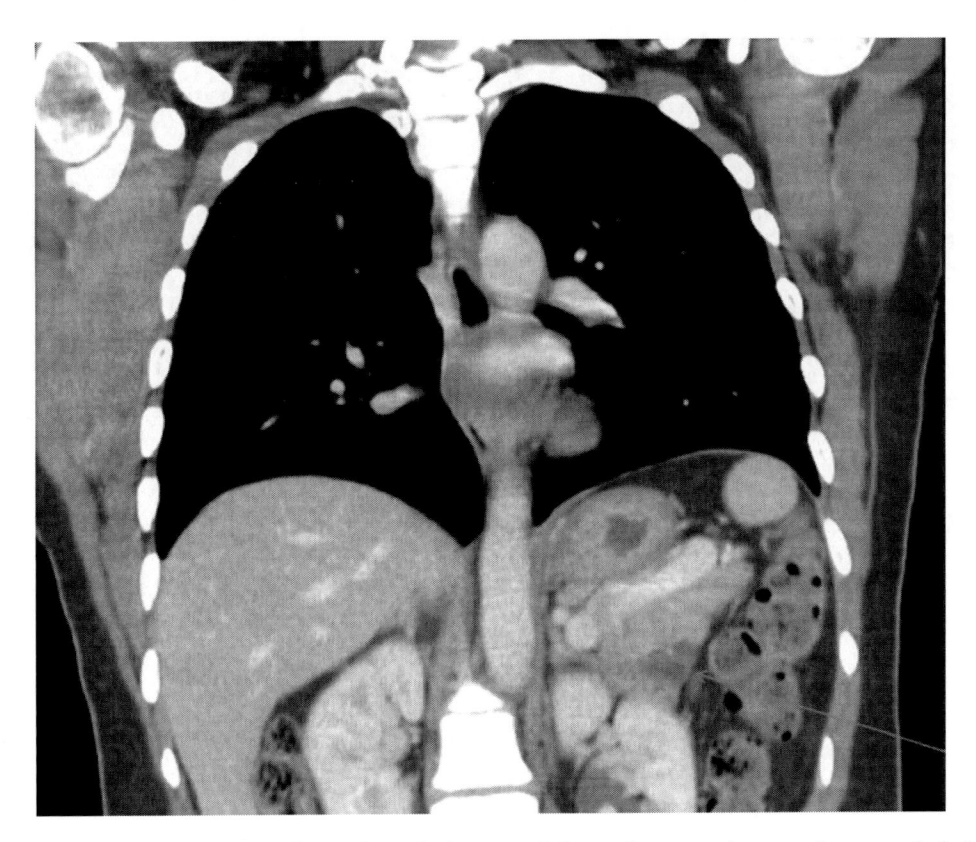

Figure 1. Coronal reformatted CT image through the upper abdomen demonstrating a cystic pancreatic lesion (arrow) compatible with the primary pancreatic carcinoma.

Soon after, in October 2012, this patient was referred to the RRRP again, this time for right knee pain. An MRI of the bilateral lower extremities was ordered by her medical oncologist to diagnose the pain. In comparison to a previous MRI scan of the pelvis, this current MRI scan showed progression of the bony metastases along the right ischium, iliac crest, acetabulum to the symphysis pubis and intertrochanteric region of the right femur. In addition, multiple femoral low density endosteal lesions were seen which, in the opinion of the radiologist, was consistent with metastatic disease. However signal abnormality was also seen extending into the right vastus lateralis, abductor magnus and vastus medialis throughout the length of the muscles (see figure 2). This abnormality was thought to be focal myositis as a presentation of paraneoplastic syndrome.

This patient arrived by ambulance to the RRRP and at that time was bed-ridden. She had a Karnofsky performance status of 40. After discussion between the radiation and medical oncologist on her situation, it was decided that her knee (region of myositis) and right hemi-pelvis which had a reoccurrence of pain, would be radiated (see figure 3).

The patient was informed of the possible side effects which included pain flare, gastrointestinal side effects, nausea, vomiting, and diarrhea and was then consented to a single radiation dose of 8 Gy, pre-medicated with Ondansetron. This treatment was prescribed in hopes of controlling the myositis in the knee region and to provide pain relief in the hemi-pelvis region.

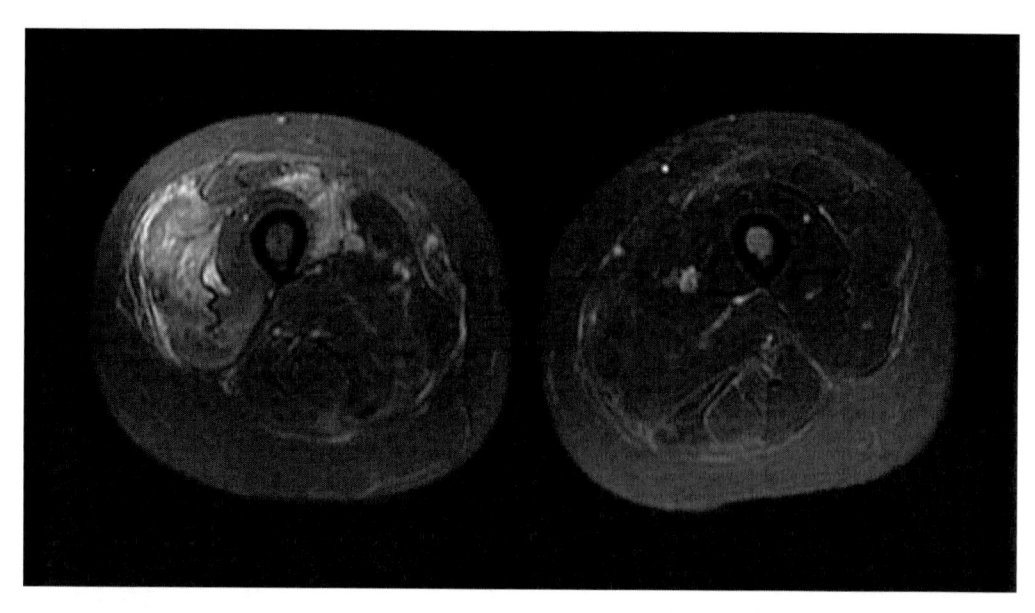

Figure 2. Axial T2 fat suppressed MR image through the bilateral femurs above the knee demonstrating increased signal compatible with edema in the right quadriceps muscle, predominately the vastus medialis and lateralis compatible with myositis.

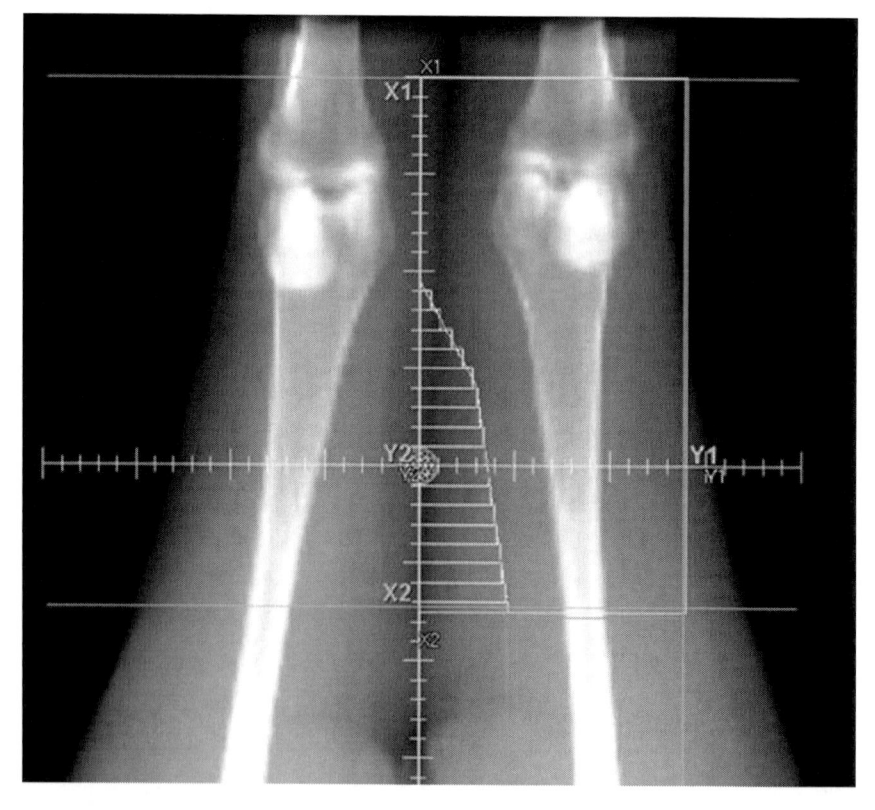

Figure 3. Anterior digitally reconstructed radiograph (DRR) depicting the radiation treatment area of the distal RT femur and knee.

Discussion

Paraneoplastic syndrome is a complex disease, with multiple manifestations and different combinations of multiple, heterogeneous clinical features, making it difficult to diagnose (1,2). It is currently estimated to be present in 8 out of 100 oncology patients; however this statistic may be under-estimated due to the difficulty in diagnosis of this syndrome (5). Conversely, the number of patients with certain symptoms manifestations which are later determined to be paraneoplastic in nature is greater. In current literature, it has been reported by Andras et al, in a small cohort of 217 patients with either DM or PM, approximately 19% of patients with DM had or were later diagnosed with malignancy (3). Similarly, in a Taiwanese cohort of 143 patients studied by Chen et al, it was found that 13% of patients with DM and PM had an associated malignancy (6). Although not significantly substantial, this percentage of patients suggests it may still be worthwhile to screen patients who have certain disorders such as DM or PM for cancer, as the disorder may later be discovered to be paraneoplastic in nature.

In the current case, focal myositis was seen in a patient with pancreatic cancer and is believed to be paraneoplastic in nature as suggested by the referring medical oncologist, radiologist and radiation oncologist.

In a case reported by Zenone et al, a 51-year-old women developed hypertrophy of her right calf prior to the diagnosis of cancer. Less than a year later, the patient presented to the same hospital with bone pain which was confirmed to be poorly differentiated adenocarcinoma of unknown primary. For this case, because of the temporal synchronicity of the two incidences, the authors believe that this focal myositis was a presentation of paraneoplastic syndrome (8).

Similar to the previous case, Naschitz et al presented a case on a 78-year-old male who presented to his doctor with a tender mass in the left forearm that had been present for 5 months. This muscle mass was found to be normal with some inflamed fibrous tissue through a biopsy. Approximately 6 months afterwards, he was diagnosed with Hodgkin's disease (9). Terrier et al. also presented a case of a 74-year-old female that was simultaneously diagnosed with both chronic lymphocytic leukemia and focal myositis of the right deltoid muscle (10). Two older case reports originally suggested the association of focal myositis with squamous cell carcinoma of the head and neck and with phaeochromocytoma of the adrenals (11,12).

Different treatment options used for patients with focal myositis in conjunction with primary malignancy have been suggested by these case reports. In the case reported by Zenone et al, prednisone was prescribed to the patient for treatment of her focal myositis (8). Alternatively, Naschitz et al. reported on surgical excision of the focal myositis followed by subsequent chemotherapy and radiation targeting the primary malignancy once it was discovered (9). In the case by Terrier et al., chemotherapy alone was used in the treatment of the focal myositis (10). In all of these cases, treatment was successful in the management of the focal myositis, with patients experiencing significant improvement (8-10).

In most of these cases, diagnoses of focal myositis either preceded or were simultaneously discovered with the primary malignancy. This similar timeline of events also occur for paraneoplastic syndrome of other manifestations. (3,13). Though this current case does not follow this timeline, it does add to the collection of evidence towards the possible paraneoplastic nature of focal myositis. As such, the knowledge and presentation of paraneoplastic syndrome can assist health care professionals in the early detection of an underlying cancer.

Acknowledgments

We thank the generous support of Bratty Family Fund, Michael and Karyn Goldstein Cancer Research Fund, Joseph and Silvana Melara Cancer Research Fund, and Ofelia Cancer Research Fund.

References

[1]   Hueber AJ, Rech J, Kallert S, Requadt C, Cavallaro A, Kalden JR, et al. Paraneoplastic syndrome, infection or arthritis: Difficulties in diagnosis. Int J Clin Pract 2006;60(10):1310-2.

[2]   Ozdogu H, Boga C, Bolat F, Kilic D, Habesoglu MA, Karatas M. Paraneoplastic syndrome associated with desquamative interstitial pneumonia mimicking lung cancer: A case report. Turkish J Cancer 2008;38(2):78.

[3]   Andras C, Csiki Z, Ponyi A, Illes A, Danko K. Paraneoplastic rheumatic syndromes. Rheumatol Int 2006;26(5):376-82.

[4]   Wood JP, Haynes AP, Cheung KL. A paraneoplastic manifestation of metastatic breast cancer responding to endocrine therapy: a case report. World J Surg Oncol 2008;6:132.

[5]   Pelosof LC, Gerber DE. Paraneoplastic syndromes: an approach to diagnosis and treatment. Mayo Clin Proc 2010;85(9):838-54.

[6]   Chen YJ, Wu CY, Shen JL. Predicting factors of malignancy in dermatomyositis and polymyositis: a case-control study. Br J Dermatol 2001;144(4):825-31.

[7]   Caldwell CJ, Swash M, Van der Walt JD, Geddes JF. Focal myositis: a clinicopathological study. Neuromuscul Disord 1995;5(4):317-21.

[8]   Zenone T, Ghadban R, Leveque-Michaud C, Chan V. Focal myositis: a paraneoplastic syndrome? Joint Bone Spine 2011;78(4):426-7.

[9]   Naschitz JE, Yeshurun D, Dreyfuss U, Best LA, Misselevich I, Boss JH. Localized nodular myositis. A paraneoplastic phenomenon. Clin Rheumatol 1992;11(3):427-31.

[10]   Terrier B, Lavie F, Miceli-Richard C, Azria A, Mariette X. Focal myositis with fasciitis and vasculitis revealing chronic lymphocytic leukaemia. Rheumatology (Oxford) 2005;44(10):1324-6.

[11]   Bhatnagar D, Carey P, Pollard A. Focal myositis and elevated creatine kinase levels in a patient with phaeochromocytoma. Postgrad Med J 1986;62(725):197-8.

[12]   McLendon CL, Levine PA, Mills SE, Black WC. Squamous cell carcinoma masquerading as focal myositis of the tongue. Head Neck 1989;11(4):353-57.

[13]   Kurzrock R, Cohen PR. Cutaneous paraneoplastic syndromes in solid tumors. Am J Med 1995;99(6):662-71.

In: Advanced Cancer
Editors: N. Thavarajah, N. Pulenzas, B. Lechner et al.

ISBN: 978-1-62808-239-5
© 2013 Nova Science Publishers, Inc.

Chapter 15

Heterotopic ossification: Mimics of other benign and malignant etiologies

Gillian Bedard, BSc(C), Liang Zeng, MD(C),
Natalie Lauzon, MRT(T), Linda Probyn, MD,
Kristopher Dennis, MD and Edward Chow, MBBS[*]

Rapid Response Radiotherapy Program, Department of Radiation Oncology,
Odette Cancer Centre, Sunnybrook Health Sciences Centre, University of Toronto,
Toronto, Ontario, Canada

Abstract

CT and MRI imaging does not always provide conclusive results and sometimes results in a differential diagnosis which can include both benign and malignant etiologies. The present case describes a twenty-seven year old male, who clinically presented with right knee pain, decreased extension and instability. The prior MRI and CT reports were in favour of heterotopic ossification; however other etiologies were included in the differential diagnosis including osteosarcoma, bizarre parosteal osteochondroma, and osteochondroma. Each of these diagnoses result in different treatment, and treating without accurate diagnosis could place the patient at a greater risk of possible malignant cell spread, as well as potentially harmful side effects of treatment. This report highlights the importance of proper diagnosis before treatment, in addition to the importance of referring a patient to an outside care facility specializing in orthopaedic oncology. Accurate diagnosis allows physicians to determine a correct course of treatment and limits patient risk.

[*] Correspondence: Professor Edward Chow MBBS, MSc, PhD, FRCPC Department of Radiation Oncology, Odette Cancer Centre, Sunnybrook Health Sciences Centre, 2075 Bayview Avenue, Toronto, ON Canada. E-mail: Edward.Chow@sunnybrook.ca.

Introduction

Heterotopic ossification (HO) is defined as the formation of lamellar bone inside soft-tissue where bone normally does not exist (1, 2). It is frequently a result of central nervous system disorders, injury, hip surgery and burns. Hereditary causes such as fibrodysplasia and Albright's hereditary osteodystrophy also exist (1). Heterotopic ossification due to musculoskeletal injury typically displays clinical signs and symptoms within 3 to 12 weeks post injury. In severe cases, HO can be treated with surgery, radiation therapy or drug treatment, although the use of one over the other is still controversial (1).

In this report, we present the case of a young man whose radiological imaging demonstrated findings suggestive of heterotopic ossification although there were some features which allowed for other diagnostic considerations. However, it was determined that this was HO and no treatment was required.

Case report

A 27 year old male injured his right knee while playing badminton in 2007. The patient stated that he moved in an abnormal direction and his knee began to hurt. The patient believed this would get better, however when it did not, he spoke with his family doctor who subsequently ordered a CT and MRI of the knee and referred him to the Rapid Response Radiotherapy Program at the Odette Cancer Centre, Sunnybrook Hospital in January 2012 (five years after the initial injury). The patient presented to clinic with complaints of pain, instability and decreased extension of the right knee. He had no significant family history and was currently taking Naprosyn and Tylenol 3 on an as needed basis.

The MRI completed in November 2011 identified a 1.7cm x 1.3cm x 1.5cm lesion at the posterior aspect of the medial tibial plateau with increased signal on T2 weighted imaging. There was no separating plane between the lesion and the underlying tibia and it was adjacent to the underlying bone (Figure 1). The differential considerations included an avulsed fragment with hypertrophic ossification and bridging callus, an osteochondroma or bizarre parosteal osteochondroma, however there was no cortical meduallary continuation or cartilaginous cap. The high T2 signal suggested edema which can be seen in heterotopic ossification although is less typical in chronic mature heterotopic ossification. Another consideration was a surface osteosarcoma (periosteal osteosarcoma) given the ongoing symptoms and edema. The lack of a stalk connecting the lesion to the underlying bone is against this possibility. The radiologist concluded that this should be further characterized with a CT scan.

The subsequent CT scan in December 2011 demonstrated a bony excrescence at the posterior aspect the medial proximal tibia (Figure 2). There was no clear continuity of the medullary space and cortex which would be expected in an osteochondroma. The lesion demonstrated trabeculation with some peripheral cortical margin suggesting heterotopic ossification although there was some sclerosis in the underlying tibia which was nonspecific and raised the possibility of a surface lesion although as previously mentioned, the lack of a stalk made a parosteal osteosarcoma less likely. The lesion was adjacent to the tibia with no separating fat plane. The question of a prior avulsion injury was raised. Four differential considerations included heterotopic ossification, parosteal osteosarcoma, osteochondroma and bizarre parosteal osteochondroma.

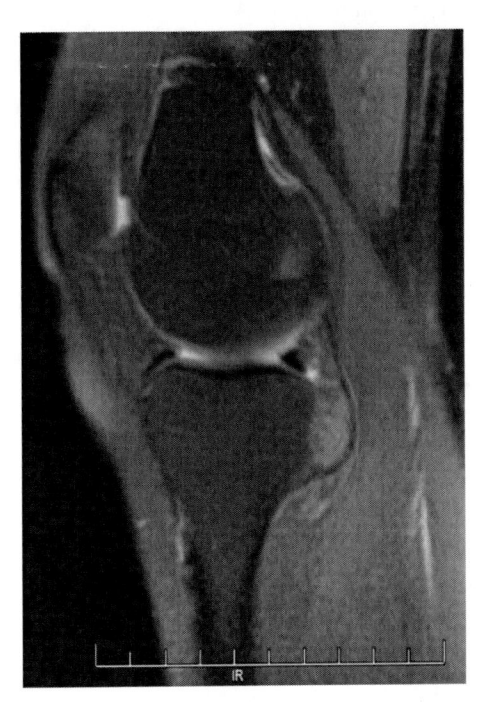

Figure 1. Sagittal T2 fat suppressed image demonstrating a 1.7cm x 1.3cm x 1.5cm lesion adjacent to the posterior aspect of the medial tibial plateau with no gap between the lesion and the underlying bone. The lesion demonstrates increased signal on T2 weighted imaging.

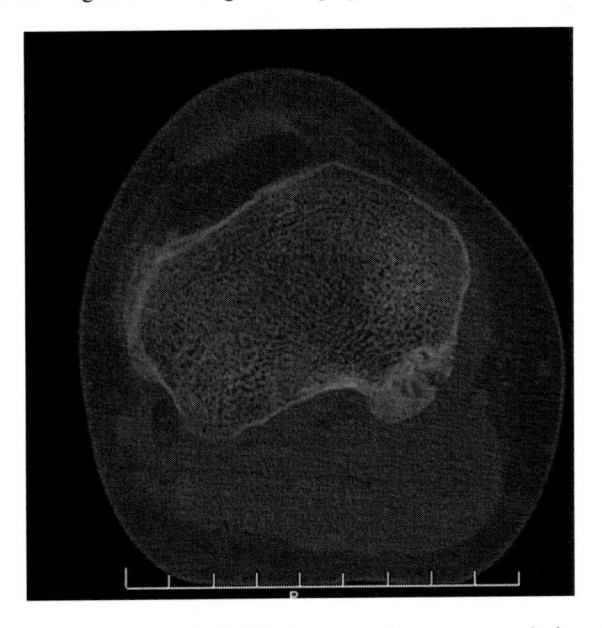

Figure 2. Axial CT image through the proximal tibia demonstrating an osseous lesion at the posterior medial tibia with no cortical medullary continuation. The lesion has trabecular formation and there is no separating plane between the lesion and the underlyingunderlyng tibia.

Given some atypical features together with the clinical history of ongoing pain, referral to a quaternary orthopaedic oncology center was recommended.

It was determined that the lesion represented heterotopic ossification and no surgery would be necessary. Given ongoing symptoms, follow-up imaging was recommended on a yearly basis.

Discussion

Heterotopic ossification is most often a consequence of trauma or a central nervous system injury. Approximately 10% of patients with this condition experience severe restriction in joint movement (3). Most patients experience decreased range of motion and pain. Although clinically this patient presented with pain and decreased range of motion, this was five years post-injury. Most often, the lesion begins to grow within one to two months post-injury and in most cases becomes smaller and less symptomatic within a year (2). This was the most likely diagnosis on imaging although there some atypical features.

Parosteal osteosarcoma was one of the potential diagnoses for this patient. This is a malignant tumor which is found in long bones and often times results in a lump on the bone. The tumor is usually found in adolescents and young adults, however there is an increase in diagnosis in those over the age of 60. Symptoms include fracture, pain, decrease in range of motion, tenderness, swelling and redness. Treatment for this type of tumor includes surgery, either limb-saving or radical, or chemotherapy (4).

The MRI of this patient also pointed to a possible osteochondroma. Osteochondromas are composed of cortical and medullar bone with an overlying hyaline cartilage cap. Usually found at the growth plates of long bones, they demonstrate continuity with the underlying parent bone cortex and medullary canal and occur when part of the growth plate forms an outgrowth on the surface of the bone, with or without a stalk (5). Deformity, fracture, vascular compromise, bursa formation, and malignant transformation are often a result. Most often painless, these types of lesions can become painful when the stalk breaks or it is located under the tendon and can cause activity related pain (5).

Bizarre parosteal osteochondroma is a benign surface based lesion that is most common in young people and in the hands and feet (6). The three major features of this lesion include: a cellular cartilaginous cap, unusual mineralized cartilaginous matrix and a fibrovascular stroma. This lesion is often confused with osteochondroma, and the key differentiation factor is the absence of continuity with the underlying medullary cavity (7).

The patient presented in this case report demonstrated some atypical features for mature or chronic heterotopic ossification. In order to accurately treat, it was best determined that the patient should be referred to an orthopaedic surgeon specializing in the oncology field. Proper referral and determination of the lesion would lead to the proper diagnosis and treatment. Physicians should make certain they make appropriate referrals in order to optimize patient care.

Conclusion

Diagnostic imaging is extremely useful although sometimes is not conclusive when there are atypical imaging features. Heterotopic ossification can sometimes display atypical findings that suggest other possible diagnoses. In these cases, referral to a center specializing in orthopaedic oncology is helpful for accurate patient diagnosis and treatment. Follow up imaging is also suggested to ensure stability especially when the patient has ongoing symptoms.

Acknowledgments

We thank the generous support of Bratty Family Fund, Michael and Karyn Goldstein Cancer Research Fund, Joseph and Silvana Melara Cancer Research Fund, and Ofelia Cancer Research Fund.

References

[1] Vanden Bossche L, Vanderstraeten G. Heterotopic ossification: A review. J Rehabil Med 2005;37:129-36.
[2] McCarthy EF, Sundaram M. Heterotopic ossification: A review. Skeletal Radiol 2005;34:609-19.
[3] Garland DE. A clinical perspective on common forms of acquired heterotopic ossification. Clin Orthop Relat Res 1991;13-29.
[4] Ta HT, Dass CR, Choong PF, Dunstan DE. Osteosarcoma treatment: State of the art. Cancer Metastasis Rev 2009;28:247-63.
[5] Murphey MD, Choi JJ, Kransdorf MJ, Flemming DJ, Gannon FH. Imaging of osteochondroma: Variants and complications with radiologic-pathologic correlation. Radiographics 2000;20:1407-34.
[6] Gruber G, Giessauf C, Leithner A, Zacherl M, Clar H, Bodo K, et al. Bizarre parosteal osteochondromatous proliferation (nora lesion): A report of 3 cases and a review of the literature. Can J Surg 2008;51:486-9.
[7] Meneses MF, Unni KK, Swee RG. Bizarre parosteal osteochondromatous proliferation of bone (nora's lesion). Am J Surg Pathol 1993;17:691-7.

SECTION TWO:
QUALITY OF LIFE ASSESSMENT TOOLS

In: Advanced Cancer ISBN: 978-1-62808-239-5
Editors: N. Thavarajah, N. Pulenzas, B. Lechner et al. © 2013 Nova Science Publishers, Inc.

Chapter 16

Quality of life measures used in radiation therapy trials for patients with Metastatic Spinal Cord Compression (MSCC)

Gunita Mitera[1], Nadil Zeiadin[1], Arjun Sahgal[1], Joel Finkelstein[2], Edward Chow[1] and Andrew Loblaw[1]*

[1]Rapid Response Radiotherapy Program, Department of Radiation Oncology, Odette Cancer Centre, Sunnybrook Health Sciences Centre, University of Toronto, Toronto, Ontario, Canada
[2]Department of Orthopaedic Surgery, Sunnybrook Health Sciences Centre, University of Toronto, Toronto, Ontario, Canada

Patient morbidity from metastatic spinal cord compression (MSCC) includes back pain, paralysis/paresis, limb weakness, sensory loss, and bowel/bladder sphincter compromise. The goal of treatment with either surgery radiation or combined treatment is to improve the patient's quality of life (QOL) through palliation of pain and neurological recovery. QOL measures are important endpoints which are not well developed and infrequently measured. Objective: To identify clinical studies for patients with MSCC where QOL has been reported as either a primary or secondary endpoint. Furthermore, our aim was to report the specific measurement tools employed used to capture QOL. Methods: A systematic literature review was conducted using the Ovid MEDLINE(R) 1950 to October 2008 database, Ovid Health and Psychosocial Instruments 1985 to October 2007 database, and EMBASE(R) 1980 to October 2008. Results: Five studies were identified. Two of the five (40%) studies employed the Schedule for Evaluation of Individualized Quality of Life (SEIQoL-DW) tool to measure QOL. The Short Form 36 (SF36) Health Survey Questionnaire, the Pediatric Quality of Life Inventory (PedsQL) 4.0 Generic Core

[*] Corresponding author: Gunita Mitera MRT(T), Department of Radiation Therapy, Odette Cancer Centre, Sunnybrook Health Sciences Centre, 2075 Bayview Avenue, Toronto, ON M4N 3M5, Canada. Tel: 416-480-6100 ext 7543; Fax: 416-480-4672; E-mail: Gunita.Mitera@sunnybrook.ca.

scale, and the Functional Assessment of Cancer Therapy (FACT-G) scales were generic QOL investigation tools that were used in the remaining three studies. Conclusions: Amongst the five studies that defined QOL as an endpoint, there was no consistency in the measure used. There appears to be no specific QOL survey tool for the MSCC population. Therefore, we identify the need to develop a tool specific for this population in order to generate meaningful data for future trials.

Introduction

Malignant spinal cord compression (MSCC) is defined as compression of the thecal sac that surrounds the spinal cord or cauda equina by an extradural tumour mass (1,2). This is a dreaded complication of advanced malignancy where neurological function may be compromised without immediate medical attention, hence, prioritizing it as an "oncological emergency" (3-5). The clinical incidence of MSCC is between 2.5% and 10% for all cancer patients (2-7), but this can be higher depending on factors such as primary cancer, disease stage and age (2). Population-based data reports that 2.5% of patients dying from cancer have at least one admission for MSCC (7). One study reports among the half a million patients who die from cancer each year, 12,700 will suffer from spinal cord compression (1) and therefore be at risk for back pain (1,3,4,8), sensory deficits, loss of mobility through paraplegia or paralysis (1,4,8-10) or incontinence (1,3,7,9).

Prognostic factors for MSCC have been reported in the literature to include the primary cancer, time interval from primary tumour diagnosis to the time of MSCC development, pre-treatment ambulatory function, time to developing motor deficits before radiation treatment, absence of visceral or other bony metastasis, and re-irradiation for in-field recurrences of MSCC (11,12-17). Life expectancy after MSCC is generally short with an expected median survival between three and six months (3,5); however, a small proportion of patients can live for years underscoring the importance of more aggressive treatment in patients with better prognosis. Radiation therapy and surgery are accepted as the primary modalities of treatment. Recently, a randomized trial has shown potential benefits in terms of neurologic recovery and survival for patients treated with a combined surgical and post-operative approach (17). However, poor performance status or surgical technical limitations render many patients ineligible for surgery and thus radiation therapy alone becomes the main treatment option. The goal of treatment is often considered to be palliation of pain, neurological recovery, and quality of life (2,3,5,9,15,18). Consequently, given the short life expectancy for these patients, it is important for them to maintain the best possible quality of life (QOL) for their remaining lifespan.

Most studies investigating treatment outcomes for spinal cord compression emphasize physical parameters, such as mobility and sphincter disturbances (8). However, according to patient reports, poor physical function is not directly associated or predictive of poor quality of life (8,20). Consequently, an increasing emphasis has been placed on QOL as an endpoint in clinical investigations. The World Health Organization defines health as "a state of complete physical, mental and social well-being and not merely the absence of disease or infirmity" (21). This multi-dimensional definition of health has encouraged health care professionals and research investigators to incorporate all aspects of health in treatment including QOL. Over the last three decades there have been numerous studies on QOL in medical literature. A Medline search using "quality of life" as a keyword reveals a significant increase in the number of articles related to the topic over a period of 30 years, from 32 in 1973 to 31,522 in 2008 (22). Interestingly, more recent publications are emphasizing the importance of the patient's perspective on QOL. According to patients, this may encompass physical, social, and cognitive levels of functioning and may have varying degrees of importance unique to the individual (9,20,23,24).

Consequently, effectiveness of treatments for MSCC patients should be evaluated from the patient's perspective. While few studies focus on QOL as a primary or secondary endpoint, we believe that research should incorporate this important outcome. Additionally, QOL measures should incorporate the unique components important to a MSCC patient population. QOL instruments help health care professionals quantify the impact of new or existing treatments on various aspects of a patient's life. For example, site-specific QOL measures have been developed to target the specific needs of each population (23,24). However, to our knowledge there are no published QOL measures specific for a MSCC population. The objective of this study was to review and document the extent to which previous studies have considered quality of life (QOL) as either a primary or secondary endpoint in MSCC study populations and document the specific measurement tool employed to capture QOL.

Literature review

A literature review was conducted in October 2008 using the Ovid MEDLINE(R) 1950 to October 2008 database, Ovid Health and Psychosocial Instruments 1985 to October 2007 database, and EMBASE(R) 1980 to October 2008 database using the terms "spinal cord compression" or "spinal compression" and "quality of life" and "cancer or neoplasm or metastasis or tumor." In the MEDLINE and EMBASE databases, we combined the terms "spinal cord compression" or "cauda equina (compression or compressed)" or "metastatic spinal cord compression" or "malignant spinal cord compression" with "quality of life" and "cancer or neoplasm or metastasis or tumor." Relevant articles and abstracts were reviewed and references from these sources were also manually searched for additional relevant publications.

The following information was extracted from the studies: the primary and secondary outcome, type and number of QOL measures used, any additional tools used, number of patients, median age and median survival, and symptom palliation. Articles were included in the literature review based on the subsequent criteria. The study population was patients diagnosed with malignant spinal cord compression or cauda equina compression; all study intervention was acceptable; randomized control trials, prospective or retrospective cohort studies were included; quality of life (QOL) measure or symptom palliation as measure of QOL were all acceptable endpoints. Articles were excluded from the literature review if they were non-English publications; testing efficacy of a treatment at prolonging development of malignant spinal cord compression or cauda equina compression or equating QOL with absence of MSCC or cauda equina compression; used performance assessment tools only; Heterogeneous study populations i.e. not exclusively MSCC or cauda equina compression patients; Individual case reports, or qualitative studies were also excluded.

Table 1. Summary of studies assessing quality of life in malignant spinal cord compression patient population

Author, Year, Trial Type	Study Purpose	N	Median Survival	QoL Assessment Tools	Performance Assessment Tool	Other Assessment Tools/ Measures	Number of instruments used to measure QoL
Conway R, Graham J, Kidd J, Levack P. 2007 P	To present further findings from the Scottish Cord Compression Study, diagnosis, management and outcome of MSCC were examined.	128	59 days (i.e. approx 2 months)	Schedule for Evaluation of Individual Quality of Life (SEIQoL – Dw)	Karnofsky Performance Status	Hospital Anxiety and Depression Scale, Visual Analogue Scale for Pain, Mobility	1
Levack P, Graham J, Kidd J. 2004 P	Examine QoL in recently diagnosed MSCC patients	180	59 days.	Schedule for the Evaluation of Individual Quality of Life (SEIQoL-Dw)	Karnosky Performance Status	Barthel Disability Index, Hospital Anxiety and Depression Scale	1
Mannion RJ, Wilby M, Godward S, Lyratzopoulos G, Lain RJC 2007 P	Prospective cohort study of metastatic cord or cauda equina compression patients treated with surgical decompression and fixation	62	13 Months	SF-36	N/A	Visual analogue pain scores, Roland Morris back pain scores.	1
Poretti A, Zehnder D, Boltshauser E, Grotzer MA 2008 P	Document effect of neurological deficits on social and psychological adjustment and quality of life of pediatric MSCC patients	28	The 10-year overall survival rate was 96%	PedsQL (Pediatric Quality of Life Inventory) 4.0 Generic Core to measure health related (HR) QoL	Functional Independence Measure (FIM) and WeeFIM	Youth Self Report (YSR) and Child Behavior Check List (CBCL)	1
Sundaresan N, Sachdev VP, Holland JF, Moore F, Sung M, et al. 1995 R	Determine results and outcome (incl. QoL) of patients with spincal metastasis treated with surgery	110	16 Months	Functional Assessment of Cancer Therapy Scale (FACT-G)	N/A	N/A	1

Notes:

R – Retrospective; P – Prospective.

What we found

Of 322 published results that manifested using the literature search criteria, only 5 studies assessed QOL as a primary or secondary endpoint and also used a QOL measure for their MSCC study populations. These studies are listed in table 1.

Schedule for Evaluation of Individualized Quality of Life (SEIQoL-DW)

Two of the five (40%) studies (8,20) employed the Schedule for Evaluation of Individualized Quality of Life (SEIQoL-DW) to measure quality of life. The SEIQoL-DW is a three-stage semi-structured, individualized interview measure from 0 (worst) to 100 (best), and has been validated for use in patients with advanced cancer (8,20,25). The questionnaire asks patients to nominate five areas of their life, termed cues, which contribute most to their QOL (20,25). Next, patients are asked to judge at which level each nominated cue is functioning by rating against a vertical visual analog scale labeled at the upper and lower extremities by the terms "as good as could possibly be" and "as bad as could possibly be" (25). In the third stage, patients provide the relative importance of each cue by "weighing" each cue relative to each other (20,25) The third stage of the SEIQoL-DW varies from that of the SEQoL in the method participants use to weight the relative importance of each QoL aspect, with the DW (direct weighing) method being more simple and direct. The SEIQoL-DW provides a global quality of life score ranging from 0 (no quality whatsoever) to 100 (perfect quality of life) as well as a personal and prioritized list of important areas of life for each patient (20,25). The SEIQoL-DW achieves high internal validity (R2= 0.88) and high internal reliability (r=0.90) (25).

The median SEIQoL score in the Conway et al (8) sample (n=128) for patients at one month after diagnosis of spinal cord compression was 72/100 and a median Karnofsky performance status of 50. In a sample of 180 patients shortly after MSCC diagnosis, Levack et al. (20) found a median SEIQoL score of 66/100 and a median KPS of 40. Both studies found a significant correlation between SEIQoL and performance status, with higher KPS associated with better SEIQoL scores (8,20). Nonetheless, physical disability was not significantly associated with SEIQoL and the effect of the physical condition on quality of life was surprisingly small (8,20). In fact, ninety-one percent of patients nominated family life as an important contributor to their quality of life. The average level of functioning of family life was 95% while the average weighting for this aspect was 30%. This means that patients determined that one third of their quality of life was determined by the level of functioning of their family life. On the other hand, health was nominated by only 44% and had an overall poor level of functioning and weighting of 20% (20).

SF36

The remaining three studies employed different quality of life measures. In one study by Mannion et al. (27), the Short Form 36 (SF36) Health Survey Questionnaire was employed as a quality of life measure in a spinal cord compression patient population. The SF36 is a widely employed general outcome measure (26,27). It attempts to capture important health dimensions common to all patients. The SF36 assesses 8 health scales to measure 3 aspects of health, functional status, well being and overall evaluation of health, and assigns individual and an overall quality of life score from 0 to 100. The SF-36 has high internal consistency, with Crohnbach alphas exceeding 0.80 and correlation coefficients of 0.55 - 0.78. Clinical validity was also established through clear and predictable differences between general and patient populations (26). Furthermore, the questionnaire has been shown to be sensitive enough to detect changes in population health. For example, a significant improvement in SF-36 scores was shown in patients three months post-surgical decompression treatment. Improvements were seen in physical function, role limitation and bodily pain (27).

Pediatric Quality of Life Inventory (PedsQL) 4.0 Generic Core

Poretti et al (28) employed the Pediatric Quality of Life Inventory (PedsQL) 4.0 Generic Core scales to measure quality of life in a pediatric population of patients with intraspinal tumors with spinal cord compression. The PedsQL is a generic health related QOL measure that can be utilized with children and adolescents between the ages of 2 and 18 across different patient populations. It is a child self-report or parent proxy-report measure. The 23-items of the PedsQL 4.0 Generic Core assess the central physical, mental and social health dimensions as defined by the World Health Organization. Additionally, it assesses school functioning. The questionnaire has been shown to be valid and reliable, with alpha scores of 0.88 for child self-report and 0.90 for parent proxy-report (28). A sample of 20 pediatric MSCC patients scored lower on the PedsQL compared to healthy controls, 79.35 and 83.00, respectively. Nonetheless, the difference was not significant. In fact, emotional functioning was the only QOL aspect significantly impaired, while social and school functioning showed no significant impairments. The quality of life scores of the PedsQL were significantly correlated with functional independence scores, paresis and neurogenic bladder and bowel dysfunction (9).

Functional Assessment of Cancer Therapy (FACT-G)

The Functional Assessment of Cancer Therapy (FACT-G) scale was employed by Sundaresan et al (29). The 33-items of the FACT-G are divided into five subscales: physical well-being, social well-being, emotional well-being, functional well-being and relationship with doctor. The FACT-G is reliable and valid given the internal consistency of the FACT-G score had an alpha value of 0.89 and test-retest correlation coefficient of 0.92. Additionally, the questionnaire is able to differentiate patients according to stage of disease ECOG performance status rating and hospitalization status. Furthermore, the questionnaire allows patients to assign personal weights to each of the five subscales, which provides an evaluation of the objective functional impairment and the perceived effect of the impairment on quality of life (29). In the Sundaresan et al (29) study, in which they analyzed the post-surgical outcome of 110 MSCC patients, the mean post-surgery score on the FACT-G was 83, corresponding to a positive outcome in terms of quality of life.

Discussion

Malignant spinal cord compression (MSCC) is an oncologic emergency and represents a major cause of morbidity in advanced cancer patients (3-5). Consequently, MSCC requires prompt diagnosis and treatment in order to preserve quality of life (4). Prognosis for MSCC patients is proven to be poor (2) and the aim of treatment is generally palliative (3-5). As such, a central aim of palliative treatment is to incorporate a combined approach of direct management of the physical symptoms as well as improving quality of life (3). However, what healthcare providers consider to be a patient's QOL may not in fact correspond to what the patient them self define as QOL (20).

The concept of QOL is inherently complex since it purposely incorporates a multitude of factors. However, the emphasis on holistic patient care which incorporates QOL has increased. This is evident by the number of health-related QOL measures that have been published in recent times (20, 22,25,26,28,30). In particular, in cancer related study populations the EORTC QLQ-C30 is the most frequently used QOL tool. This measure is a general QOL measure that uses 30 core questions in attempt to assess overall QOL (20,31).

However, studies measuring the efficacy of treatment for MSCC often do not incorporate quality of life as an endpoint (8). Most studies of treatment outcome focus on physical parameters such as motor function, functional status, local tumor control, ambulatory status and survival (12,13, 15,29). Additionally, it has been reported that healthcare providers associate a patient's physical health to their quality of life, however, from the patient's perspective this may not be true (8). For example, in three of the five studies which examined multiple components of QOL, the physical condition had an unremarkable effect on quality of life (8,9,20). Indeed, patients which had major physical disability such as decreased mobility and neurological dysfunction rated their quality of life scores as good (8,20) or not significantly different from their healthy counterparts (9). Therefore, to ensure patients continue to have both quality and meaning during their remaining life, it is important to consider improvements in quality of life from the patient's perspective when measuring treatment outcome (27).

Physical functioning is only one component of quality of life. Other main components assessed by the quality of life measures used on the MSCC patient population include social well-being, mental well-being and emotional well-being (26,28,29). As such, it is important to incorporate a more holistic approach to the study of quality of life in general and specifically in the MSCC research field. Furthermore, in order to account for the individualistic property of quality of life, QOL measures should also incorporate a subjective component to allow patients to report their perceived level of QOL. Our analysis revealed only two measures that have been applied in the MSCC patient population which incorporate an individualistic approach to QOL (5,8,20).

The SEIQoL questionnaire allows patients to nominate their own components of QOL as well as report the level of functioning and importance of each component (8,20,25). Congruent with the idea that physical functioning is not the most important aspect of QOL; family life was most frequently nominated and was generally given the highest importance for determining QOL (20). The FACT-G questionnaire allows patients to assign personal importance to each QOL components assessed in the measure, which allows for a simultaneous evaluation of functional impairment and its perceived effect (29).

Due to the complexities of the concept of QOL (20), it is important to approach the assessment of QOL in a multi-dimensional manner which incorporates the subjective dimension. However, it is also important to employ a measure which is easy to administer in the MSCC population. For example, only a fraction of patients were able to complete the SEIQoL (64% of sample alive at one month follow-up) (8) or the SF-36 (29% of sample alive at one month follow-up) (27), because of the burden of their disease. Overall, we found that all of the QOL measures used in the MSCC patient population were general QOL measures and assessed multiple components of QOL that may or may not be relevant to this population (5,8,9,20,27). Furthermore, we also found that MSCC patients have a better level of QOL than would be assumed based on the physical condition (8,9,20). Finally, our analysis revealed that QOL is important to this population and can be measured from the patients' perspective using appropriate QOL tools (5,9, 27). Consequently, considerations should be given to develop a QOL module specific for MSCC patients to be used in future studies incorporate quality of life as a primary endpoint when assessing treatment efficacy.

Conclusion

Our findings show that despite the increased attention in recent years on quality of life of patients, only a small amount of research has investigated QOL in malignant spinal cord compression patients. Also, no consistent QOL measure was used across the studies for this group, which makes it difficult to compare findings or understand the relative meaning of a score on a measure. Furthermore, the concept of QOL must be expanded beyond just the physical condition to include cognitive and emotional aspects as well as unique subjective components of the patient. Only two measures incorporated all of these aspects (5,8,20). However, these measures tended to be quite demanding on patients to complete (8,20) and did not capture the unique, disease-specific components of this patient population. As such, future research should focus on designing an assessment tool for QOL in the MSCC patient population that is both easy to administer and incorporates physical, emotional, social, cognitive and subjective dimensions.

References

[1]   Abrahm, JL. Assessment and treatment of patients with malignant spinal cord compression. J Support Oncol 2004;2(5): 377-401.
[2]   Prasad D, Schiff D. Malignant spinal-cord compression. Lancet Oncol 2005;6(1):15-24.
[3]   Aass N, Fossa SD. Pre- and post-treatment daily life function in patients with hormone resistant prostate carcinoma treated with radiotherapy for spinal cord compression. Radiat Oncol 2005; 74:259-65.
[4]   Penas-Prado M, Loghin ME. Spinal cord compression in cancer patients: Review of diagnosis and treatment. Curr Oncol Rep 2008; 10(1):78-85.
[5]   Sundaresan N, Sachdev VP, Holland JF, Moore F, Sung M, et al. Surgical treatment of spinal cord compression from epidural metastasis. J Clin Oncol 1995;13(9): 2330-5.
[6]   Jawahar A, Ampil F, Reddy PK, Harman GH, Sathyanarayana S, Nanda A. Analysis of outcome and prognostic factors in metastatic cauda equina compression: A 20-year single institution experience. Neurosurg Quart 2002;12(2):108-13.

[7] Loblaw DA, Laperriere NJ, Mackillop WJ. A Population-based study of malignant spinal cord compression in Ontario. Clin Oncol 2003; 15:211-7.

[8] Conway R, Graham J, Kidd J, Levack P. What happens to people after malignant spinal cord compression? Survival, function, quality of life, emotional well-being and place of care 1 month after diagnosis. Clin Oncol 2007;19:56-62.

[9] Poretti A, Zehnder D, Boltshauser E, Grotzer MA. Long-term complications and quality of life in children with intraspinal tumors. Pediatr Blood Cancer 2008;50(4):844-8.

[10] Tang V. Harvey D. Park Dorsay J. Jiang S. Rathbone MP. Prognostic indicators in metastatic spinal cord compression: using functional independence measure and Tokuhashi scale to optimize rehabilitation planning. Spinal Cord 2007;45(10):671-7.

[11] Helweg-Larsen S, Sorensen P, Kreiner S. Prognostic factors in metastatic spinal cord compression: A prospective study using multivariate analysis of variables influencing survival and gait function in 153 patients. Int J Radiat Oncol Biol Phys 2000;46(5):1163-9.

[12] Rades D, Fehlauer F, Veninga T, Stalpers LJ, Basic H, et al. Escalation of radiation dose beyond 30Gy in 10 fractions for metastatic spinal cord compression. Int J Radiat Oncol Biol Phys 2007;67(2):525-31.

[13] Rades D, Fehlauer F, Veninga T, Stalpers LJ, Basic H, et al. Functional outcome and survival after radiotherapy of metastatic spinal cord compression in patients with cancer of unknown primary. Int J Radiat Oncol Biol Phys 2007;67(2):532-7.

[14] Rades D, Heidenreich F, Bremer M, Karstens J. Time of developing motor deficits before radiotherapy as a new and relevant prognostic factor in metastatic spinal cord compression: Final results of a retrospective analysis. Eur Neurol 2001;45:266-9.

[15] Rades D, Rudat V, Veninga T, Stalpers LJ, Hoskin PJ, Schild SE. Prognostic factors for functional outcome and survival after reirradiation for in-field recurrences of metastatic spinal cord compression. Cancer 2008;113(5):1090-6.

[16] Rades D, Stalpers LJA, Veninga T, Rudat V, Schults R, Hoskin PJ. Evaluation of functional outcome and local control after radiotherapy for metastatic spinal cord compression in patients with prostate cancer. J Urol 2006;175:552-6,9.

[17] Venkitaraman R, Barbachano Y, Dearnaley DA, Parker CC, Khoo V, Huddart RA, Eeles R, Horwich A, Sohaid A. Outcome of early detection and radiotherapy for occult spinal cord compression. Radiother Oncol 2007;85:469-72.

[18] Patchell RA, Tibbs PA, Regine WF, Payne R, Saris S, Kryscio RJ, Mohiuddin M, Young B. Direct decompressive surgical resection in the treatment of spinal cord compression caused by metastatic cancer: a randomised trial. Lancet 2005;366(9486):643-8.

[19] Kovner F, Shulem S, Rider I, et al. Radiation therapy of metastatic spinal cord compression. J Neurooncol 1999;42:85-92.

[20] Levack P, Graham J, Kidd J. Listen to the patient: Quality of life of patients with recently diagnosed malignant cord compression in relation to their disability. Palliat Med 2004;18(7):594-601.

[21] World Health Organization. http://www.who.int/en/

[22] Schoeggl A, Reddy M, Matula C. Neurological outcome following laminectomy in spinal metastases. Spinal Cord 2002;40:363-6.

[23] Tharmalingam S, Chow E, Harris K, Hird A, Sinclair E. Quality of life measurement in bone metastases: A literature review. J Pain Res, in press.

[24] Wong J, Hird A, Kirou-Mauro A, Napolskikh J, Chow E. Quality of life in brain metastases radiation trials: a literature review. J Curr Oncol 2008;15(5):25-45.

[25] Waldron D, O'Boyle CA, Kearney M, Moriarty M, Carney D. Quality-of-life measurement in advanced cancer: Assessing the individual. J Clin Oncol 1999;17(11):3603-11.

[26] Garratt AM, Ruta DA, Abdalla MI, Buckingham JK, Russell IT. The SF36 health survey questionnaire: an outcome measure suitable for routine use within the NHS? BMJ 1993;306(6890):1440-4.

[27] Mannion RJ, Wilby M, Godward S, Lyratzopoulos G, Lain RJC. The surgical management of metastatic spinal disease: Prospective assessment and long-term follow-up. Br J Neurosurg 2007;21(6): 593-8.

[28] Varni JW, Seid M, Knight TS, Uzark K, Szer IS. The PedsQL 4.0 Generic Core Scales: Sensitivity, responsiveness, and impact on clinical decision-making. J Behav Med 2002;25(2):175-93.

[29] Cella DF, Tulsky DS, Gray G, Sarafian B, Linn E, et al. The functional assessment of cancer therapy scale: Development and validation of the general measure. J Clin Oncol 1993;11(3):570-9.

[30] Rades D, Walz J, Schild SE, Veninga T, Dunst J. Do bladder cancer patients with metastatic spinal cord compression benefit from radiotherapy alone?. Urology 2007; 69(6):1081-5.

[31] Aaronson NK, Ahmedzai S, Bergman B, et al. The European Organisation for Research and Treatment of Cancer. QLQ-C30: a quality of life instrument for use in international clinical trials in oncology. J Natl Cancer Inst 1993;85:365-76.

In: Advanced Cancer
Editors: N. Thavarajah, N. Pulenzas, B. Lechner et al.

ISBN: 978-1-62808-239-5
© 2013 Nova Science Publishers, Inc.

Chapter 17

The Palliative Performance Scale: Examining its correlation to the Karnofsky Performance Scale in an outpatient palliative radiation oncology clinic

Sarah Campos, Liying Zhang, Emily Sinclair, May Tsao,
Elizabeth A Barnes, Cyril Danjoux, Arjun Sahgal, Philiz Goh,
Shaelyn Culleton, Gunita Mitera and Edward Chow[*]

Rapid Response Radiotherapy Program, Department of Radiation Oncology, Odette Cancer Centre, Sunnybrook Health Sciences Centre, University of Toronto, Toronto, Ontario, Canada

The Palliative Performance Scale (PPS) was developed in 1996 to modernize the Karnofsky Performance Scale (KPS), an established tool for measurement of patient performance status. Although the reliability of the KPS is well established, there has been little research done on the reliability of the PPS, despite its wide use in Canada. Furthermore, only limited research has been done correlating the PPS with other performance status tools such as the KPS. Purpose: To examine the correlation between the KPS and the PPS in patients with advanced cancer. Methods: KPS and PPS were recorded for 421 patients seen in the Rapid Response Radiotherapy Program (RRRP) at the Odette Cancer Centre in Toronto, Ontario, between July 2007 and March 2008. KPS and PPS scores of patients were then examined using the Pearson correlation. This study was approved by the research ethics board at Sunnybrook Health Sciences Centre. Results: Good overall correlation was observed between KPS and PPS of the patients enrolled in this study (r = 0.87). The correlation between KPS and PPS was higher when

[*] Corresponding author: Edward Chow, MBBS, PhD, FRCPC, Department of Radiation Oncology, Odette Cancer Centre, Sunnybrook Health Sciences Centre, 2075 Bayview Avenue, Toronto, ON M4N 3M5, Canada. Tel: 416-480-4998; Fax: 416-480-6002; E-mail: Edward.Chow@sunnybrook.ca.

the performance status of the patient fell within the middle portion of the scales at 50-80 ($r>0.5$; $p< 0.05$). Conclusion: PPS showed good correlation with the well-established KPS and thus is a reliable measure of patient performance status.

Introduction

Performance status is defined by the National Cancer Institute as "A measure of how well a patient is able to perform ordinary tasks and carry out daily activities" (1). Reliable measurement of performance status is useful for clinicians to quantitatively measure and track patients' disease and symptom progression to ensure appropriate treatment. Performance status can often help determine which treatment course is appropriate for an individual patient. It is also used to determine the level of supportive care patients may require and may determine their eligibility for enrolment into clinical trials. Lastly, performance status can be a useful tool in predicting patient prognosis.

Karnofsky and Burchenal (1949) recognized the need for a standard quantifier of performance status and developed the Karnofsky Performance Scale (KPS, Figure 1) (2). The KPS has since been established as an accurate measure of performance status with good inter-rater reliability (3). Today, it is still considered a good predictor of survival in patients with advanced cancer and is used very commonly in clinical practice (4-8).

Index	Specific Criteria
100	Normal, no complaints, no evidence of disease
90	Able to carry on normal activity, minor signs of symptoms of disease
80	Normal activity with effort, some signs or symptoms of disease
70	Cares for self, unable to carry on normal activity or to do work
60	Requires occasional assistance from others but able to care for most needs
50	Requires considerable assistance from others and frequent medical care
40	Disabled, requires special care and assistance
30	Severely disabled, hospitalization indicated, death not imminent
20	Very sick, hospitalization necessary, active supportive treatment necessary
10	Moribund
0	Dead

The KPS was developed in 1948 for the purpose of assessing performance status in patients with inoperable lung cancer undergoing palliative treatment.

Figure 1. The Karnofsky Performance Scale (2).

In 1996, the Victoria Hospice Society developed the Palliative Performance Scale (PPS, Figure 2) as a tool designed to expand on and modernize the existing KPS. The PPS was developed for the purpose of accurately assessing and communicating a patient's functional level, describing the workload needed for their care, and assisting in prognosis (9). It includes several different categories, which cumulatively predict a patient's ability to carry out their activities of daily living (ADLs). The PPS assesses ambulation, activity, evidence of level of disease, self-care, intake, and consciousness (9). Like the KPS, the score is a quantitative measure with a scale ranging from 0 (death) to 100 (normal activity), but evaluates some clinically important criteria not included in the KPS, such as ambulation and nutritional intake. This additional information may provide a more accurate reflection of patient physical status and therefore overall performance status (10).

PPS Level	Ambulation	Activity & Evidence of Disease	Self-Care	Intake	Conscious Level
100%	Full	Normal activity & work No evidence of disease	Full	Normal	Full
90%	Full	Normal activity & work Some evidence of disease	Full	Normal	Full
80%	Full	Normal activity *with* Effort Some evidence of disease	Full	Normal or reduced	Full
70%	Reduced	Unable Normal Job/Work Significant disease	Full	Normal or reduced	Full
60%	Reduced	Unable hobby/house work Significant disease	Occasional assistance necessary	Normal or reduced	Full or Confusion
50%	Mainly Sit/Lie	Unable to do any work Extensive disease	Considerable assistance required	Normal or reduced	Full or Confusion
40%	Mainly in Bed	Unable to do most activity Extensive disease	Mainly assistance	Normal or reduced	Full or Drowsy +/- Confusion
30%	Totally Bed Bound	Unable to do any activity Extensive disease	Total Care	Normal or reduced	Full or Drowsy +/- Confusion
20%	Totally Bed Bound	Unable to do any activity Extensive disease	Total Care	Minimal to sips	Full or Drowsy +/- Confusion
10%	Totally Bed Bound	Unable to do any activity Extensive disease	Total Care	Mouth care only	Drowsy or Coma +/- Confusion
0%	Death	-	-	-	-

The PPS was developed by the Victoria Hospice Society for the purpose of assessing performance status in palliative care patients in Victoria, B.C. This version replaces the original PPS, developed in 1996. This is reproduced with the permission of the Victoria Hospice Society.

Figure 2. The Palliative Performance Scale (PPSv2) (9).

Cancer Care Ontario (CCO), a Canadian provincial cancer authority, has recently implemented a plan to standardize patient assessment tools in order to improve integration and co-ordination of care across the province (11). As part of an initiative launched in 2006 to improve palliative care services in Ontario, CCO began collecting PPS data for patients seen in cancer clinics province-wide, using a common database (11). In a recent review of prognostication tools, Lau and colleagues remark on the value of the PPS as a communication, as well as prognostic tool for palliative patients. These authors suggest that the PPS may eventually replace the KPS as a component of other predictive tools (12).

In a palliative medicine review of prognostication, Glare and colleagues also suggest that the PPS may be better fit to measure performance status in today's contemporary health care system (13). Despite the remarkable enthusiasm in embracing the PPS as the standard performance status measurement tool instead of the well-established KPS, only one study to date has compared the two tools (14). The primary objective of this study was to determine the degree of correlation between these two measurement tools in an outpatient palliative radiation oncology clinic.

Our study

Patients referred for palliative radiotherapy with a pathological diagnosis of cancer and documented evidence of symptomatic metastases were eligible. The patients' PPS scores were determined by the attending radiation oncologist upon initial patient evaluation, while the KPS score was determined concurrently by the research assistant. Demographic data was also collected, including reason for referral to the RRRP (Rapid Response Radiotherapy Program), primary cancer site, the location from which the patient came to the consultation from (i.e. home, hospital) and whether or not they came by ambulance. Ethics approval for this study was obtained from the hospital research ethics board.

Correlation between PPS and KPS was calculated using Pearson correlation and a linear regression model. Correlation was also calculated between corresponding levels of KPS and PPS. Patients were grouped by KPS level, and the Pearson correlation conducted for each group's KPS and PPS scores. For example, correlation between KPS and PPS scores of patients having KPS =20, =30, =40, =50, =60, =70, =80, =90 and =100 were calculated. Similarly, correlation between KPS and PPS of patients having KPS of <20, <30, <40, <50, <60, <70, <80, <90 and <100 were calculated to determine at which specific levels better correlation existed. Correlation coefficients with p values <0.05 were considered statistically significant results.

Our findings

Between July 2007 and March 2008, 421 patients were seen in the Rapid Response Radiotherapy Program (RRRP) at the Odette Cancer Center of the Sunnybrook Health Sciences Centre in Toronto, Ontario, Canada. Approximately 45% of patients studied were female, and 55% were male. The median age was 69 years (range, 26-100 years). The majority of patients had either: lung (36%), prostate (19%), or breast cancer (17%) (Table 1). Patients varied in the reason for referral to RRRP, but were mostly referred for palliation of their painful bone metastases (55%), or brain metastases (21%) (see table 2). Most patients (72%) received radiotherapy after consultation; 8% of patients required further investigation before treatment, 6% were referred for treatment other than radiotherapy, 5% were asymptomatic, and 3% declined treatment. The majority of patients were outpatients living at home, and the minority of patients traveled to their appointments by ambulance (Table 1). Of the 421 patients, the mean KPS and PPS scores were both 60 with a standard deviation of 20. Similarly, median KPS and PPS scores were 60. Both sets of scores ranged from 10-100.

Pearson correlation of the relationship between KPS and PPS scores reported a highly significant, positive correlation (r=0.84; p<0.0001). Table 3 shows the cross-analysis of KPS and PPS scores. There is good correlation between KPS and PPS, and most patients had identical KPS and PPS scores.

The correlation between KPS and PPS was further analyzed by comparing correlation of different levels of the tools. Patients were broken down into groups based on KPS score, and their KPS and PPS scores were subsequently correlated. The aim of this test was to determine whether correlation between the two tools varied according to patients' level of performance status. Table 4 shows correlation coefficients for patients grouped into separate KPS levels. KPS and PPS were best correlated at levels 50, 60, 70 and 80 (r>0.5; p< 0.05). When analyzing the correlation between the KPS and PPS of patients who fell within the KPS range of 10 to 40, inclusively (n = 48), no significant relationship was found. Similarly, no significant correlation was found in patients whose KPS fell within the range of 90 to 100, inclusively (n = 53). It should be noted, however, that KPS scores for this patient population were relatively centralized in the middle of both scales, so the lack of significant correlation could likely be due to the small sample of patients on either extreme end of performance status.

Despite observed variation in correlation between levels of KPS and PPS, the overall relationship between these variables is a strongly positive one, as shown in the General Linear Model plotted in Figure 3. Although a few outliers are present, the plot is generally well distributed on the regression line (PPS = 6.85 + 0.89(KPS)).

Table 1. Patient demographics (n = 421)

Age		
	Median	69 years
	Range	26 – 100 years
Sex		
	Female	191 (45 %)
	Male	230 (55 %)
Primary Cancer Site		
	Lung	152 (36 %)
	Prostate	80 (19 %)
	Breast	74 (18 %)
	Genitourinary	44 (11 %)
	Gastrointestinal	40 (10 %)
	Others	18 (4 %)
	Unknown	13 (3 %)
Patient from		
	Outpatient	314 (75 %)
	Inpatient in Hospital	103 (24 %)
	Others	4 (<1 %)
Ambulance		
	Yes	90 (21 %)
	No	329 (79 %)
	Unknown	2 (<1 %)

Table 2. Reason for referral to the Rapid Response Radiotherapy Clinic (n = 421)

Reason for Referral	n (%)
Painful Bony Metastases	232 (55%)
Brain Metastases	92 (22 %)
Others (i.e. reduction of mass, spinal cord compression, fracture, bleeding)	97 (23%)

Table 3. Cross table of KPS and PPS

KPS	PPS 10	20	30	40	50	60	70	80	90	100	Total KPS
10	0	1	0	0	0	0	0	0	0	0	1
20	2	4	3	0	0	0	0	0	0	0	9
30	1	0	19	6	2	0	0	1	0	0	29
40	0	0	5	23	5	2	0	0	0	0	35
50	0	0	1	17	43	11	2	1	1	1	77
60	0	1	0	1	11	61	17	3	1	0	95
70	0	0	0	0	0	12	43	11	3	0	69
80	0	0	0	1	0	4	15	35	5	0	60
90	0	0	0	0	0	2	3	5	30	2	42
100	0	0	0	0	0	0	0	0	1	2	3
Total PPS	3	6	28	48	61	92	80	56	41	5	420

The above table shows the number of patients at each KPS level (rows), crossed with the number of patients at the corresponding PPS level (columns). The bolded numbers show the number of patients at each level who had identical KPS and PPS values.

Table 4. Pearson Correlation between KPS and PPS by level of KPS

	Correlation based on KPS above a certain level	Correlation based on KPS below a certain level
	KPS ≥ 20	**KPS < 20**
n	515	1
r (p-value)	0.87 (< 0.0001)	-
	KPS ≥ 30	**KPS < 30**
n	502	14
r (p-value)	0.86 (< 0.0001)	0.048 (0.90)
	KPS ≥ 40	**KPS < 40**
n	468	48
r (p-value)	0.84 (< 0.0001)	0.47 (0.0023)
	KPS ≥ 50	**KPS < 50**
n	424	92
r (p-value)	0.80 (< 0.0001)	0.58 (< 0.0001)
	KPS ≥ 60	**KPS < 60**
n	327	189
r (p-value)	0.75 (< 0.0001)	0.66 (< 0.0001)
	KPS ≥ 70	**KPS < 70**
n	216	300
r (p-value)	0.63 (< 0.0001)	0.76 (< 0.0001)
	KPS ≥ 80	**KPS < 80**
n	126	390
r (p-value)	0.55 (< 0.0001)	0.82 (< 0.0001)
	KPS ≥ 90	**KPS < 90**
n	53	463
r (p-value)	0.29 (0.055)	0.84 (< 0.0001)
	KPS ≥ 100	**KPS < 100**
n	4	512
r (p-value)	-	0.87 (< 0.0001)

The above table analyzes the correlation between KPS and PPS based on the level of KPS into which the patient falls. KPS and PPS were best correlated at levels 50, 60, 70 and 80 ($r > 0.5$; $p < 0.05$).

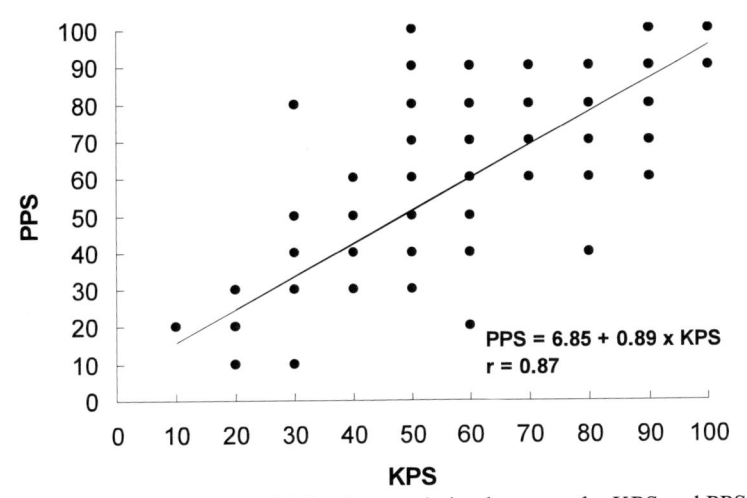

The above figure plots the regression model for the correlation between the KPS and PPS scales.

Figure 3. General Linear Model of Pearson Correlation between KPS and PPS.

Discussion

Our study found an excellent correlation between KPS and PPS (r= 0.87), suggesting that both tools are similarly accurate in assessing performance status in this palliative cancer population. In a 2004 description of the PPS, Wilner and Arnold comment on the need for further studies analyzing the correlation of the PPS with other commonly used prognostic tools and symptom assessment scales (15). Although much research has been done on the KPS, only one study to date has compared it with the PPS scale. Morita et al. undertook a study using PPS to predict survival in terminally ill cancer patients in Japan in 1999. The authors analyzed the relationship between KPS and PPS scores for 588 patient samples as a secondary objective of the study. They too found an excellent correlation between KPS and PPS (r = 0.93) (14), which supports the more detailed results obtained in this study.

An important difference to consider when interpreting the results obtained by Morita et al. when compared to our study lies in the patient demographics. The majority of our population consisted of outpatients, living in their own homes, not requiring ambulance services, and being treated with a palliative intent at the time of consultation. Patients included in the study by Morita et al. consisted of hospitalized terminally ill patients with a low performance status score (14). Eighty-one percent of patients in Morita et al.'s study had a PPS of =50 (14), compared to 35% in our study. Morita et al.'s study was able to correlate low PPS and KPS scores, whereas the patients in our population provided a wider scope of the two scales.

One apparent limitation of our study design lies in the method of assessment. KPS scores were rated by the research assistant, while PPS scores were formulated by the attending physician. This is a direct result of CCO's requirement that all PPS scores entered into their database be rated by a physician. The research assistant routinely rates KPS scores for all patients seen in the clinic, which are then entered into the clinical database. Furthermore, de Borja et al. studied the relationship between both KPS and ECOG scores assigned by various health care providers including physicians, nurses, radiation therapists and radiation therapy students (16). This study found moderate correlation of radiation therapist and physician scores (r = 0.57, p = 0.002), very good correlation of nurse and physician scores (r = 0.77, p<0.0001), and very good correlation of radiation therapy student and physician scores (r = 0.81, p<0.0001). Additionally, a study done by Liem et al. compared KPS assessments assigned by resident and attending physicians and found an excellent correlation (r = 0.85, p<0.01) between them (17). This demonstrates the similarity of performance status scores determined by all health care providers working with a particular patient. The research assistant, as a member of a multidisciplinary clinical team, was thereby named an accurate rater of performance status, and her KPS scores were deemed valid for the purpose of this study.

Despite the lack of research validating the PPS as a reliable performance status tool, much literature exists on the role of the PPS in predicting patient survival. PPS has been shown to be an independent prognostic factor in many studies (7,18-23), and is at least as good at predicting survival as the Eastern Co-operative Oncology Group (see Figure 4) (24) and the KPS scales (19). Although the PPS is useful overall as a predictive tool, one study showed it to produce some discrepancies between patients of different performance status (21). Like the results produced by our study, suggesting different correlation of KPS and PPS at different levels of performance status, Lau and Downing reported the PPS to be better at calibrating expected survival of patients at 10, 20, 30 and 40%, as compared to higher levels of PPS (21). Correlation between KPS and PPS tended to be higher in patients with a better performance status, signifying that the PPS can isolate distinct changes in lower performance status patients that are not measured by the KPS scale. This suggests that the PPS is unique in grouping patients with low performance status, and can fairly reliably predict their survival accordingly. A systematic review of the literature by Lau and colleagues also suggests that the PPS is useful for predicting 1-6 month survival (12), which is the range typically expected for low performance status patients.

ECOG PERFORMANCE STATUS	
Grade	**ECOG**
0	Fully active, able to carry on all pre-disease performance without restriction
1	Restricted in physically strenuous activity but ambulatory and able to carry out work of a light or sedentary nature, e.g., light house work, office work
2	Ambulatory and capable of all self-care but unable to carry out any work activities. Up and about more than 50% of waking hours
3	Capable of only limited self-care, confined to bed or chair more than 50% of waking hours
4	Completely disabled. Cannot carry on any self-care. Totally confined to bed or chair
5	Dead

The ECOG scale was developed in 1982 as part of criteria developed to assess toxicity and response to treatment. It is now widely used to assess performance status in cancer patients in clinical settings as well as in clinical trials and studies.

Figure 4. The Eastern Cooperative Oncology Group (ECOG) Scale (22).

The PPS was developed by the Victoria Hospice Society with the intention of modernizing the KPS. The KPS, although well established, does not reflect the shift of resources to community and outpatient settings that have recently come into play in Canadian healthcare (10,25). Hospitalization is a vital part of KPS criteria, but is no longer an integral part of a patient's performance status given that many palliative patients are able to access adequate home care. Furthermore, many patients now choose available end-of-life care to allow them to die in their own homes. The PPS is advantageous in that it does not use information regarding patient hospitalization, but instead takes into account patients' levels of ambulation, oral intake and consciousness: criteria that clinical experience has shown to be very important in performance status evaluation (9).

In a study of survival predictors, Vigano and Bruera chose to measure performance status using the Eastern Co-Operative Oncology Group (ECOG) scale (see Figure 4) (24) due to the incorporation of patient ambulation status (26). Had this study been performed after the PPS was released, the PPS might have been a more reliable choice due to the additional attention it gives to nutritional intake and consciousness. PPS is also the performance status tool used in the Palliative Prognostic Index: a tool developed by Morita that used performance status and the presence or absence of four symptoms to predict survival in terminally ill cancer patients (27).

Most research evaluating the PPS, as a survival tool or otherwise, involves patients in inpatient palliative care, hospice or hospital studies. Only one study evaluated PPS in patients from a tertiary care setting (22). Furthermore, the majority of studies in the literature look at patient populations with low median PPS. This suggests that PPS is only being analyzed in palliative care patients who have been admitted to hospice settings and are very near t o death (20).

Conclusion

The PPS showed good correlation to the KPS overall in this primary outpatient palliative patient population. In particular, the PPS was highly correlated to the KPS for patients within the intermediate range of the scales (50-80), which applies to the majority of patients enrolled in the study. The PPS has the further advantage of accounting for clinically relevant variables applicable to modern outpatient palliative healthcare, and adequately assesses patients' ability to perform the activities of daily living.

PPS was reliable in assessing patients at intermediate levels of the scale, but shows some variance in measuring the performance status of nearly moribund patients. Studies evaluating the reliability of the PPS in populations with more evenly distributed performance status scores are necessary in determining the consistency of the scale as a whole.

Although we were able to measure the reliability of the PPS scale in terms of its correlation to the KPS, the value of this tool also greatly depends on its use in clinical practice. In light of the recent "closer to home" (25) shift in Canadian healthcare as well as the use of the PPS by Canadian authorities in cancer care, the usability of this tool by health care professionals and patients is crucial to its value. Further research is needed to ensure it is easy to understand and produces consistent, reliable results in a variety of settings.

Our study concludes that the PPS is reliable in predicting the performance status of outpatients with advanced cancer; however more research is needed to validate the PPS as a performance status tool in more heterogeneous populations.

Acknowledgments

This project was funded by Michael and Karyn Goldstein Cancer Research Fund. Conflicts of Interest Notification: None

References

[1]   Definition of Performance Status - NCI Dictionary of Cancer Terms. 2008; Available at:http://www.cancer.gov/dictionary/?searchTxt=performance+status&sgroup=Starts+with&lang=&btnGo.x=9&btnGo.y=3. Accessed 2009 Jan 3.

[2]   Karnofsky DA, Abelmann WH, Craver LF, Burchenal JH. The use of the nitrogen mustards in the palliative treatment of carcinoma. With particular reference to bronchogenic carcinoma. Cancer 1948; 1(4):634-56.

[3]   Yates JW, Chalmer B, McKegney FP. Evaluation of patients with advanced cancer using the Karnofsky performance status. Cancer 1980;45(8):2220-4.

[4]   Chow E, Harth T, Hruby G, Finkelstein J, Wu J, Danjoux C. How accurate are physicians' clinical predictions of survival and the available prognostic tools in estimating survival times in terminally ill cancer patients? A systematic review. Clin Oncol (R Coll Radiol) 2001;13(3):209-18.

[5]   Chow E, Fung K, Panzarella T, Bezjak A, Danjoux C, Tannock I. A predictive model for survival in metastatic cancer patients attending an outpatient palliative radiotherapy clinic. Int J Radiat Oncol Biol Phys 2002;53(5):1291-1302.

[6]   Maltoni M, Nanni O, Pirovano M, Scarpi E, Indelli M, Martini C, et al. Successful validation of the palliative prognostic score in terminally ill cancer patients. Italian Multicenter Study Group on Palliative Care. J Pain Symptom Manage 1999;17(4):240-7.

[7]   Sloan JA, Loprinzi CL, Laurine JA, Novotny PJ, Vargas-Chanes D, Krook JE, et al. A simple stratification factor prognostic for survival in advanced cancer: the good/bad/uncertain index. J Clin Oncol 2001;19(15):3539-46.

[8]   Wigren T. Confirmation of a prognostic index for patients with inoperable non-small cell lung cancer. Radiother Oncol 1997; 44(1):9-15.

[9]   Downing GM, Wainwright W. Palliative Performance Scale (PPSv2) Version 2. Medical care of the dying, 4th ed. Victoria, BC: Victoria Hospice Society Learning Centre Palliat Care, 2006.

[10]   Anderson F, Downing GM, Hill J, Casorso L, Lerch N. Palliative performance scale (PPS): a new tool. J Palliat Care 1996;12(1):5-11.

[11]   Palliative care strategy: Improving the quality of palliative care services for cancer patients in Ontario. Toronto, ON: Cancer Care Ontario, 2006.

[12]   Lau F, Cloutier-Fisher D, Kuziemsky C, Black F, Downing M, Borycki E, et al. A systematic review of prognostic tools for estimating survival time in palliative care. J Palliat Care 2007; 23(2):93-112.

[13]   Glare PA, Sinclair CT. Palliative Medicine Review: Prognostication. J Palliat Med 2008;11(1):84-103.

[14]   Morita T, Tsunoda J, Inoue S, Chihara S. Validity of the palliative performance scale from a survival perspective. J Pain Symptom Manage 1999;18(1):2-3.

[15]   Wilner LS, Arnold RM. The Palliative Performance Scale #125. J Palliat Med 2006;9(4):994.

[16]   de Borja MT, Chow E, Bovett G, Davis L, Gillies C. The correlation among patient and health care professionals in assessing functional status using the karnofsky and eastern cooperative oncolog group performance status scales. Support Cancer Ther 2004;2(1):59-63.

[17] Liem BJ, Holland JM, Kang MY, Hoffelt SC, Marquez CM. Karnofsky Performance Status Assessment: resident versus attending. J Cancer Educ 2002;17(3):138-41.

[18] de Miguel Sanchez C, Elustondo SG, Estirado A, Sanchez FV, de la Rasilla Cooper,C.G., Romero AL, et al. Palliative performance status, heart rate and respiratory rate as predictive factors of survival time in terminally ill cancer patients. J Pain Symptom Manage 2006; 31(6):485-92.

[19] Harrold J, Rickerson E, Carroll JT, McGrath J, Morales K, Kapo J, et al. Is the palliative performance scale a useful predictor of mortality in a heterogeneous hospice population? J Palliat Med 2005; 8(3):503-9.

[20] Head B, Ritchie CS, Smoot TM. Prognostication in hospice care: can the palliative performance scale help? J Palliat Med 2005; 8(3):492-502.

[21] Lau F, Downing GM, Lesperance M, Shaw J, Kuziemsky C. Use of Palliative Performance Scale in end-of-life prognostication. J Palliat Med 2006;9(5):1066-75.

[22] Olajide O, Hanson L, Usher BM, Qaqish BF, Schwartz R, Bernard S. Validation of the palliative performance scale in the acute tertiary care hospital setting. J Palliat Med 2007;10(1):111-7.

[23] Virik K, Glare P. Validation of the palliative performance scale for inpatients admitted to a palliative care unit in Sydney, Australia. J Pain Symptom Manage 2002;23(6): 455-7.

[24] Oken MM, Creech RH, Tormey DC, Horton J, Davis TE, McFadden ET, et al. Toxicity and response criteria of the Eastern Cooperative Oncology Group. Am J Clin Oncol 1982;5(6):649-55.

[25] Seaton PD, et al. Closer to home. Report of the British Columbia Royal Commission on health care and costs. Victoria, BC: British Columbia Min Health, 1991.

[26] Vigano A, Bruera E, Jhangri GS, Newman SC, Fields AL, Suarez-Almazor ME. Clinical survival predictors in patients with advanced cancer. Arch Intern Med 2000;160(6):861-8.

[27] Morita T, Tsunoda J, Inoue S, Chihara S. The Palliative Prognostic Index: a scoring system for survival prediction of terminally ill cancer patients. Support Care Cancer 1999;7(3):128-33.

In: Advanced Cancer   ISBN: 978-1-62808-239-5
Editors: N. Thavarajah, N. Pulenzas, B. Lechner et al.   © 2013 Nova Science Publishers, Inc.

Chapter 18

Confirmatory factor analysis of Brief Pain Inventory (BPI) functional interference clusters in patients with bone metastases

Edward Chow[1]*, Jennifer James[2], Andrea Barsevick[3], William Hartsell[4], Sarah Ratcliffe[5], Charles Scarantino[6], Robert Ivker[7], John Suh[8], Ivy Petersen[9], Andre Konski[3], William Demas[10] and Deborah Bruner[11]

[1]Odette Cancer Centre, Toronto, Canada,
[2]RTOG Statistical Center, Philadelphia, Pennsylvania, US
[3]Fox Chase Cancer Center, Cheltenham, Pennsylvania, US
[4]Good Samaritan Cancer Center, Downers Grove, Illinois, US
[5]University of Pennsylvania School of Medicine,
Philadelphia, Pennsylvania, US
[6]Rex Healthcare Cancer Center, Raleigh, North Carolina, US
[7]Newark Beth Israel Medical Center, Newark, New Jersey, US
[8]Cleveland Clinic Foundation, Cleveland, Ohio, US
[9]Mayo Clinic, Rochester, Minnesota, US
[10]Akron City Hospital Cancer Care Center, Akron, Ohio, US
[11]Abramson Cancer Center, Philadelphia, Pennsylvania, US

To determine which of the previously proposed functional interference cluster models is most appropriate in patients with bone metastases. Methods: Breast and prostate cancer patients treated with palliative radiotherapy between May 2003 to January 2007 assessed

* Corresponding author: Edward Chow, MBBS, PhD, FRCPC, Department of Radiation Oncology, Odette Cancer Centre, Sunnybrook Health Sciences Centre, 2075 Bayview Avenue, Toronto, ON M4N 3M5, Canada. Tel: 416-480-4998; Fax: 416-480-6002; E-mail: Edward.Chow@sunnybrook.ca.

using Brief Pain Inventory at baseline, 4, 8 and 12 weeks post radiation treatment. The baseline cluster structure of the confirmatory dataset was compared to each of the previously proposed baseline cluster models. Maximum likelihood CFA was used to account for possible correlation amongst the factor components. A MIMIC model was used to determine the invariance of the cluster models between responders and non-responders during follow-up. Results: A total of 169 eligible patients were analysed. There were 91 male and 78 female patients with a median age of 68 years. The median KPS was 70. A single 8 Gy and 20 Gy in 5 fractions were used in 97% of all analysed patients. The RTOG model, in which relationships with others and sleep comprised the mood-related interference cluster and walking ability and normal work comprised the physical-interference cluster, provides the best fit for the sample data. The follow-up cluster structure is not similar across the responder groups indicating that cluster structures shift following radiation treatment, as evidenced by pain response. Conclusion: Although differing slightly this analysis confirms pretreatment symptom clusters exist for patients with bone metastases from breast or prostate cancer based on the RTOG 9714 data. This could help formulate symptom management interventions at initial diagnosis.

Introduction

Bone metastases are common in patients with breast and prostate cancers. Bone metastases not only cause pain and skeletal related events such as hypercalcemia, pathological fracture and spinal cord compression, but also functional interference in a lot of patients (1). The Brief Pain Inventory (BPI) developed by Cleeland and colleagues measures general activity, normal work, walking ability, mood, sleep, relations with others and enjoyment of life (2,3). Previous research involving heterogeneous groups of cancer patients in United States, Europe and Asia has shown that the seven functional interference items in BPI can be grouped into two clusters: activity-related interference and mood-related interference (4-6). An exploratory factor analysis of RTOG 9714 patients (7) limited to breast and prostate cancer patients treated at US/Canadian institutions showed similar clusters, but with different items in each cluster (8) (see table 1). Walking ability, normal work, and relationship with others were consistent across each of the cluster models. The models differed in the assignment of sleep and mood to the mood-related interference cluster and the assignment of general activity to the activity-related interference cluster. The primary objective of this study was to conduct a confirmatory factor analysis in an independent homogeneous patient population to determine which, if any, of the previously proposed functional interference cluster models is most appropriate. The secondary objective was to determine if the cluster structures identified at baseline differed between responders and non-responders following palliative radiotherapy.

Our study

Pain and functional interference assessment

The Brief Pain Inventory consists of a worst pain score and 7 functional interference items on a scale of 0-10 with 0 indicating no pain or no interference and 10 indicating unimaginable pain and maximal interference (2,3). Pain response was categorized as the following: 1) complete response, post-treatment pain score of 0; 2) partial response, post-treatment improvement of at least 2 points; 3) stable response, post-treatment pain score within 1 point of the initial pain score, or 4) progressive response, a post-treatment increase of at least 2 points (7). Patients with complete or partial response were considered responders; patients with stable or progressive response were considered non-responders.

Patient population

The confirmatory test data set consists of breast and prostate cancer patients treated at Rapid Response Radiotherapy Program (9) at Odette Cancer Centre, Sunnybrook Health Sciences Centre with palliative radiotherapy for bone metastases between May 2003 to January 2007. Patient demographics, Karnofsky performance status (KPS), analgesic intake converted into total daily oral morphine equivalent, sites and dose of radiation treatment were collected. Patients were excluded if there was prior radiation therapy or palliative surgery to the planned radiation treatment site, pathological or impending fracture, spinal cord or cauda equina compression. Worst pain and functional interference scores were assessed using BPI at baseline, 4, 8 and 12 weeks post radiation treatment.

Statistical methods

Spearman's correlation coefficients were calculated to compare the association between the baseline BPI functional item scores. Principal component analysis (PCA) with varimax rotation was used to determine relationships between the functional items at baseline for all patients, and at subsequent follow-up for non-responders and responders. The highest factor score determined the assignment of a functional item to a component. Functional items with high factor scores (>0.40) in multiple components were not assigned. Components with at least two factors were retained. The final communality details the percent of variance of each BPI item that was explained by the retained components. Cronbach's alpha was used to determine the internal consistency and reliability of each component at baseline.

Confirmatory Factor Analysis (CFA)

The cluster structure of the confirmatory dataset was compared to each of the previously proposed cluster models. Maximum likelihood CFA was used to account for possible correlation amongst the factor components. A consensus goodness of fit measure has not been established; rather several measures are used jointly to determine which model best fits the data (10). The chi-square statistic is very sensitive to sample size, and will frequently reject valid models simply due to large samples (n>100). The adjusted goodness of fit index (AGFI) ranges from 0 to 1 with values greater than 0.8 indicating a good fit. The standardized root mean square residual (SRMR) ranges from 0 to 1 with values lower than 0.08 indicating a good fit. Bentler's comparative fit index (CFI) ranges from 0 to 1 with values greater than 0.95 indicating a good fit. The root mean square error of approximation (RMSEA) is greater than 0 with values lower than 0.06 indicating a good fit. After determining the most appropriate cluster structure for the BPI functional items at baseline (all patients), a MIMIC model (11), commonly referred to as CFA with covariates, was used to determine the invariance between the responder and non-responder groups at 4, 8, and 12 weeks post-treatment. Although only comparing two groups, a MIMIC model was used instead of the more popular multiple groups CFA due to the small sample sizes in each resultant subgroup. The fit indices to evaluate the invariance of the cluster factor model are the same ones used to evaluate the baseline cluster factor models. All data were analyzed using SAS (version 9.2 for Windows, SAS institute, Cary, NC).

Our findings

A total of 169 patients from the Rapid Response Radiotherapy Program were analyzed. There were 91 male and 78 female patients with a median age of 68 years (range 30 – 91). The median KPS was 70 (range 30 – 90). The most commonly irradiated sites were spine (31%), hips (20%), and pelvis (17%). A single 8 Gy and 20 Gy in 5 fractions were used in 97% of all patients (Table 2). The median worst pain score was 7.4 (range 0 to 10). The median functional item scores were 2 for relations with others, 4 for sleep, 5 for mood, 7 for walking ability, enjoyment of life, and general activity, and 8 for normal work. Each functional item score ranged from 0 to 10. The correlation between each BPI item was highly significant at baseline ($p<0.001$). The correlation between normal work and general activity was the highest (0.65); whereas the correlation between walking ability and sleep were the lowest (0.27). The follow up rates at 4, 8, and 12 weeks were 71%, 61%, and 51% respectively. The response rates at each follow up were 68%, 63% and 72% respectively.

Table 1. BPI Functional Item Clusters Previously Identified

Research Team	Patient Population	Mood-Related Interference Cluster	Activity-Related Interference Cluster	Non-cluster Items
[4]Cleeland et al, 1996	(n=1843) All cancers USA, France, Philippines, China	Mood Relations w/ others Enjoyment of life	Walking ability General activity Normal work	Sleep
[5]Saxena et al, 1999	(n=200) All cancers, majority cervical North India	Mood Relations w/ others Enjoyment of life	Walking ability General activity Normal work	Sleep
[6]Klepstad et al, 2002	(n=235) All cancers, majority breast/prostate Norway	Mood Relations w/ others Enjoyment of life Sleep	Walking ability General activity Normal work	None
[8]Chow et al, 2009	(n=909) Breast/prostate cancer only USA/Canada	Relations w/ others Sleep	Walking ability Normal work	Mood Enjoyment of Life General activity

Table 2. Patient characteristics (n = 169)

Characteristics	n (%)
Gender	
Male	91 (54)
Female	78 (46)
Age at consultation (years)	
Mean ± SD	66.2 ± 12.9
Median (range)	68 (30 – 91)
Primary cancer site	
Breast	87 (51)
Prostate	82 (49)
Karnofsky Performance Status	
Mean ± SD	71.5 ± 13.4
Median (range)	70 (30 – 90)
Total Daily Oral Morphine Equivalent (mg)	
Mean ± SD	98 ± 252
Median (range)	12 (0 – 2600)
Site of radiotherapy	
Spine	53 (31)
Hips	33 (20)
Pelvis	28 (17)
Ribs	9 (5)
Others	46 (27)
Radiation Dose cGy/fraction number(s)	
800/1	116 (69)
2000/5	48 (28)
Others	5 (3)

Table 3. Principal components analysis Baseline factor loadings

Item	Physical Interference Cluster (Component 1)	Psychosocial Interference Cluster (Component 2)	Final Communality
Normal Work	**0.81**	0.27	**0.72**
General Activity	**0.79**	0.31	**0.72**
Walking Ability	**0.78**	0.11	0.61
Enjoyment of Life	0.72	0.43	0.70
Relations with Others	0.12	**0.88**	**0.78**
Mood	0.35	**0.75**	**0.69**
Sleep	0.45	0.50	0.45
Variance	55%	12%	
Cronbach's alpha	0.79	0.70	

Table 4. Principal Components Analysis Follow-up Factor Loadings

	Week 4		Week 8		Week 12	
	Component 1	Component 2	Component 1	Component 2	Component 1	Component 2
Non-Responders	Gen activity Mood Walk ability Normal work	Sleep	Walk ability	Relationships Sleep	Gen activity Walk ability Sleep	Mood Relationships
Variance	*65%*	*14%*	*64%*	*13%*	*55%*	*17%*
Alpha	*0.86*	*--*	*--*	*0.47*	*0.70*	*.80*
Responders	Sleep	Mood Relationships	Gen activity Walk ability Normal work Enjoy life	Sleep	Walk ability Relationships	Sleep
Variance	*70%*	*13%*	*72%*	*11%*	*68%*	*11%*
Alpha	*--*	*0.87*	*0.96*	*--*	*0.78*	*--*

* Principal components analysis with varimax rotation.

Principal components which had eigenvalues greater than 1 or explained more than 10% of the variance were retained (see table 3). The two baseline clusters accounted for 67% of the total variance. The first cluster (physical interference) included normal work, general activity, and walking ability which accounted for 55% of the total variance. The second cluster (psychosocial interference) included relations with others and mood which accounted for 12% of the total variance. The internal reliabilities of each cluster based on the Cronbach's alpha statistic were 0.79 and 0.70, respectively. Final communality estimates ranged from 0.45 for sleep to 0.78 for relations with others.

Confirmatory Factor Analysis (CFA)

The fit indices for each of the previously proposed models based on the test dataset are detailed in Table 5. The Cleeland et al. and Saxena et al. models (4, 5) have low AGFI values (0.8835) and high RMSEA values (0.1194) indicating a poor fit for the sample data. The Klepstad et al. model (6) has similar AGFI (0.9909) and RMSEA (0.1002) values also indicating a poor fit. The Chow et al. model (8), which was determined using the most similar patient population, provides the best fit for the sample data with optimal AGFI (0.9745), SRMR (0.0143), RMSEA (0.0365), and CFI (0.9983) values. After determining that the Chow et al. model provided the best fit for functional status at baseline; the model fit during radiation follow-up was evaluated. Table 6 details the invariance of the model across the responder and non-responder subgroups at each follow-up assessment. The poor fits at each follow-up—AGFI <0.80, SRMR>0.08, RMSEA>0.06, CFI <0.95— indicate that the baseline cluster structure is not similar across the groups and that cluster structures shift following radiation treatment, as evidenced by pain response (Table 4).

Table 5. Fits provided by competing cluster models Baseline BPI Functional Items

Proposed Model	X^2 (df)	Adjusted Goodness of Fit Index (AGFI)	Standardized Root Mean Square Residual (SRMR)	Root Mean Square Error of Approximation (RMSEA)	Bentler's Comparative Fit Index (CFI)
[4]Cleeland et al, 1996	38.13 (8)	0.8835	0.0443	0.1194	0.9539
[5]Saxena et al, 1999	38.13 (8)	0.8835	0.0443	0.1194	0.9539
[6]Klepstad et al, 2002	47.44 (13)	0.9009	0.0431	0.1002	0.9542
[6]**Chow et al, 2009**	**1.351 (1)**	**0.9745**	**0.0143**	**0.0365**	**0.9983**

AGFI > 0.80; SRMR <0.08; CFI >0.95; RMSEA <0.06 indicate good fit.

Table 6. Invariance of cluster model fits across response status groups*
Follow-up BPI Functional Items

Follow-up	χ^2 (df)	Adjusted Goodness of Fit Index (AGFI)	Standardized Root Mean Square Residual (SRMR)	Root Mean Square Error of Approximation (RMSEA)	Bentler's Comparative Fit Index (CFI)
Week 4	482.2 (6)	-0.0502	0.3061	0.5483	0.2013
Week 8	408.1 (6)	0.0329	0.3047	0.5039	0.1063
Week 12	475.0 (6)	0.0406	0.3182	0.5441	0.0209

*Chow et al, 2009 cluster model. Responders vs. non-responders as defined by complete or partial response based on BPI worst pain score.

AGFI > 0.80; SRMR <0.08; CFI >0.95; RMSEA <0.06 indicate model invariance.

Discussion

Four previously proposed factor models were evaluated using the CFA (4-6, 8). Two models proposed a mood-related interference cluster—mood, relations with others, enjoyment of life—and an activity-related interference cluster—walking ability, general activity, normal work— in which sleep was not a cluster component (4, 5). A third model proposed a similar cluster structure in which sleep was included in the mood-related interference cluster (6). The fourth model proposed a mood-related interference cluster—relations with others, sleep—and an activity-related interference cluster—walking ability, normal work— in which mood, enjoyment of life, and general activity were not cluster components (8).

Functional interference clusters are dependent on the composition of the patient population. The RTOG 9714 only enrolled bone metastases patients with breast and prostate cancers. The confirmatory dataset employed in this study consisted of patients with again breast and prostate cancers. The composition of functional interference items at baseline was most similar to the clusters identified in the RTOG study. Why different cancer composition results in different clusters would be of interest in future studies.

In our exploratory RTOG study, we examined the interactions of the functional interference clusters with radiation treatment. Components of functional interference changed over time in that sample. We hypothesized changes in these components could be due to treatment response. The same observation was noted in our confirmatory study, strengthening our hypothesis.

Clinical implications of this work include identification of pretreatment clusters which may help improve symptom interventions beyond the focus of RT on pain alone and assist with monitoring changes in clusters after RT is delivered. For example, while clinicians monitor pain related to bone metastasis closely, the impact on general activities or mood are variably assessed. Testing protocols that intervene on all three symptoms simultaneously with, for example, a home care or hospice consult to ensure general daily activities are safe and met and a short term antidepressant for mood disturbances until the pain is under control, would be a reasonable trial. Closer monitoring of sleep disturbances and how they impact mood and activities may be necessary in both responders and nonresponders and has been widely overlooked in the literature.

In conclusion, cancer clusters are dynamic constructs that may provide guidance for management protocols that recognize the potential synergy among clusters to worsen quality of life. The early identification of these clusters would provide hypotheses for protocols to treat symptoms simultaneously rather than in isolation and potentially improve outcomes and improve them sooner than would occur with current standard of care.

Acknowledgments

We thank Ms Stacy Lue for secretarial assistance. Conflicts of interest: None. This publication is supported in part by grants RTOG U10 CA 21661 and CCOP U 10 CA37422 from the National Cancer Institute. Its contents are solely the responsibility of the authors and do not necessarily represent the official views of the National Cancer Institute.

References

[1]   Hoskin P, Makin W. Oncology for palliative medicine. New York: Oxford Univ Press, 2003:271-89.

[2]   Cleeland CS, Nakamura Y, Mendoza TR, Edwards KR, Douglas J, Serlin RC. The dimensions of pain: a multidimensional scaling comparison of cancer patients and healthy volunteers. Pain 1989; 37(1):23-32.

[3]   Cleeland CS, Ryan KM. Pain assessment: Global use of the Brief Pain Inventory. Ann Acad Med Singapore 1994;23(2):129-38.

[4]   Cleeland CS, Nakamura Y, Mendoza TR, Edwards KR, Douglas J, Serlin RC. Dimensions of the impact of cancer pain in a four country sample: New information from multidimensional scaling. Pain 1996; 67(2-3):267-73.

[5]   Saxena A, Mendoza T, Cleeland CS. The assessment of cancer pain in North India: The validation of the Hindi Brief Pain Inventory - BPI-H. J Pain Symptom Manage 1999;17(1):27-41.

[6]   Klepstad P, Loge JH, Borchgrevink PC, Mendoza TR, Cleeland CS, Kaasa S. The Norwegian Brief Pain Inventory questionnaire: translation and validation in cancer pain patients. J Pain Symptom Manage 2002;24(5):517-25.

[7]   Hartsell W, Scott C, Bruner D, Scarantino C, Ivker R, Roach M, Suh J, Demas W, Movasas B, Petersen I, Konski A, Cleeland C, Janjan N, DeSilvio M. Randomized trial of short-versus long-course radiotherapy for palliation of painful bone metastases. J Natl Cancer Inst 2005;97(11):798-804.

[8]   Chow E, James J, Barsevick A, Hartsell W, Ratcliffe S, Scarantino C, Ivker R, Roach M, Suh J, Peterson I, Konski A, Demas W, Bruner D. Functional interference clusters in cancer patients with bone metastases: A secondary analysis of RTOG 9714, Int J Radiat Oncol Biol Phys 2008;72(Suppl 1):141.

[9]   Danjoux C, Chow E, Hayter C, Tsao M, Barnes E, Holden L, Sinclair E, Drossos A, Farhadian M. An innovative Rapid Response Radiotherapy Program to reduce waiting time for palliative radiotherapy. Support Care Cancer 2006;14(1):38-43.

[10]   Brown TA. Confirmatory factor analysis for applied research. New York: Guilford, 2006.

[11]   Joreskog KG, Goldberger AS. Estimation of a model with multiple indicators and multiple causes of a single latent variable. J Am Statist Assoc 1975;70:631-9.

In: Advanced Cancer
ISBN: 978-1-62808-239-5
Editors: N. Thavarajah, N. Pulenzas, B. Lechner et al.   © 2013 Nova Science Publishers, Inc.

Chapter 19

Correlation of the Palliative Performance Scale with the Karnofsky Performance Status in an outpatient palliative radiotherapy clinic

Shaelyn Culleton, Kristopher Dennis, Kaitlin Koo, Liying Zhang,
Liang Zeng, Justin Kwong, Janet Nguyen, Florencia Jon,
Lori Holden, Elizabeth Barnes, May Tsao, Cyril Danjoux,
Arjun Sahgal and Edward Chow[*]

Rapid Response Radiotherapy Program, Department of Radiation Oncology, Odette
Cancer Centre, Sunnybrook Health Sciences Centre, University of Toronto,
Toronto, Canada

Performance scales are important predictors of response to therapy and survival. Both the Palliative Performance Scale (PPS) and the Karnofsky Performance Status (KPS) measure ambulation, evidence of disease and self-care abilities. However the two measures differ in that PPS has incorporated oral intake and level of consciousness into their measure. The purpose of this study was to determine the level of agreement between the PPS and the KPS in evaluating patients with advanced cancer referred for palliative radiotherapy (RT). Patients treated with palliative RT for metastases to brain, bone or lung, or advanced lung cancer from 2007-2010 were assigned KPS and PPS scores at baseline. KPS was scored by a trained research assistant and PPS scores were assigned by a radiation oncologist. Spearman correlations and general linear regression analysis were used to assess the correlation between KPS and PPS scores for patients. A total of 1,002 patients receiving RT to bone (n=698), brain (n=257) and lung (n=47) sites were evaluated. The median KPS scores for patients with bone, brain and lung disease were 60, 70, and 60 respectively. The median PPS score for patients with bone, brain and lung

[*] Corresponding author: Edward Chow, MBBS, PhD, FRCPC, Department of Radiation Oncology, Odette Cancer Centre, Sunnybrook Health Sciences Centre, 2075 Bayview Avenue, Toronto, ON M4N 3M5, Canada. E-mail: Edward.Chow@sunnybrook.ca.

disease was 60 for all 3 groups. Highly significant correlations between KPS and PPS score were found in all 3 groups; lung (r=0.94), bone (r=0.91) and brain (r=0.89). Despite measuring different patient parameters in order to evaluate performance status, the KPS and PPS assigned scores highly correlated final scores. Either scale can be employed effectively in an outpatient palliative radiotherapy setting.

Introduction

Assessing patients' performance status in oncology has long been an important part of clinical practice. It has been used to assess patient needs, individualize treatment plans, track disease progression, aid in survival prediction, and has been incorporated into the inclusion criteria for many clinical trials (1,2). Many tools for assessing performance status have been developed over the years, with the first well-established tool being the Karnofsky Performance Status (KPS) which was initially developed in 1948 for chemotherapy trials. Since then, other tools have been derived from the KPS, including Eastern Cooperative Oncology Group performance status (ECOG-PS) and the Palliative Performance Scale (PPS) (1,2). The KPS and ECOG-PS are the most utilized in oncology today and have demonstrated great validity and reliability (1,3-6). The more widespread use of the KPS and ECOG-PS over the PPS is in part due to the fact that both tools were created and established well before the PPS.

The PPS was created in 1996 by the Victoria Hospice Society in an effort to modernize the KPS and make it more relevant to the palliative population. The PPS was initially developed for a subset of palliative care patients that were closer to the end-of life. The majority of these patients died within the hospice unit at approximately 7 days post admission; and of those patients that were discharged, the average time to death was approximately 11 days (7).

The same 11-point rating scale, spanning from 0% (dead) to 100% (normal, no complaints or evidence of disease) was used in the construction of the PPS; however two additional parameters were added to further qualify performance scores, and some of the wording of the original KPS was changed.

In addition to the three physical functioning related categories of the KPS which were ambulation, activity and evidence of disease, and self-care; the PPS added intake and level of consciousness. The qualification of the KPS where it states that 'hospital admission is required' (levels 20-30%) was removed in the PPS in order to reflect the contemporary model of palliative care where patients receive more care from home than in previous years. The PPS was initially piloted in both the hospice and community settings, and it was found to be a valuable tool for assessing, communicating and planning care for palliative patients (7). It has since been validated and tested for its reliability primarily in these settings (1,2,8-11).

The KPS and PPS were designed in separate eras for different target populations, and use slightly different patient measures to assign performance. This study sought to evaluate the correlation between KPS and PPS scores in patients receiving palliative radiotherapy in an outpatient radiotherapy clinic to determine the correlation in how the two scales rate these patients.

Our study

A retrospective review was conducted on patients that attended a rapid response palliative radiotherapy clinic between January 2007 and July 2010. It operates five days a week and is staffed by a radiation oncologist, a research assistant, nurse and radiation therapist. As part of patients' clinical visit, KPS and PPS scores were routinely collected and recorded in a clinical database during the study period. Only patients with completed KPS and PPS scores; as well as patients treated for symptomatic brain metastases, bone metastases or advanced or metastatic lung disease were included in this study. The KPS scores were determined by the trained clinical research assistant and the PPS scores were assigned by one of the five staff radiation oncologists who rotate through the clinic. Approval was obtained from the research ethics board of Sunnybrook Health Sciences Centre for this retrospective review.

Statistical methods

Demographics were summarized in patients with bone metastases, brain metastases, and advanced lung primary/metastases, and all cohorts combined. Results were expressed as mean, standard deviation (SD), median, and range for continuous variables (i.e. age, KPS, PPS); as proportions for categorical variables (gender, primary caner site, primary reason for referral). A cross-table between KPS and PPS was also conducted to see the score distributions. To determine the correlation between the KPS and PPS scales, two different methods were applied for patients with advanced disease to bone, brain and lung sites, and for all cohorts combined. The first method used for correlation was the Spearman rank correlation coefficient (r). An r value of 1 was considered as a perfect positive correlation, whereas r values of 0 or negative 1 were indicative of no relationship or a perfect negative correlation respectively. The classification for r values in between this range were defined as follows: $r \leq 0.2$ was a poor correlation; $0.2 < r \leq 0.4$ was a fair correlation, $0.4 < r \leq 0.6$ was a moderate correlation, $0.6 < r \leq 0.8$ was a good correlation, $0.8 < r \leq 1.0$ was an excellent correlation (10). The second method of determining the correlation between KPS and PPS scales was general linear regression analysis. In this statistical test, KPS was considered as the outcome variable and PPS was the independent variable. In both statistical tests, a p-value of < 0.05 was considered statistically significant. All results were conducted by Statistical Analysis Software (SAS version 9.2 for Windows).

Our findings

During the study period, 1002 patients had a complete set of KPS and PPS scores and received palliative radiotherapy to either bone (n=698), brain (n=257) or lung (n=47) sites. The average age for all patients was 67 years and slightly more males (55.2%) than females (44.8%) were treated. The most common primary cancer types seen were lung (33%), breast (24%) and prostate (20%). The median KPS and PPS were 60% (range 10-100). All other demographic information can be found in Table 1. In 63.2% of patients, KPS and PPS scores were identical. The percentage of patients who had PPS and KPS scores that differed by

± 10% was found to be 32.6%. All additional KPS and PPS data can be found in Table 2 and Figure 1.

Spearman correlation coefficients demonstrated excellent correlation between KPS and PPS scores when determined for the entire cohort (all 1002 patients) (r=0.91). When broken down by bone, brain or lung site, primary or metastatic lung disease had the highest correlation (r=0.94) followed by bone metastases (r=0.93) and brain metastases (r=0.90) (Table 3). All these coefficients demonstrated highly significant positive correlations between the KPS and the PPS (p<0.0001). General linear regression analysis also demonstrated highly significant correlation (p<0.0001) between KPS and PPS in all patients as well as in all three sites (Table 4).

Table 1. Patient demographics

	Bone Metastases		Brain Metastases		Advanced lung Primary/Metastases		All Patients	
N=	698		257		47		1002	
Percent of overall	69.7%		25.6%		4.7%		100%	
% Male	57.5		47.5		63.8		55.2	
Age (mean ± SD)	68 ± 12		65 ± 12		69 ± 13		67 ± 12	
KPS (mean ± SD)	61.5 ± 17		62.9 ± 18		59.1 ± 18		61.8 ± 17	
Median	60		70		60		60	
Range	10-100		10-100		20-90		10-100	
PPS (mean ± SD)	60.7 ± 17		62.0 ± 18		59.1 ± 18		60.9 ± 17	
Median	60		60		60		60	
Range	10-100		10-100		20-90		10-100	
Primary Cancer Site (n=; %)								
Lung	167;	23.9%	136;	52.9%	31;	66.0%	334;	33.3%
Breast	177;	25.4%	57;	22.2%	1;	2.1%	235;	23.5%
Prostate	197;	28.2%	4;	1.6%		---	201;	20.1%
Gastrointestinal	40;	5.7%	17;	6.6%	9;	19.2%	66;	6.6%
Renal Cell	52;	7.5%	7;	2.7%	3;	6.4%	62;	6.2%
Unknown	26;	3.7%	19;	7.4%		---	45;	4.5%
Genitourinary	21;	3.0%	2;	0.8%	1;	2.1%	24;	2.4%
Skin	2;	0.3%	8;	3.1%	1;	2.1%	11;	1.1%
Others	16;	2.3%	7;	2.7%	1;	2.1%	24;	2.4%
Primary Reason for Referral (n=; %)								
Bone Pain	659;	94.4%	10;	3.9%	7;	14.9%	676;	67.5%
Brain Metastases		---	245;	95.3%	2;	4.3%	247;	24.7%
Lung symptoms	1;	0.1%		---	26;	55.3%	27;	2.7%
Post-op RT	15;	2.2%		---		---	15;	1.5%
Mass	2;	0.3%		---	11;	23.4%	13;	1.3%
Others	21;	3.0%	2;	0.8%	1;	2.1%	24;	2.4%

Table 2. Detailed KPS and PPS data per site

	Exact Match between KPS and PPS (%)	+/- 10% between KPS and PPS (%)
All Patients	63.2	32.6
Bone Metastases	63.3	32.5
Brain Metastases	63.4	31.5
Advanced lung Primary/Metastases	59.6	40.4

KPS \ PPS	0	10	20	30	40	50	60	70	80	90	100
0											
10			2	2							
20		1	7	3							
30			2	47	14	3					
40			1	14	45	22		1			
50				2	37	97	25	3			
60					5	32	154	31	6		
70						3	51	132	26		
80						1	5	36	97	11	
90						1	1	9	17	48	2
100										2	4

Figure 1. KPS and PPS cross-table.

Table 3. Spearman Correlation Analysis

	Spearman Correlation between KPS/PPS (r=)	P-value for Spearman Correlation
All Patients	0.91	<0.0001
Bone Metastases	0.91	<0.0001
Brain Metastases	0.89	<0.0001
Advanced lung Primary/Metastases	0.94	<0.0001

Table 4. Linear Regression Analysis

	Coefficient	Standard Error between KPS/PPS	T-value	P-value (Probability > T-value)
All Patients	0.93	0.0132	70.31	<0.0001
Bone Metastases	0.92	0.0158	58.43	<0.0001
Brain Metastases	0.94	0.0272	34.47	<0.0001
Advanced lung Primary/Metastases	0.91	0.0490	18.60	<0.0001

Discussion

This is the largest study to date comparing KPS and PPS scores in patients receiving palliative radiotherapy for symptomatic bone, brain or lung sites. This study has shown an extremely high significant correlation ($p < 0.0001$) between the two performance scales using both Spearman correlation and linear regression analysis.

The approaches to palliative care have changed since 1996 where it is no longer exclusively synonymous with end-of-life care. It is now considered as part of a broader context where earlier access to palliative treatments is made as soon as possible in the disease trajectory of any chronic and fatal illness. Early referral to palliative care services, like palliative radiotherapy, helps to improve a patient's quality of life and reduce their symptom burden (16). As such, patients with advanced cancer are being referred earlier to palliative care services and are living longer as a result of improved palliative systemic therapies and interventions (12, 16). At our outpatient palliative radiotherapy clinic, we typically were referred patients with higher performance status than those seen in a hospice or palliative care facility. The average and median KPS and PPS scores for our patients were approximately 60%; meaning these patients may be unable to work and had some difficulty ambulating, but could care for most of their personal needs. In contrast, most of the patients admitted to hospice or palliative care facilities have lower KPS and PPS scores between 30-40% which indicates that these patients cannot perform self-care, have rapidly progressing disease, and remain mainly bedbound (1, 7, 11, 17).

The KPS and PPS both heavily rely on parameters including ambulation, self care and disease status. The only significant difference the additional items exert within the PPS is between levels 10-30% where the scores in this range are solely dictated by intake level (normal or reduce, minimal to sips, or mouth care only) and level of consciousness (full, drowsy or comatose with or without confusion). In our outpatient palliative radiotherapy clinic, less than one tenth of the patients had scores that would be affected by the changes made in the 10-30% range of the PPS scale (7, 18). In addition, the items of intake and consciousness were arbitrarily included based on observations made by the initial developers of the PPS with respect to hospice and home care based populations of palliative patients. Other factors, most notably dyspnoea (which has been shown to have modest correlation with both survival and performance status in several studies) is just one example of a parameter that could have been of benefit to the PPS but was not included (9, 13, 15, 19).

With the excellent correlation demonstrated between the KPS and PPS in our patient population ($r=0.9062$), the modifications applied by the PPS do not seem to provide any more insight to the performance status of patients in our outpatient facility when only the final score of PPS being reported. Two other studies have used the Spearman correlation coefficients between KPS and PPS in other facilities with the same rater assessing both scales. Morita et al. (8) demonstrated excellent correlation between the two scales ($r=0.94$; $p<0.001$) in 245 patients within a palliative care unit where the average performance score was 40%. Another study by Myers et al. (1) which collected KPS and PPS from a broad range of 134 palliative care patients in outpatient, inpatient and a palliative care facilities also found excellent correlation between the two scales ($r = 0.9628$; $p<0.0001$). Both these studies consisted mainly of advanced cancer patients and further demonstrate that there is very little variability between the two scales. Of note, clinical trials that collect either KPS or PPS in higher performance status outpatients can be compared to one another with a relatively high degree of corroboration. Overall, both tools are relatively simple and easy to use and demonstrate good validity and reliability (1,3-6,8,10,24).

Briefly with respective to survival trends as predicted by the KPS and PPS, several studied have evaluated survival curves in the advanced cancer setting; however the majority of these studies employed the PPS. Two earlier studies that used the KPS in advanced cancer patients found that generally KPS scores below 50% predicted lower rates of survival (less than 6 months). The study populations were not limited to patients in a hospice or inpatient setting and therefore both these studies were more reflective of our outpatient population. The average KPS in both studies was 60% and 70% (5, 13). In contrast to the studies using KPS, the vast majority of the PPS studies looked at survival of palliative patients in hospices or palliative care units with average PPS scores around 20-40% (9,17,19-23). Smaller studies that included between 261-446 patients with PPS scores found that there were unique survival groupings below 50-60% but not above these cut-offs (somewhat similar to the results reported in the KPS studies) (8, 9, 21); however a larger study and meta-analysis of 6066 and 1808 patients respectively found that there were unique survival curves at each PPS level between 10-70% (19,22). Because the focus of the PPS studies were on patients closer to the end-of-life, it is difficult to say whether PPS is more accurate tool for prognostication in all palliative care patients. In addition, Lau et al (22) commented that the survival curves for stable versus critically ill palliative patients can be quite different and these survival predictions are not generalizable across all palliative populations.

A few limitations of this study should be noted. One may question that a trained research assistant scored the KPS and a radiation oncologist scored the PPS. This could have resulted in some inter-rater reliability issues however our results are still very similar to other studies that used the same rater for both KPS and PPS scores (1, 8). Moreover our previous reported studies revealed high inter-rater correlations in both KPS and PPS (10, 25). The correlation found between the KPS and PPS may also not be generalizable in all settings, and it is recommended that further research be done to assess the differences between lower KPS and PPS scores. It is also not known to what extent intake and level of consciousness correlate with performance status or whether including other factors such as dyspnoea may be more useful in a performance status tool for palliative patients. Further research is also recommended in this area.

To conclude, the KPS and PPS are highly correlated and therefore either scale can be employed effectively in an outpatient palliative radiotherapy clinic similar to ours. The PPS may provide a prognostic and communicative advantage for palliative patients closer to the end-of-life; however the KPS seems adequate in our outpatient palliative radiotherapy clinic looking after patients with relatively higher performance status.

Acknowledgments

The study was supported by the Michael and Karyn Goldstein Cancer Research Fund and we thank Mrs. Stacy Yuen for assistance.

References

[1] Myers J, Gardiner K, Harris K, Lilien T, Bennett M, Chow E et al. Evaluating correlation and interrater reliability for four performance scales in the palliative care setting. J Pain Symptom Manage 2010;39:250-8.

[2] Zimmermann C, Burman D, Bandukwala S, Seccareccia D, Kaya E, Bryson J, et al. Nurse and physician inter-rater agreement of three performance status measures in palliative care outpatients. Support Care Cancer 2010;18:609-16.

[3] Verger E, Salamero M, Conill C. Can Karnofsky performance status be transformed to the eastern cooperative oncology group scoring scale and vice versa? Eur J Cancer 1992;28:1328-30.

[4] Schag CC, Heinrich RL, Ganz PA. Karnofsky performance status revisited: reliability, validity, and guidelines. J Clin Oncol 1984;2:187-93.

[5] Yates JW, Chalmer B, McKegney FP. Evaluation of patients with advanced cancer using the Karnofsky performance status. Cancer 1980;45:2220-4.

[6] Taylor AE, Olver IN, Sivanthan T, Chi M, Purnell C. Observer error in grading performance status in cancer patients. Support Care Cancer 1999;7:332-5.

[7] Anderson F, Downing GM, Hill J, Casorso L, Lerch N. Palliative performance scale (PPS): a new tool. J Palliat Care 1996;12:5-11.

[8] Morita T, Tsunoda J, Inoue S, Chihara S. Validity of the palliative performance scale from a survival perspective. J Pain Symptom Manage 1999;18:2-3.

[9] Olajide O, Hanson L, Usher BM, Qaqish BF, Schwartz R, Bernard S. Validation of the palliative performance scale in the acute tertiary care hospital setting. J Palliat Med 2007;10:111-7.

[10] Campos S, Zhang L, Sinclair E, Tsao M, Barnes EA, Danjoux C, et al. The palliative performance scale: examining its inter-rater reliability in an outpatient palliative radiation oncology clinic. Support Care Cancer 2009;17:685-90.

[11] Virik K, Glare P. Validation of the palliative performance scale for inpatients admitted to a palliative care unit in Sydney, Australia. J Pain Symptom Manag 2002;23:455-7.

[12] Canadian Cancer Society's Steering Committee. Canadian cancer statistics 2010. Canadian Cancer Society, editor. Toronto: Canadian Cancer Society, 2010.

[13] Hwang SS, Scott CB, Chang VT, Cogswell J, Srinivas S, Kasimis B. Prediction of survival for advanced cancer patients by recursive partitioning analysis: role of Karnofsky performance status, quality of life, and symptom distress. Cancer Invest 2004;22:678-87.

[14] Friendlander AH, Ettinger RL. Karnofsky performance status scale. Special Care Dentistry 2009;29:147-8.

[15] Schnadig ID, Fromme EK, Loprinzi CL, Sloan JA, Mori M, Li H, et al. Patient-physician disagreement regarding performance status is associated with worse survivorship in patients with advanced cancer. Cancer 2008;113:2205-14.

[16] Sepulveda C, Marlin A, Yoshida T, Ullrich A. Palliative care: the world health organization's global perspective. J Pain Symptom Manage 2002;24:91-6.

[17] Head B, Ritchie CS, Smoot TM. Prognostication in hospice care: Can the palliative performance scale help? J Palliat Med 2005;8:492-502.

[18] Grieco A, Long CJ. Investigation of the Karnofsky performance status as a measure of quality of life. Health Psychol 1984;3:129-42.

[19] Downing M, Lau F, Lesperance M, Karlson N, Shaw J, Kuziemsky C, et al. Meta-analysis of survival prediction with palliative performance scale. J Palliat Care 2007;23:245-52.

[20] Lau F, Downing GM, Lesperance M, Shaw J, Kuziemsky C. Use of palliative performance scale in end-of-life prognostication. J Palliat Med 2006;9:1066-75.

[21] Harrold J, Rickerson E, Carroll JT, McGrath J, Morales K, Kapo J, et al. Is the palliative performance scale a useful predictor of mortality in a heterogeneous hospice population? J Palliat Med 2005;8:503-9.

[22] Lau F, Downing M, Lesperance M, Karlson N, Kuziemsky C, Yang J. Using the palliative performance scale to provide meaningful survival estimates. J Pain Symptom Manage 2009;38: 134-44.

[23] Lau F, Maida V, Downing M, Lesperance M, Karlson N, Kuziemsky C. Use of the palliative performance scale (PPS) for end-of-life prognostication in a palliative medicine consultation service. J Pain Symptom Manage 2009;37:965-72.

[24] Mor V, Laliberte L, Morris JN, Wiemann M. The karnofsky performance status scale an examination of its reliability and validity in a research setting. Cancer 1984;53:2002-7.

[25] de Borja M, Chow E, Bovett G, Davis L, Gilles C. The correlation among patients and health care professionals in assessing functional status using the Karnofsky and Eastern Cooperative Oncology Group performance status scales. Support Cancer Ther 2004;2:59-63.

In: Advanced Cancer
Editors: N. Thavarajah, N. Pulenzas, B. Lechner et al.

ISBN: 978-1-62808-239-5
© 2013 Nova Science Publishers, Inc.

Chapter 20

Comparison of baseline quality of life scores in patients with bone and brain metastases as assessed using the EORTC QLQ-C30

Michael Poon[1], Liang Zeng[1], Liying Zhang[1], Ling-Ming Tseng[2], Ming-Feng Hou[3], Alysa Fairchild[4], Vassilios Vassiliou[5], Reynaldo Jesus-Garcia[6], Mohamed A Alm El-Din[7], Aswin Kumar[8], Fabien Forges[9,10], Wei-Chu Chie[11], Arjun Sahgal[12], Erin Wong[1] and Edward Chow[1*]

[1]Department of Radiation Oncology, Odette Cancer Centre, Sunnybrook Health Sciences Centre, University of Toronto, Toronto, Ontario, Canada
[2]Department of Surgery, Taipei Veterans General Hospital, National Yang-Ming University, Taipei, Taiwan
[3]Department of Gastroenterologic Surgery, Kaohsiung Medical University Hospital, Kaohsiung, Taiwan
[4]Department of Radiation Oncology, Cross Cancer Institute, Edmonton, Alberta, Canada
[5]Department of Radiation Oncology, Bank of Cyprus Oncology Centre, Nicosia, Cyprus
[6]Department of Orthopedic Oncology, Federal University of Sao Paulo, Sao Paulo, Brazil
[7]Department of Clinical Oncology, Tanta University Hospital, Tanta Faculty of Medicine, Tanta, Egypt
[8]Division of Gynaecology and Genitourinary Oncology, Department of Radiation Oncology, Regional Cancer Center, Trivandrum, Kerala, India
[9]Inserm CIE3, Saint Etienne University Hospital, Saint-Etienne, France

* Corresponding author: Professor Edward Chow, MBBS, MSc, PhD, FRCPC, Department of Radiation Oncology, Odette Cancer Centre, Sunnybrook Health Sciences Centre, 2075 Bayview Avenue, Toronto, Ontario, Canada M4N 3M5. E-mail: edward.chow@sunnybrook.ca.

[10]Unit of Clinical Research, Innovation, and Pharmacology,
Saint Etienne University Hospital, France
[11]Department of Public Health and Institute of Epidemiology
Preventative Medicine, National Taiwan University, Taipei, Taiwan
[12]Department of Radiation Oncology, Princess Margaret Hospital,
University of Toronto, Toronto, Ontario, Canada

In advanced cancer patients, quality of life (QOL) is often a more meaningful clinical endpoint as patients often have shorter life expectancies and treatment intent is palliative in nature. Since 1993, the European Organization for Research and Treatment of Cancer Core 30 Questionnaire (EORTC QLQ-C30) has been widely used to study cancer-specific health-related quality of life. This study seeks to compare EORTC QLQ-C30 scores in patients with bone and brain metastases. Methods: The EORTC QLQ-C30 was used to assess QOL internationally in patients with bone metastases. A univariate linear regression model (GLM) was applied to detect significant differences between both groups on each QLQ-C30 scale at baseline. To normalize the distribution, natural log-transformations were applied for each C30 summary scale. Results: KPS, gender, marital status, and primary cancer site were found to be significantly different between the two groups (p < 0.005). After accounting for these confounding factors, three EORTC-C30 scales found to be significantly different between patients with bone and brain metastases: physical functioning (p < 0.0001), role functioning (p < 0.0004), and pain scale (p < 0.0001). Bone metastases patients reported worse pain and physical functioning, while brain metastases exhibited greater role functioning deficits. Conclusion: Patients with bone metastases have more pain and reduced physical functioning. However, patients with brain metastases have more severe role functioning deficits. The use of disease-specific assessment modules such as the QLQ-BM22 and QLQ-BN20 will enhance the capture of relevant QOL in these populations.

Introduction

Quality of life (QOL) is a subjective, multidimensional measurement that reflects physical symptoms, functional ability, psychosocial aspects and health perceptions of patients (1). In advanced cancer patients, QOL is often a more meaningful clinical endpoint for clinical trials as due to shorter patient life expectancies; traditional endpoints such as survival are less relevant (2). In most cases, QOL assessments are performed in the form of questionnaires, completed by either the patient themselves, or via proxy. These assessments tools can provide information about patient's responsiveness and effectiveness of treatment (1).

Bone metastases are a frequent complication of advanced cancer. Breast and prostate carcinomas commonly metastasize to bone, occurring in their disease trajectory in up to 70% of patients (3). In addition, 15% to 30% of lung, thyroid, and renal cell carcinomas metastasize to bone (3). Although the exact incidence of bone metastases is unknown, it is estimated that 70% to 85% of cancer patients have bone metastases at the time of autopsy (4). Bone metastases are a common cause of intractable pain as well as skeletal related events (SREs). Traditionally, primary outcomes in clinical trials examining bone metastases have focused on objective endpoints of these SREs, such as pathological fractures, spinal cord compression, analgesic use, or hypercalcemia (5). However, patient's health-related quality of life has recently garnered increased focus (6).

Brain metastases (BN) are the most common intracranial neoplasm in adults. The majority of BN originate from primary lung (40–50%), breast (15–25%) or skin (5–20%) cancer (7,8). BN occurs in 10–15% of patients with advanced cancer (9,10), and depending on the location may cause patients to present with a wide range of neurological symptoms including headaches, focal weakness, mental disturbances, behavioural changes, seizures, speech difficulties, and ataxia (11). While survival and local brain tumour control are important endpoints, quality of life (QOL) is arguably the more relevant given the prognosis of this patient population (12).

Since 1993, the European Organization for Research and Treatment of Cancer core questionnaire (EORTC QLQ-C30) has been widely used in the study of cancer-specific QOL (13, 14). It is an internationally validated questionnaire which is commonly used to assess QOL in advanced cancer patients, such as patients with bone or brain metastases. This instrument can be administered with relative ease, which can reduce the burden on patients and avoid unnecessary hospital appointments. To date, comparisons with the palliative cancer patient setting among broad patient subgroups have not been made. This study seeks to compare EORTC QLQ-C30 scores in bone and brain metastases patients and delineate how these conditions affect patients' QOL.

Our study

Patients with bone metastases were accrued internationally from March 2010 until January 2011, under the supervision of the EORTC QOL module development group for the development of the bone metastases module (the QLQ-BM22) (6). These patients were recruited from Edmonton, Alberta, Canada; Kaohsiung, Taiwan; Kerala, India; Nicosia, Cyprus; Sao Paulo, Brazil; Taipei, Taiwan; Tanta, Egypt; and Toronto, Ontario, Canada. Patients were required to be aged 18 years with histological confirmation of their primary cancer and radiologic evidence of bone metastases. To be included the patients also had to be cognitively able to complete the questionnaire and must understand the language used in the questionnaire. All EORTC questionnaires were translated into the region's primary language by at least 2 fluent translators to ensure accuracy. Languages used in the current included Arabic, English, French, Greek, Malayalam, Mandarin (Taiwan), and Portuguese (Brazil).

Within the same time period, patients undergoing whole-brain radiotherapy (WBRT), radiosurgery/gamma knife and/ or neurosurgical resection for their brain metastases from Sunnybrook Odette Cancer Centre were approached. To be eligible patients were required to be aged 18 years and speak English with documented single or multiple brain metastases. Both studies received ethics approval from their respective hospital ethics boards.

EORTC QLQ-C30

The QLQ-C30 is a 30-item quality of life instrument validated for the assessment of QOL in patients with advanced cancer (13). It contains five subscales: physical functioning, role functioning, emotional functioning, cognitive functioning and social functioning (13). It also entails six single-item symptom scales (sleep disturbance, constipation, diarrhoea, dyspnoea, appetite loss and financial issues), three symptom scales (fatigue, pain and nausea) and a single global health status scale (13).

Items were rated on a 4 point Likert scale from 1 'not at all' to 4 'very much' with the exception of the last two items assessing overall health and overall QOL which were scored from 1 (very poor) to 7 (excellent). The responses for each scale and single item were translated according to published manuals into scores from 0-100 (14). In symptom scales, a high score is reflective of greater severity. In contrast, on the functional scales and the global QOL scale, higher scores indicate greater functional ability.

Statistical analyses

Descriptive analysis was conducted in all patients, in patients with bone or brain metastases, respectively. The mean, standard deviation (SD), median, and ranges were calculated for continuous demographic variables, and categorical variables were expressed as proportions of patients. To compare baseline characteristics, between patients with bone metastases and patients with brain metastases, Chi-squared tests were applied for categorical variables and the Wilcoxon rank-sum test was performed for age and KPS. A two-sided p-values of <0.05 was considered statistically significant.

A simple univariate linear regression model (GLM) was applied to detect significant differences between patient groups on each QLQ-C30 scale (after scoring). Each unscored subscales was compared between both patient groups using a Chi-square test. To normalize the distribution, natural log-transformations were applied for each QLQ-C30 summary scale. The outcomes were natural log scales of each QLQ-C30 scale and the independent variable was treated as binary (1=bone metastases, 0=brain metastases). No confounding factors were considered at this step.

The coefficient, standard error (SE) of the coefficient, p-value and mean square error (MSE) of the model were calculated. The MSE refers to the estimate of error variance: residual sum of squares divided by the number of degrees of freedom. Relative to the smaller estimated error variance, MSE was close to zero. Positive coefficient of a group indicated that patients with bone metastases have higher score than patients with brain metastases.

The scored QLQ-C30 results were further analyzed adjusting for confounding factors previously identified in the comparison of demographics between both groups. To see which QLQ-C30 scales had statistical significant differences between patients with bone and brain metastases, after accounting for the confounders (KPS, gender, married status, and primary cancer site), each confounding factor was treated as a categorical variable. For gender, 1 indicated female and 0 male; for marital status, 1 indicated married and 0 indicated others. Primary cancer site was treated as an unordered categorical variable (breast, lung, prostate, gastrointestinal, renal cell, and other). Simple univariate linear regression analysis was performed. The outcome was a natural log scale of each C30 scale. The independent variables were the binary variable of group (1=BM, 0=BN) and 4 the confounders. Therefore, the model used was: $ln(C30\ scale) = a + b\times(Group) + c\times(KPS) + d\times(Gender) + e\times(Married) + f\times(Primary\ Cancer\ Site)$. To account for multiple comparisons, a Bonferroni adjusted p-value of p< 0.002 (0.05/30 items) was considered statistically significant. Analyses were performed using Statistical Analysis Software (SAS version 9.2 for Windows) and PROC GLM was applied for modelling.

Our findings

A total of 47 patients with brain metastases and 400 patients with bone metastases were enrolled. Among the 400 patients with bone metastases, 3 patients were missing responses for some of the QLQ-C30 items and were excluded from the analysis. Baseline patient characteristics of the two study populations are summarized in Table 1.

Table 1. Demographics in Patients with Bone Metastases and in Patients with Brain Metastases

	Total N=444	Bone Metastases N=397	Brain Metastases N=47	p-value*
Age (years)				0.1012
Mean (SD)	58.3 (12.9)	58.0 (13.0)	60.6 (11.9)	
Median (range)	57 (24-95)	57 (26-95)	61 (24 – 86)	
KPS at baseline				**<0.0001**
Mean (SD)	81.9 (16.9)	83.2 (16.8)	70.4 (13.3)	
Median (range)	80 (30-100)	80 (30-100)	70 (40-100)	
Gender				**0.0067**
Female	328 (73.87%)	301 (75.82%)	27 (57.45%)	
Male	116 (26.13%)	96 (24.18%)	20 (42.55%)	
Married status				**<0.0001**
Married	149 (66.82%)	114 (64.77%)	35 (74.47%)	
Widowed	27 (12.11%)	21 (11.93%)	6 (12.77%)	
Single	20 (8.97%)	15 (8.52%)	5 (10.64%)	
Other	27 (12.11%)	26 (14.77%)	1 (2.13%)	
Primary cancer site				<0.0001
Breast	287 (64.64%)	271 (68.26%)	16 (34.04%)	
Lung	48 (10.81%)	31 (7.81%)	17 (36.17%)	
Prostate	45 (10.14%)	45 (11.34%)	0 (0.00%)	
Gastrointestinal	16 (3.60%)	10 (2.52%)	6 (12.77%)	
Renal Cell	11 (2.48%)	9 (2.27%)	2 (4.26%)	
Other	37 (8.33%)	31 (7.81%)	6 (12.77%)	
Patients status				0.1191
Outpatient	404 (91.20%)	364 (91.92%)	40 (85.11%)	
Inpatient	39 (8.80%)	32 (8.08%)	7 (14.89%)	
Previous systemic treatment				0.6047
Yes	154 (69.06%)	123 (69.89%)	31 (65.96%)	
No	69 (30.94%)	53 (30.11%)	16 (34.04%)	

* P-value was obtained by Chi-squared test for categorical variables and Wilcoxon rank-sum test for age and KPS.

Comparison of baseline characteristics

In a comparison of the demographics of both groups, KPS, gender, marital status, and primary cancer site were found to be significantly different between the two groups (P < 0.005). In patients with bone metastases the most common primary cancer sites were the breast (68%), followed by the prostate (11%), while in the brain metastases study population the most common primary cancers were of the lung (36%) and breast (34%). A greater proportion of patients with primary breast or prostate cancer and lower proportions of patients with primary lung, gastrointestinal or renal cell sites were seen in bone metastases patients compared to the brain metastases. The bone metastases patient group also had higher KPS scores, more females, smaller proportions with married status when compared to patients with brain metastases. No significant differences between patient status, gender, age of patients who completed the assessment or proportion of patients whom received previous systemic therapy were found (p > 0.005).

Baseline quality of life

Patients with bone metastases reported average functional scores (mean ± standard deviation) from 58.3 to 73.4 (Table 2). Cognitive functioning was found to be the best (highest average score) within this patient population and role functioning the worst (lowest average score). Overall, cognitive and emotional functioning were found to be better than physical, social, or role functioning. Symptom scores ranged between 14.0 ± 21.61 and 49.3 ± 32.46 in the BM patient group. Pain (49.3 ± 32.46), fatigue (46.1 ± 27.83), and insomnia (40.9 ± 33.65) were the most severe symptoms, while nausea/ vomiting and diarrhoea were the least severe with scores of 14.0 ± 21.61 and 10.9 ± 19.80, respectively.

Similar results were seen within patients with brain metastases. This group reported functional scores between 55.1 ± 28.73 (role functioning) and 73.4 ± 23.74 (cognitive functioning). The EORTC QLQ-30 symptom scores ranged between 4.3 ± 16.47 and 44.1 ± 28.36. In this group, fatigue was the most severe symptom (44.1 ± 28.36)   , followed by insomnia (39.7 ± 27.49). Diarrhoea was the least severe symptom (4.3 ± 16.47).

Overall QOL scores were found to be slightly better in patients with brain metastases than patients with bone metastases, with scores of 57.4 ± 18.02 versus 50.3 ± 23.31 respectively.

Comparison of EORTC QLQ-C30 scores unadjusted for confounders

The findings of the simple univariate linear regression model are summarized in Table 3. Only the C30 symptom scale of pain was found to be significantly different (p < 0.0001). Patients with bone metastases had more pain compared to patients with brain metastases (average scale score of 49.3 vs. 29.8). Significant differences between BM and BN in other scales were not seen (p > 0.002).

Table 2. Converted Functional and Symptom Scores between Bone and Brain Metastases Patients at Baseline

		N	Mean	Std	Median	Min	Max
Functional Scales							
Physical Functioning	Group BM-C30	390	63.6	27.90	66.7	0	100
	BN-C30	46	65.8	24.02	66.7	13	100
Role Functioning	Group BM-C30	396	58.3	35.13	66.7	0	100
	BN-C30	46	55.1	28.73	50.0	0	100
Emotional Functioning	Group BM-C30	397	66.2	24.71	66.7	0	100
	BN-C30	47	66.5	24.36	66.7	17	100
Cognitive Functioning	Group BM-C30	397	73.4	23.74	83.3	0	100
	BN-C30	47	73.4	23.74	83.3	17	100
Social Functioning	Group BM-C30	397	61.9	32.14	66.7	0	100
	BN-C30	47	59.2	29.04	66.7	0	100
Global health status / QOL	Group BM-C30	397	50.3	23.31	50.0	0	100
	BN-C30	46	57.4	18.02	58.3	25	100
Symptom Scales							
Fatigue	Group BM-C30	396	46.1	27.83	44.4	0	100
	BN-C30	46	44.1	28.36	38.9	0	100
Nausea / Vomiting	Group BM-C30	397	14.0	21.61	0.0	0	100
	BN-C30	47	14.2	17.71	0.0	0	67
Pain	Group BM-C30	397	49.3	32.46	50.0	0	100
	BN-C30	47	29.8	29.27	33.3	0	100
Dyspnoea	Group BM-C30	395	22.6	26.35	33.3	0	100
	BN-C30	46	17.4	21.93	0.0	0	67
Insomnia	Group BM-C30	397	40.9	33.65	33.3	0	100
	BN-C30	47	39.7	27.49	33.3	0	100
Appetite loss	Group BM-C30	396	29.5	33.15	33.3	0	100
	BN-C30	47	32.6	32.96	33.3	0	100
Constipation	Group BM-C30	396	27.1	31.65	33.3	0	100
	BN-C30	47	27.0	30.80	33.3	0	100
Diarrhoea	Group BM-C30	396	10.9	19.80	0.0	0	100
	BN-C30	47	4.3	16.47	0.0	0	100
Financial Problems	Group BM-C30	396	23.9	30.57	0.0	0	100
	BN-C30	47	29.8	32.03	33.3	0	100

BM-C30: Patients with bone metastases, BN-C30: patients with brain metastases.

Table 3. Comparing both groups by Univariate Linear Regression Analysis: without accounting for Confounders

At Baseline	Coefficient	SE	p-value *	MSE
Global Health Status	-0.308	0.139	0.0273	0.798
Physical Functioning	-0.198	0.150	0.1853	0.921
Role Functioning	-0.205	0.233	0.3789	2.239
Emotional Functioning	-0.073	0.112	0.5170	0.531
Cognitive Functioning	-0.049	0.104	0.6395	0.456
Social Functioning	-0.165	0.196	0.4015	1.619
Fatigue	0.103	0.176	0.5608	1.282
Nausea / Vomiting	-0.164	0.264	0.5338	2.921
Pain	**1.070**	**0.226**	**<0.0001**	**2.142**
Dyspnoea	0.315	0.294	0.2832	3.551
Insomnia	-0.236	0.275	0.3901	3.173
Appetite loss	-0.233	0.306	0.4473	3.935
Constipation	-0.035	0.303	0.9079	3.854
Diarrhoea	0.675	0.246	0.0062	2.534
Financial Problems	-0.354	0.301	0.2402	3.800

Natural log-transformation was applied for each C30 scale. MSE = Mean square error; *Bonferroni adjusted p-value < 0.002 was considered statistical significant.

Table 4. Comparing both groups by Univariate Linear Regression Analysis: accounting for Confounders

At Baseline	p-value of Group (bone vs. brain)	p-value of Confounders					MSE
		KPS	Gender	Married Status	Primary Cancer Site		
Global Health Status	0.0040	0.0004	0.4876	0.2500	0.4287		0.778
Physical Functioning	**<0.0001**	<.0001	0.2246	0.5015	0.5432		0.631
Role Functioning	**0.0004**	<.0001	0.0072	0.6439	0.0207		1.589
Emotional Functioning	0.0416	<.0001	0.8024	0.4256	0.5986		0.479
Cognitive Functioning	0.1066	0.0011	0.0157	0.1766	0.0143		0.436
Social Functioning	0.0037	<.0001	0.0057	0.7747	0.2703		1.362
Fatigue	0.1109	<.0001	0.2296	0.9093	0.9650		1.102
Nausea / Vomiting	0.8496	0.4646	0.0638	0.8062	0.2882		2.924
Pain	**<0.0001**	<.0001	0.9134	0.5854	0.5589		1.816
Dyspnoea	0.5150	0.0544	0.5112	0.0198	0.9200		3.542
Insomnia	0.9222	0.0047	0.8198	0.4667	0.1865		3.095
Appetite loss	0.3281	<.0001	0.4048	0.4850	0.1238		3.554
Constipation	0.4674	<.0001	0.9498	0.2227	0.7708		3.625
Diarrhoea	0.0132	0.4190	0.9807	0.2575	0.9102		2.544
Financial Problems	0.4677	0.0001	0.3495	0.0851	0.0004		3.463

Natural log-transformation was applied for each C30 scale. MSE = Mean square error; * Bonferroni adjusted p-value < 0.002 was considered statistical significant.

Comparison of EORTC QLQ-C30 scores adjusting for confounders

After accounting for the confounding factors of KPS, gender, marital status, and primary cancer site, two other scales were found to be significantly different as well (Table 4). The three EORTC-C30 scales found to be significantly different between patients with bone metastases and patients with brain metastases were physical functioning ($p < 0.0001$), role functioning ($p = 0.0004$), and pain scale ($p < 0.0001$). Patients with brain metastases reported better physical functioning, with an average score of 65.8 compared to 63.6. However, patients with bone metastases are more likely to have better role functioning, with average scores of 58.3 and 55.1 respectively.

As previously seen in the comparison of EORTC QLQ-C30 scores without confounding factor adjustment, patients with bone metastases had more problems on only one symptom scale, pain, compared to patients with brain metastases. Other scales had no significant difference between patient groups after adjusting for confounders ($p > 0.002$).

Following analysis, the confounders of gender and married status were no longer significant; primary cancer site was only significant associated with financial problems. KPS was still significantly related to all C30 scales, except for nausea/vomiting, dyspnoea, and diarrhoea.

Discussion

Quality of life is an important endpoint, especially in advanced cancer patient clinical trials. To our knowledge, this is the first study to compare baseline EORTC QLQ-C30 baseline scores of patients with brain metastases to patients with bone metastases. After adjusting for confounding factors (KPS, gender, marital status, and primary cancer site), patients with bone metastases were found to have significantly greater pain than those with brain metastases. These patients also had significantly better role functioning. In comparison, patients with brain metastases functioned better physically than those with bone metastases. Other scores were not found to be significantly different. This may be a result of how both patient groups experience these symptoms and have similar functional difficulties.

Localized pain commonly presents itself in bone metastases patients, occurring in 75% of patients (15). Therefore, the significantly greater pain in bone metastases patients found upon analysis was expected. It is for this reason, in a study of QOL with bone metastases, thirty-nine of all forty-seven studies measured the intensity and frequency of bony pain (16). Similarly, reduced physical functioning was expected in patients with bone metastases. Along with SREs, decreased mobility and spinal instability are common symptoms that manifest over the course of bone disease (17,18). These symptoms would equate to higher raw scores of items 1-5 of the QLQ-C30, indicating reduced physical functioning, as patients would be unable to do strenuous activity and would have reduced ambulatory capabilities.

The clinical presentation of brain metastases is similar to that of any intracranial mass lesions. Two thirds of patients with brain metastases develop neurological symptoms during the course of their illness (19). Signs and symptoms of brain metastases can be divided into a "generalized" category and a "focal" variety. Typically, generalized symptoms refer to symptoms secondary to cerebral edema and/or increased intracranial pressure; this includes symptoms such as headaches, nausea/vomiting, and cognitive problems (20). The "focal" variety, which frequently results from localized compression or destruction of brain tissue, usually manifests as weakness, numbness, speech disturbance, or seizures (20). It was expected that the domain of cognitive functioning would be different in patients with bone and brain metastases. Although cognitive functioning was the most impacted, our analysis shows no such indication, with similar scores in both patient groups. The similar cognitive functional deficits experienced by both patient groups may be resulting from different symptoms. In patients with bone metastases, deficits may be caused by pain, which can limit cognitive aspects such as concentration (21, 22). On the QLQ-C30, this could result in a similar score to what brain metastases patients experience because of dizziness or other neurological symptoms. Although more validation is necessary and compliance issues need to be minimized, specific modules tailored to symptoms of brain metastatic disease such as the FACT-BR or EORTC QLQ-BN20 should be employed to accurately distinguish the root of difficulties experienced (23,24). This would limit the ambiguity and focus assessments on issues of importance to patients.

A similar conclusion can be drawn from how lower role functioning was found in patients with brain metastases. From only the two role functioning items in the QLQ-C30, it is difficult to pinpoint why patients are unable to perform their regular daily activities. It is likely a result of the aforementioned generalized and focal symptoms, in particular fatigue and nausea/ vomiting (25). However, in the analysis, no significant differences in these symptom scales were found between brain and bone metastases patients. Nonetheless, this difference may still be a result of fatigue and nausea due to the heterogeneity in patients' understanding of these symptoms (26). Patients can refer to nausea as a brief episode lasting mere seconds or a prolonged period of symptoms that can last hours or days (27). In many cases, nausea episodes are ambiguous and symptoms can be mistaken or confused by patients. Future studies should seek to evaluate how individual symptoms correlate and affect patients' ability to maintain their norm activities.

This study is primary limited as patients are selected for inclusion by their reason for referral. This means that in the patient populations, patients were not excluded if they had other illnesses or metastases so long as the reason for their referral was for treatment of their brain or bone metastases. If a patient required palliative radiotherapy for painful bone metastases but also had brain metastases for which they previously were treated, they would be included solely in the bone metastases group, which may confound our findings. Heterogeneity within the two subgroups is also likely to be present. While patient status was accounted for, we are unable to comment as to where patients were on the continuum of disease trajectory. This may potentially influence our analysis as symptoms experienced by patients increase in severity with reduced survival. The patient population size was also vastly different, with almost eight times the patient population in the bone metastases group than the brain metastases group. Perhaps within a larger brain metastases population, more significant differences between these two subgroups would be exhibited.

In conclusion, the difficulties bone and brain metastases patients experience are different in several ways. Patients with bone metastases have more pain and reduced physical functioning. However, patients with brain metastases have more severe role functioning deficits. With use of the QLQ-C30, it is also found that there is ambiguity regarding the root of patient issues. Future studies that require more comprehensive disease-specific findings should include disease-specific assessment modules such as the QLQ-BM22 and QLQ-BN20.

Important domains such as the minimal clinically important difference should also be established in individual subgroups of patients to assist in clinical trial design.

Acknowledgments

We thank the generous support of Bratty Family Fund, Michael and Karyn Goldstein Cancer Research Fund, Joseph and Silvana Melara Cancer Research Fund, and Ofelia Cancer Research Fund.

References

[1]   Chow E, Hoskin P, van der Linden Y, Bottomley A, Velikova G. Quality of life and symptom end points in palliative bone metastases trials. Clin Oncol (R Coll Radiol) 2006;18(1):67-9.

[2]   Zeng L, Chow E, Zhang L, Tseng LM, Hou MF, Fairchild A, et al. An international prospective study establishing minimal clinically important differences in the EORTC QLQ-BM22 and QLQ-C30 in cancer patients with bone metastases. Support Care Cancer 2012 May 6.

[3]   Mundy GR. Metastasis to bone: causes, consequences and therapeutic opportunities. Nat Rev Cancer 2002;2(8):584-93.

[4]   Soni MK, Cella D. Quality of life and symptom measures in oncology: an overview. Am J Manag Care 2002;8(18 Suppl):S560-73.

[5]   Major PP, Cook R. Efficacy of bisphosphonates in the management of skeletal complications of bone metastases and selection of clinical endpoints. Am J Clin Oncol 2002;25(6 Suppl 1):S10-8.

[6]   Chow E, Nguyen J, Zhang L, Tseng LM, Hou MF, Fairchild A, et al. International field testing of the reliability and validity of the EORTC QLQ-BM22 module to assess health-related quality of life in patients with bone metastases. Cancer 2012;118(5):1457-65.

[7]   Schouten LJ, Rutten J, Huveneers HA, Twijnstra A. Incidence of brain metastases in a cohort of patients with carcinoma of the breast, colon, kidney, and lung and melanoma. Cancer 2002;94(10):2698-2705.

[8]   Barnholtz-Sloan JS, Sloan AE, Davis FG, Vigneau FD, Lai P, Sawaya RE. Incidence proportions of brain metastases in patients diagnosed (1973 to 2001) in the Metropolitan Detroit Cancer Surveillance System. J Clin Oncol 2004;22(14):2865-72.

[9]   Chamberlain MC. Brain metastases: a medical neuro-oncology perspective. Expert Rev Neurother 2010;10(4):563-73.

[10] Sperduto PW, Chao ST, Sneed PK, Luo X, Suh J, Roberge D, et al. Diagnosis-specific prognostic factors, indexes, and treatment outcomes for patients with newly diagnosed brain metastases: a multi-institutional analysis of 4,259 patients. Int J Radiat Oncol Biol Phys 2010;77(3):655-61.

[11] Posner JB. Management of central nervous system metastases. Semin Oncol 1977;4(1):81-91.

[12] Caissie A, Nguyen J, Chen E, Zhang L, Sahgal A, Clemons M, et al. Quality of Life in Patients With Brain Metastases Using the EORTC QLQ-BN20+2 and QLQ-C15-PAL. Int J Radiat Oncol Biol Phys 2012;83(4):1238-45.

[13] Aaronson NK, Ahmedzai S, Bergman B, Bullinger M, Cull A, Duez NJ, et al. The European Organization for Research and Treatment of Cancer QLQ-C30: a quality-of-life instrument for use in international clinical trials in oncology. J Natl Cancer Inst 1993;85(5):365-76.

[14] Fayers P, Aaronson N, Bjordal K, Groenvold M, Curran D, Bottomley A editors. The EORTC QLQ-C30 scoring manual (3rd edition). Brussels: European Organisation for Research and Treatment of Cancer, 2001.

[15] Wagner G. Frequency of pain in patients with cancer. Recent Results Cancer Res 1984;89:64-71.

[16] Tharmalingam S, Chow E, Harris K, Hird A, Sinclair E. Quality of life measurement in bone metastases: A literature review. J Pain Res 2008;1:49-58.

[17] Nielsen OS, Munro AJ, Tannock IF. Bone metastases: pathophysiology and management policy. J Clin Oncol 1991;9(3):509-24.

[18] Goetz MP, Callstrom MR, Charboneau JW, Farrell MA, Maus TP, Welch TJ, et al. Percutaneous image-guided radiofrequency ablation of painful metastases involving bone: a multicenter study. J Clin Oncol 2004;22(2):300-6.

[19] Cairncross JG, Kim JH, Deck MD, Posner JB. Radiation therapy of brain metastases. Trans Am Neurol Assoc 1979;104:252-5.

[20] Shaffrey ME, Mut M, Asher AL, Burri SH, Chahlavi A, Chang SM, et al. Brain metastases. Curr Probl Surg 2004;41(8):665-741.

[21] Kenefick AL. Pain treatment and quality of life: reducing depression and improving cognitive impairment. J Gerontol Nurs 2004;30(5):22-9.

[22] Padilla GV, Ferrell B, Grant MM, Rhiner M. Defining the content domain of quality of life for cancer patients with pain. Cancer Nurs 1990;13(2):108-15.

[23] Lien K, Zeng L, Nguyen J, Cramarossa G, Cella D, Chang E, et al. FACT-Br for assessment of quality of life in patients receiving treatment for brain metastases: a literature review. Expert Rev Pharmacoecon Outcomes Res 2011;11(6):701-8.

[24] Leung A, Lien K, Zeng L, Nguyen J, Caissie A, Culleton S, et al. The EORTC QLQ-BN20 for assessment of quality of life in patients receiving treatment or prophylaxis for brain metastases: a literature review. Expert Rev Pharmacoecon Outcomes Res 2011;11(6):693-700.

[25] Bower JE, Ganz PA, Desmond KA, Rowland JH, Meyerowitz BE, Belin TR. Fatigue in breast cancer survivors: occurrence, correlates, and impact on quality of life. J Clin Oncol 2000;18(4):743-53.

[26] Olver I, Molassiotis A, Aapro M, Herrstedt J, Grunberg S, Morrow G. Antiemetic research: future directions. Support Care Cancer 2011;19(Suppl 1):S49-55.

[27] Dennis K, Maranzano E, De Angelis C, Holden L, Wong S, Chow E. Radiotherapy-induced nausea and vomiting. Expert Rev Pharmacoecon Outcomes Res 2011;11(6):685-92.

In: Advanced Cancer
Editors: N. Thavarajah, N. Pulenzas, B. Lechner et al.

ISBN: 978-1-62808-239-5
© 2013 Nova Science Publishers, Inc.

Chapter 21

Comparison of baseline quality of life scores in patients with bone and brain metastases as assessed using the EORTC QLQ-C15-PAL

Julia Di Giovanni, BSc(C)[1], Liang Zeng, MD(C)[1],
Liying Zhang, PhD[1], Vassilios Vassiliou, MD[2],
Takefumi Satoh, MD[3], Palmira Foro, MD[4], Brigette BY Ma, MD[5],
Wei-Chu Chie, MD[6], Arjun Sahgal, MD[1], Michael Poon, BSc(C)[1]
and Edward Chow, MBBS[1]

[1]Rapid Response Radiotherapy Program, Department of Radiation Oncology,
Odette Cancer Centre, Sunnybrook Health Sciences Centre,
University of Toronto, Toronto, Ontario, Canada
[2]Department of Radiation Oncology, Bank of Cyprus Oncology Centre,
Nicosia, Cyprus; [3]Department of Urology,
Kitasato University School of Medicine, Kanagawa, Japan
[4]Hospital de l'Esperança, Sant Josep de la Muntanya, Barcelona, Spain
[5]Department of Clinical Oncology, Prince of Wales Hospital, Shatin,
New Territories, Hong Kong, SAR
[6]Department of Public Health and Institute of Epidemiology
and Preventative Medicine, National Taiwan University,
Taipei, Taiwan

* Correspondence: Professor Edward Chow MBBS, MSc, PhD, FRCPC, Department of Radiation Oncology, Odette Cancer Centre, Sunnybrook Health Sciences Centre, 2075 Bayview Avenue, Toronto, ON, Canada M4N 3M5. E-mail: Edward.Chow@sunnybrook.ca.

Abstract

From February 2009 to May 2010, patients receiving treatment for bone or brain metastases from five cancer centers across the world completed the EORTC QLQ-C15-PAL. Demographic information as well as various disease characteristics was recorded. To compare baseline QLQ-C15-PAL scores between patients with bone and brain metastases, univariate linear regression analysis was performed with or without confounders. A Bonferroni adjusted p-value < 0.003 (0.05/15 items) was considered statistically significant. A total of 109 patients with brain metastases and 233 patients with bone metastases completed the QLQ-C15-PAL. As expected, primary cancer site and previous systemic treatments were different between groups: there was a significantly greater number of patients with prostate and renal cell cancers and fewer patients with lung or gastrointestinal cancers with bone metastases, compared to patients with brain metastases (p<0.005). Prior to accounting for these two confounding factors, there were two QLQ-C15-PAL symptom scales significantly different between patients with bone metastases and patients with brain metastases. Patients with bone metastases had greater severity in pain (baseline mean score: 53.7 vs. 22.8; p<0.001) and fatigue (47.8 vs. 40.4; p=0.0029), compared to those with brain metastases. After accounting for confounders, only pain was significantly different (p<0.0001). Patients with bone metastases experience more pain at baseline compared to those with brain metastases. Patients with either bone or brain metastases otherwise experienced similar QOL profiles as assessed by the QLQ-C15-PAL. Supplementing of QLQ-C15-PAL by disease-specific instruments such as the QLQ-BM22 or QLQ-BN20 is therefore recommended in future trials depending on patient population included.

Introduction

Advanced cancer patients often have significant symptom burden and poor performance status. It has previously been shown that symptoms increase in severity with reduced survival (1). As patients have shorter life expectancies, traditional clinical trial endpoints such as survival are no longer appropriate in this population and therefore, clinicians tend to focus more on quality of life (QOL) (2). QOL is commonly assessed using validated self-administered questionnaires. The European Organization for Research and Treatment of Cancer (EORTC) offers a core module (QLQ-C30) along with more disease specific modules, such as the QLQ-BM22 for patients with bone metastases (5). However, these questionnaires can be cumbersome, especially if multiple assessments are required. Shorter questionnaires may therefore be beneficial as they can reduce patient burden (3). For this reason, a shorter, palliative version of the core module was developed, the QLQ-C15-PAL (4).

The QLQ-C15-PAL contains 15-items originally from the QLQ-C30 that was identified to be most representative of subscales within the core module itself (8). A previous study conducted by Steinman et al which used the QLQ-C15-PAL for patients with brain metastases found this instrument reduced the burden of repeated questionnaire completion for patients with advanced disease. Patients themselves even favored this instrument over the longer QLQ-C30 (7). Bone metastases are a common cause of intractable pain in the advanced cancer population, and cause skeletal related events (SREs) including pathological fractures, bone pain requiring radiotherapy, surgery to bone, spinal cord compression and hypercalcaemia (7). Brain metastases constitute the most common intracranial neoplasm in adults, occurring in 10-15% of patients with advanced cancer (6, 9). Depending on the location of the brain metastases, patients may present with a range of neurological symptoms such as headaches, focal weakness, mental disturbance, behavioral changes, seizures, speech difficulty, and ataxia (10). Although the QLQ-C15-PAL has been successfully shortened through rigorous statistical means, its adoption has been relatively slow in the palliative setting. Few prospective studies have detailed its use in the population. To date, comparisons among broad patient subgroups within the palliative cancer patient setting have not been made. The purpose of the present study was to compare QLQ-C15-PAL scores in patients with brain metastases to those with bone metastases.

Our study

From February 2009 to May 2010, patients receiving treatment for bone or brain metastases from cancer centers in Canada (three sites in total: Odette Cancer Centre, Toronto; Cross Cancer Institute, Edmonton; Tom Baker Cancer Centre, Calgary; Japan, Hong Kong, Cyprus and Taiwan) completed the QLQ-C15-PAL at baseline. Demographic information along with various disease characteristics was recorded. All research was conducted after approval from all local research ethics boards.

QLQ-C15-PAL

All items of the QLQ-C15-PAL are rated on a 4 point Likert scale from 1-4. The items are then scored as single or multi-item scales in the following domains: physical functioning, emotional functioning, fatigue, nausea/vomiting, pain, dyspneoa, insomnia, appetite loss, constipation and overall quality of life. For functional scales and the global QOL scale, a higher score indicates better function whereas for symptom scales, a higher score indicates a greater severity.

Statistical analyses

Demographic results were expressed as mean, standard deviation (SD), median and ranges for continuous demographics, and proportions for categorical values. To compare baseline characteristics in patients with bone and brain metastases, the Chi-square test was performed for categorical variables and the Wilcoxon rank-sum test for age and KPS. A two-sided p-value of <0.05 was considered statistically significant.

Individual items (un-scored subscales) were compared between both patient groups (brain vs. bone metastases) using the Chi-square test. A Bonferroni adjusted p-value < 0.003 (0.05/15 items) was determined and therefore considered statistically significant. To compare baseline QLQ-C15-PAL scores between patients with bone and brain metastases (BM and BN), univariate linear regression model (GLM) was performed. To normalize the distribution, natural log-transformation was applied for each score. A Bonferroni adjusted p-value < 0.003 was used for this step. After adjusting for confounding factors (i.e., significant demographics between groups, in this case, previous systemic treatment and primary cancer site), univariate linear regression analysis was performed to compare QLQ-C15-PAL baseline scores in patients with BM or with BN as well. In this step, the outcome was natural log scale of each QLQ-C15-PAL scale, the independent variables were the binary variable of group (1=BM, 0=BN), and 2 confounders, such as *ln (QLQ-C15-PAL scale) = a + b×Group + c×previous systemic treatment + d×Primary Cancer Site.* All analyses were conducted using Statistical Analysis Software (SAS version 9.2 for Windows).

Our findings

A total of 109 patients with brain metastases and 233 patients with bone metastases were enrolled (Table 1). Genders were balanced (51% female). Overall in all patients, the median age and Karnofsky Performance Status (KPS) were 62 years (range: 22-87) and 80 (range: 10-100), respectively. The most common primary cancers were of the breast (n=107, 31%), lung (n=99, 29%) and prostate (n=65; 19%).

**Table 1. Demographics in Patients with Bone Metastases (BM)
and in Patients with Brain Metastases (BN)**

	Total N=342	BM N=233	BN N=109	p-value *
Age (years)				0.2467
Mean (SD)	61.3 (11.7)	61.8 (11.9)	60.2 (11.2)	
Median (range)	62 (22-87)	62.5 (28-87)	61 (22 – 83)	
KPS at baseline				0.1105
Mean (SD)	75.9 (14.8)	75.0 (14.9)	77.7 (14.4)	
Median (range)	80 (0-100)	80 (0-100)	80 (40-100)	
Gender				0.9583
Female	175 (51.17%)	119 (51.07%)	56 (51.38%)	
Male	167 (48.83%)	114 (48.93%)	53 (48.62%)	
Married status				0.3338
Married	222 (67.89%)	153 (69.86%)	69 (63.89%)	
Widowed	22 (6.73%)	17 (7.76%)	5 (4.63%)	
Single	36 (11.01%)	23 (10.50%)	13 (12.04%)	
Partner	11 (3.36%)	10 (4.57%)	1 (0.93%)	
Other	36 (11.01%)	16 (7.31%)	20 (18.52%)	
Primary cancer site				<0.0001
Breast	107 (31.29%)	88 (37.77%)	19 (17.43%)	
Lung	99 (28.95%)	36 (15.45%)	63 (57.80%)	
Prostate	65 (19.01%)	65 (27.90%)	0 (0.00%)	
Gastrointestinal	20 (5.85%)	13 (5.58%)	7 (6.42%)	
Renal Cell	14 (4.09%)	11 (4.72%)	3 (2.75%)	
Others	37 (10.82%)	20 (8.58%)	17 (15.60%)	
Patients status				0.6210
Outpatient	312 (91.50%)	212 (90.99%)	100 (92.59%)	
Inpatient	29 (8.50%)	21 (9.01%)	8 (7.41%)	
Previous systemic treatment				<0.0001
Yes	261 (77.45%)	193 (83.91%)	68 (63.55%)	
No	76 (22.55%)	37 (16.09%)	39 (36.45%)	

* P-value was obtained by Chi-squared test for categorical variables and Wilcoxon rank-sum test for age and KPS. Bold indicates statistical significance.

Table 2. Mean Symptom Scores between Bone and Brain Metastases Patients at Baseline

		N	Mean	Std	Median	Min	Max
Overall QOL	group						
	BM-PAL15	230	54.8	25.28	50.0	0	100
	BN-PAL15	107	61.4	25.04	66.7	0	100
Physical Functioning	group						
	BM-PAL15	231	57.7	28.89	60.0	0	93
	BN-PAL15	107	69.5	27.06	73.3	0	93
Emotional Functioning	group						
	BM-PAL15	229	71.5	27.33	66.7	0	100
	BN-PAL15	106	73.8	23.41	75.0	0	100
Fatigue	group						
	BM-PAL15	228	47.8	27.09	44.4	0	100
	BN-PAL15	105	40.4	28.25	33.3	0	100
Nausea / Vomiting	group						
	BM-PAL15	230	15.1	27.40	0.0	0	100
	BN-PAL15	108	9.7	21.02	0.0	0	100
Pain	group						
	BM-PAL15	231	53.7	31.12	50.0	0	100
	BN-PAL15	108	22.8	29.59	16.7	0	100
Dyspnea	group						
	BM-PAL15	231	19.3	27.12	0.0	0	100
	BN-PAL15	108	18.5	25.51	0.0	0	100
Insomnia	group						
	BM-PAL15	231	36.2	35.59	33.3	0	100
	BN-PAL15	107	34.0	35.46	33.3	0	100
Appetite loss	group						
	BM-PAL15	230	27.7	35.54	0.0	0	100
	BN-PAL15	107	20.2	31.31	0.0	0	100
Constipation	group						
	BM-PAL15	231	27.4	32.88	0.0	0	100
	BN-PAL15	107	17.8	28.34	0.0	0	100

Descriptive statistics on QLQ-C15-PAL scores for patients with bone and brain metastases at baseline are available in Table 2. For patients with bone metastases, emotional functioning was better (mean score: 71.5±27.33) than physical functioning (57.7±28.89). Pain was the most severe symptom (53.7±31.12) while nausea/vomiting was least (15.1 ± 27.4). For bone metastases patients emotional functioning (mean score: 73.8±23.41) was also better than physical functioning (69.5 ± 27.06). Fatigue was the most severe symptom (40.4 ±28.25) while nausea was the least severe symptom (9.7 +/-21.02). Overall QOL was slightly better in patients with brain metastases compared to patients with bone metastases (61.4 and 54.8 respectively).

Comparison of baseline characteristics

Primary cancer site and previous systemic treatment were significantly different between the two groups and as a result were included in additional analyses as confounding factors. Patients from bone metastases have higher proportions with previous systemic treatment, in comparison to patients with brain metastases (83.9% vs. 63.6%). In the patients with bone metastases, there were higher proportions of patients with breast, prostate or renal cell cancer site and lower proportions of patients with lung or GI, compared to patients with brain metastases (P<0.0001). There were no significant differences between the age of patients who completed the assessment, the KPS, the gender, married status, or patient status.

Comparison of QLQ-C15-PAL scores unadjusted for confounders

Table 3 summarizes findings of the simple univariate linear regression model. There were two QLQ-C15-PAL symptom scales significantly different between patients with bone metastases and patients with brain metastases, namely, fatigue (47.8 vs. 40.4; p=0.0029) and pain (53.7 vs. 22.8; p<0.0001). Patients with bone metastases reported greater severity in pain and fatigue, compared to those with brain metastases.

Table 3. Comparing baseline QLQ-C15-PAL scores in patients with BM and in patients with BN by univariate linear regression analysis without accounting for confounders

At Baseline	Coefficient	SE	p-value *	MSE
Overall QOL	-0.154	0.107	0.1520	0.840
Physical Functioning	-0.284	0.107	0.0085	0.839
Emotional Functioning	-0.106	0.096	0.2721	0.671
Fatigue	0.421	0.140	0.0029	1.413
Nausea / Vomiting	0.390	0.195	0.0464	2.799
Pain	1.713	0.178	<.0001	2.321
Dyspnea	-0.013	0.219	0.9524	3.540
Insomnia	0.121	0.234	0.6044	3.994
Appetite loss	0.425	0.234	0.0696	3.988
Constipation	0.633	0.229	0.0060	3.832

A Bonferroni adjusted p-value < 0.003 was considered statistical significant.

Comparison of QLQ-C15-PAL scores adjusting for confounders

After accounting for previous systemic treatment and primary cancer sites as confounders, results were similar (Table 4). Only pain symptom scale was significantly different between both groups. Patients with bone metastases had more pain than those with brain metastases. The average pain scale was 53.7 for patients with bone metastases, compared to 22.8 for those with brain metastases (p<0.0001). Other scales were not significantly different after adjusting for confounders.

Table 4. Comparing baseline QLQ-C15-PAL scores in patients with BM and in patients with BN by univariate linear regression analysis with accounting for confounders

At Baseline	p-value of Group (BM vs. BN)	*p-value of Confounders* Previous Systemic Treatment	Primary Cancer Site	MSE
Overall QOL	0.2477	0.6858	0.0014	0.816
Physical Functioning	0.0047	0.5102	0.6081	0.852
Emotional Functioning	0.1614	0.8278	0.5538	0.684
Fatigue	0.0159	0.9113	0.8821	1.449
Nausea / Vomiting	0.0562	0.8881	0.8058	2.810
Pain	<0.0001	0.4863	0.7702	2.341
Dyspnea	0.3867	0.6311	0.0030	3.394
Insomnia	0.2723	0.2355	0.7733	4.021
Appetite loss	0.0636	0.5992	0.9124	4.041
Constipation	0.0106	0.1869	0.3477	3.832

A Bonferroni adjusted p-value < 0.003 was considered statistical significant.

The confounders of previous systemic treatment was not significant related to any QLQ-C15-PAL score; primary cancer site was only significantly associated with overall QOL (p = 0.0014).

Discussion

Few studies have reported on the use of the QLQ-C15-PAL for patients with advanced cancer. The present study assessed whether the QLQ-C15-PAL scores were significantly different between patients with bone and brain metastases. In the palliative setting when facing treatment decisions for patients with poor prognosis, symptom control and QOL become arguably the most important goals of care rather than the traditional endpoint of survival. There have been several editorials discussing the use of QLQ-C15-PAL along with several papers discussing the planned use of QLQ-C15-PAL in upcoming studies. Furthermore, as the QLQ-C15-PAL extracts items already included in the QLQ-C30, this instrument is available in many languages (7).

After adjusting for confounders, patients with bone metastases had significantly greater pain than those with brain metastases; as the majority of patients with bone metastases present the existence of pain. We did not find other scores to be significantly different and this may be due to the fact that both groups of patients were experiencing these issues, albeit possibly due to different causes. For example, physical functioning deficits may be observed in patients with bone metastases due to pain whereas, for those with brain metastases, due to dizziness or other neurologic symptoms. We would however, expect other domains not assessed by the QLQ-C15-PAL, such as cognitive functioning to be different in patients with bone and brain metastases. Unfortunately, these items were removed when the QLQ-C30 was shortened. Therefore, we recommend that future trials involving patients with brain metastases elect to supplement core instruments such as the QLQ-C15-PAL in conjunction with disease specific instruments such as the QLQ-BN20 to assess these domains.

In a similar study done on QLQ-C15-PAL symptoms in advanced cancer patients, it was found that domains of physical and emotional functioning, pain, and appetite loss were significant predictors of overall QOL in these patients with advanced cancer (7). Both appetite loss and emotional functioning were independently predictive of overall QOL in patients with bone metastases (n = 190). In patients with brain metastases (n = 150), independent predictors of overall QOL included physical and emotional functioning as well as fatigue. The QLQ-C15-PAL domains of physical and emotional functioning, pain and appetite loss were significant predictors of overall QOL in this cohort of patients with advanced cancer (7). Similarly to our study in which it was found that patients with bone metastases were primarily affected by pain and in brain metastases patients by fatigue. Overall QOL on average was slightly better in patients with brain metastases, but both were affected by these symptoms.

A limitation in this study is that patients were grouped by their reason for referral. If a patient requires palliative radiotherapy for painful bone metastases but also previously had brain metastases, they would be included in the bone metastases group only. This therefore may confound our findings. In addition, although we divided patients by treatment for bone or brain metastases, significant heterogeneity may still exist for patients included in these subgroups. Previously it has been shown that symptoms increase in severity with reduced survival (1). However, no information as to patients' disease trajectory was collected and we are unable to comment on this potential confounding factor in our analysis (1). Overall, the QLQ-C15-PAL demonstrated the ability to detect QOL issues expected in patients with bone and brain metastases. Future studies requiring more disease-specific findings should include disease-specific tools such as the QLQ-BM22 and QLQ-BN20.

Acknowledgments

We thank the generous support of the Bratty Family Fund, Michael and Karyn Goldstein Cancer Research Fund, Joseph and Silvana Melara Cancer Research Fund, and the Ofelia Cancer Research Fund. The authors have no conflicts of interest to disclose.

References

[1]   Zeng L, Zhang L, Culleton S, Jon F, Holden L, Kwong J, Khan L, Tsao M, Danjoux C, Sahgal A, Barnes E, Chow E. Edmonton symptom assessment scale as a prognosticative indicator in patients with advanced cancer. J Palliat Med 2011;14(3):337-42.
[2]   Zeng L, Chow E, Zhang L, Tseng LM, Hou MF, Fairchild A, Vassiliou V, Jesus-Garcia R, El-Din MA, Kumar A, Forges F, Chie WC, Bedard G, Bottomley A. An international prospective study establishing minimal clinically important differences in the EORTC QLQ-BM22 and QLQ-C30 in cancer patients with bone metastases. Support Care Cancer 2012;20(12):3307-13.
[3]   Lien K, Zeng L, Bradley N, Culleton S, Popovic M, Di Giovanni J, Jamani R, Cramarossa G, Nguyen J, Koo K, Jon F, Chow E. Poor accrual in palliative research studies: An update from the Rapid Response Radiotherapy Program. World J Oncol 2011t;2(5):217-24 .

[4]   Groenvold M, Petersen MA, Aaronson NK, Arraras JI, Blazeby JM, Bottomley A, Fayers PM, de Graeff A, Hammerlid E, Kaasa S, Sprangers MA, Bjorner JB. The development of the EORTC QLQ-C15-PAL: a shortened questionnaire for cancer patients in palliative care. Eur J Cancer 2006;42(1): 55-64.

[5]   Chow E, Hird A, Velikova G, Johnson C, Dewolf L, Bezjak A, Wu J, Shafiq J, Sezer O, Kardamakis D, van der Linden Y, Mak B, Castrol M, Foro Arnalot P, Ahmedzai S, Clemons M, Hoskin P, Yee A, Brundage M, Bottomley A. The European Organization for Research and Treatment of Cancer Quality of Life Questionnaire for patients with bone metastases: The EORTC QLQ-BM22. Eur J Cancer 2009;45:1146-52.

[6]   Diagnostics of central nervous system metastatic disease. Arch Oncol 2006;14(1):41-3.

[7]   Caissie A, Culleton S, Nguyen J, Zhang L, Zeng L, Holden L, Dennis K, Chan E, Jon F, Tsao M, Danjoux C, Sahgal A, Barnes E, Koo K, Chow E. What QLQ-C15-PAL symptoms matter most for overall quality of life in patients with advanced cancer? World J Oncol 2011;2(4):166-74.

[8]   Lien K, Zeng L, Nguyen J, Cramarossa G, Culleton S, Caissie A, Lutz S, Chow E. Comparison of the EORTC QLQ-C15-PAL and the FACIT-Pal for assessment of quality of life in patients with advanced cancer. Expert Rev Pharmacoecon Outcomes Res 2011;11(5):541-7.

[9]   Schiff D, Kesari S, Wen PY. Cancer neurology in clinical practice. Brain 2004;127(3):714.

[10]   Cheng J, Zhang X, Liu B. Health-related quality of life in patients with high-grade glioma. Neuro Oncol 2009;11(1):41–50.

In: Advanced Cancer   ISBN: 978-1-62808-239-5
Editors: N. Thavarajah, N. Pulenzas, B. Lechner et al.   © 2013 Nova Science Publishers, Inc.

Chapter 22

Review of brain metastases research in the Rapid Response Radiotherapy Program (RRRP)

Natalie Pulenzas, BSc(C), Breanne Lechner, BSc(C),
Nemica Thavarajah, BSc(C) and Edward Chow, MBBS[*]*
Rapid Response Radiotherapy Program, Department of Radiation Oncology,
Odette Cancer Centre, Sunnybrook Health Sciences Centre,
University of Toronto, Toronto, Ontario, Canada

Abstract

Brain metastases develop in approximately 20-40% of patients, and are frequently treated with whole brain radiation therapy (WBRT) for patients ineligible for aggressive treatment. The Rapid Response Radiotherapy Program (RRRP) provides timely radiotherapy for palliative cancer patients, focusing on quality of life (QOL) as an important endpoint. In this chapter we review the past research conducted in the RRRP on brain metastases patients. QOL studies have used a wide variety of assessment tools and determined that the effect of WBRT on QOL is widely variable, ranging from decreased QOL to improvement. There is not a current standardized QOL questionnaire which has been created and validated in the brain metastases population. Research in the RRRP is lacking in other treatment options for brain metastases such as stereotactic radiosurgery (SRS), likely due to the palliative nature of our patients. Future research should focus on creating a standard QOL instrument, measuring QOL following SRS, and better determining prognostic factors of brain metastases patients before treatment.

[*] Correspondence: Profesor Edward Chow MBBS, MSc, PhD, FRCPC, Department of Radiation Oncology, Odette Cancer Centre, Sunnybrook Health Sciences Centre, 2075 Bayview Avenue, Toronto, ON Canada. E-mail: Edward.Chow@Sunnybrook.ca.

Introduction

Brain metastases develop in approximately 20-40% of cancer patients and are frequently treated by whole brain radiotherapy (WBRT), and more aggressively stereotactic radiosurgery (SRS), or neurosurgical resection. Candidates for more aggressive treatments such as SRS or resection, typically have a solitary brain metastasis, controlled disease elsewhere and good performance status (1). Median survival is typically one month with no intervention, and in some cases up to 3-6 months with the addition of WBRT (2). Patients may experience a reduction in symptoms while receiving corticosteroids as these medications can reduce cerebral edema. The primary objective of WBRT is to achieve some magnitude of symptom relief, allow for tapering off of corticosteroids, so as to avoid potentially debilitating long term side effects, and to possibly increase survival (1,3). Brain metastases most commonly develop from primary lung and breast cancers (1-4). The standard practice of WBRT is 2000cGy in 5 fractions in the Rapid Response Radiotherapy Program (RRRP) (2,4,5).

There have been many studies focusing on brain metastases patients in the RRRP at the Sunnybrook Odette Cancer Centre, which is a specialized clinic developed in 1996 to provide timely palliative radiotherapy with the purpose to improve or maintain quality of life (QOL) (6). This chapter reviews the past research in the RRRP investigating brain metastases. A significant limitation of many brain metastases studies is a low compliance and high attrition rate due to progression of disease and neurological deficits. Questionnaires conducted in brain metastases patients can create a large patient burden, especially when these lengthy questionnaires may contain up to 50 items (3,7).

The efficacy of WBRT for treating patients with active extracranial disease and limited survival has been questioned (8). Physician expectations of the results from treatment to brain metastases are important as these physicians refer patients to the RRRP, which may lead to inappropriate treatment (5). The main focus of the past research in the RRRP is the measurement of QOL and improvement of patient-rated symptoms (2).

Methods

A retrospective review was conducted of research involving brain metastases from 2004 – present. Any research including brain metastases from the RRRP focused on QOL, prognostic factors, and use of corticosteroids was included.

Results

Doyle et al (7) examined QOL in patients after receiving WBRT. Patient evaluations used the Functional Assessment of Cancer Therapy-Brain (FACT-BR) questionnaire at baseline, one month, and two months following completion of treatment. This assessment was originally developed in patients with primary brain cancer, and includes the general questionnaire (FACT-G) (7,9). In 2012 the FACT-BR content was successfully validated for patients with brain metastases by health care professionals (HCPs) and patients. Generally, the content was considered relevant, and patients did not report items being difficult, upsetting, or irrelevant (10). An endpoint of the study by Doyle et al (7) was to assess the discrepancy between patient or proxy reported QOL, which was only analyzed at baseline due to small sample size at follow-ups. Sixty patients and their caregivers were enrolled. At one month post treatment only 45% of patients completed the one month follow-up, and 25% completed the two month follow up, which occurs frequently in long term studies involving this population (7). Low completion rate occurred due to various reasons such as death and deterioration in health. There was no significant difference seen in any comparisons of the Eastern Cooperative Oncology Group (ECOG) performance status between baseline, one month and two month follow-ups. Agreeability between patient and proxy rated scales was deemed to be poor, suggesting a factor to take into account in future studies using proxy questionnaires. Patient's QOL showed a non-significant trend of deterioration over time. This trend was likely clinically significant however, as the high attrition was majorly due to deterioration or death (7).

Caissie et al (9) examined the effect of radiation to brain metastases on QOL using the 20-item European Organisation for Research and Treatment of Cancer Quality of Life Questionnaire-Brain Neoplasm (EORTC QLQ-BN20) and the EORTC Quality of Life Questionnaire - Core 15 Palliative (QLQ-C15-PAL) (9). A limitation of QOL studies in brain metastases patients is the patient burden that arises from the use of lengthy questionnaires such as the combination of the EORTC Quality of Life Questionnaire (QLQ-C30) and QLQ-BN20, which contains 50 items in total. Studies observing the combination of these two questionnaires have concluded that poor compliance and high attrition rates limit the effectiveness of these questionnaires (7,11,12). The assessment tool used by Doyle et al, FACT-BR, has also been reported to have high patient burden leading to low compliance and difficulty with data collection (7,12). Therefore the QLQ-C15-PAL was developed to help decrease patient burden, and two additional items assessing cognitive function (concentration and memory) were added to create the QLQ-BN20+2 since this was absent from shortening the QLQ-C30 (3,9). Nguyen et al (13) successfully conducted content validation of the BN20+2 by interviewing brain metastases patients receiving radiation treatment and consulting HCPs about the relevance of each item. Majority of patients and HCPs reported all items were relevant to brain metastases patients except seizures, hair loss, and incontinence (>50% patients); itchy skin (15% HCPs); and future uncertainty (12% HCPs) were rated as irrelevant (13).

Caissie et al (9) conducted field testing of the combination of the 37 item BN20+2 and C15-PAL, and reported 65% of the cohort completed the one month follow up (9). When compared with a previous study which conducted follow-ups using the BN20 and C-30, there was a 67% compliance rate at one month, therefore the use of the C15-PAL was shown to be successful in this population, though did not show an increase in compliance rate (14). Post treatment of WBRT, maintenance of QOL occurred in this study, which may be explained due to the wide range of KPS (median 80, range 40-100), as this included poor prognosis and good performance status patients alike (9). Wong et al (2) conducted a study from 2005-2007 which utilized the validated Spitzer Quality of Life Index in 129 patients to assess QOL, symptom severity, and neurological function for up to three months following WBRT (2). As examined previously, benefit from WBRT would have been evident if QOL and neurological function improved, and symptom severity decreased. However, approximately half of the study cohort experienced symptom relief, as 43% had stable or improved fatigue, and 47%

improved neurological function. Similar trends were seen in improvement of daily living (29%), and health (54%). Therefore, objectives of WBRT may be appropriate to focus on the prevention of worsening or progression of symptom severity and QOL because of the general stabilization of symptoms that were found in this study (2).

A systematic review of the literature by Wong et al (1) was conducted from 1950 to 2007 focusing on QOL outcome after WBRT. Sixty-one trials were included in the review that fit the inclusion criteria. Twenty-four QOL assessments were used including the Edmonton Symptom Assessment Scale (ESAS), QLQ-C30, BN20, FACT-G and FACT-BR. The authors concluded there is no standardized QOL instrument used consistently with brain metastases patients as stated in multiple studies, which demonstrates the importance of creating a questionnaire to be validated in brain metastases patients (1,3,11). Wong and colleagues determined that in the majority of studies, there is deterioration in at least one domain of QOL after radiotherapy (1). Three important studies highlighted in the review included patients with good performance status and/or satisfactory prognosis, and observed that certain domains of QOL improved following WBRT with follow-up time points extending up to six months. Radiation Therapy Oncology Group (RTOG) Recursive Partitioning Analysis (RPA) class I and II, or KPS of 70 or greater, formed the majority of patient groups in these three studies, suggesting better prognosis patients do benefit from radiotherapy (1). Another study randomized nineteen patients to WBRT or no additional intervention following surgery or radiotherapy. Majority of this cohort had good performance status, with one patient in RPA Class III. No change in QOL was reported in either of the arms, which could promote the notion that better prognosis patients benefit from radiotherapy, as there was no decline in QOL (1).

QOL is an important outcome to maintain or improve in patients receiving palliative radiation for brain metastases (7). All of the studies reported in this review thus far have focused on WBRT as the treatment for brain metastases.

Prognostic factors

A prospective study by Lock et al (15) in 2004 investigated prognostic variables in brain metastases patients to determine if a certain subgroup, particularly poor prognostic status, would not benefit from WBRT. There were 275 patients with brain metastases assessed over a two year period from two cancer centers, and the median overall survival was 5.3 months (15). The rationale for this study was that patients with a poor expected survival may not achieve any symptom relief from WBRT, and their symptoms may be managed effectively by corticosteroids alone. It is demonstrated in the literature that the purpose of WBRT is generally for symptom control and it does not significantly increase survival (2,15). The patient population that would not benefit from WBRT, as defined by this study, was those with a life expectancy of less than 8 weeks. RTOG RPA is a method of determining performance status through division into three classes. RPA Class I includes patients with KPS ≥70, age <65 years, no extracranial metastases, and primary tumor controlled. RPA Class III are patients with KPS <70, and Class II encompasses the remaining patients (2). Number of metastatic sites, other than brain, and performance status, as measured by RTOG RPA, were determined to be significant predictors of survival. The study was unsuccessful in creating a model to accurately predict which patients would not benefit from WBRT (15).

Wong et al (1) conducted a study between 2005 and 2007 and found that when compared with their opposite counterparts, patients; age <60 years, KPS≥70, and RPA Class I or II, were all significantly associated with a longer survival. Two domains of QOL (activity and daily living), vomiting, and neurological function were all associated with survival, as worse scores corresponded with poor survival (2). Chow et al (8) also concluded that KPS≥70 was associated with longer survival. A literature review of brain metastases research was conducted by Wong and colleagues (1) in 2008, which reviewed studies that reported the Spitzer Index was superior in survival prediction when compared to KPS (1). Chow et al determined that KPS was the most significant predictor of survival in their study; however the questionnaire used was ESAS (8).

Though there are factors which assist in determining patient prognosis, there is no consensus on how to determine which patients would not be suitable for WBRT (15). Barnes et al (5) reported referring physicians overestimate the benefit of WBRT, therefore may be more likely to improperly refer patients for treatment (5). Further analysis into factors contributing to prognosis can contribute to reducing unnecessary treatment for poor prognosis patients, and aid in guiding physician expectations of survival and treatment.

Corticosteroids

A common limitation of many brain metastases studies is the inability to determine if the effects are due to WBRT, corticosteroids, or a combination of both. This was experienced in a QOL study by Wong et al (2) conducted from 2005-2007 in which 35% of patients at one month, and 29% at two months following WBRT, could not be tapered off of corticosteroids (2). Corticosteroids are commonly used to first treat brain metastases, and are usually associated with the presence of symptom response. However, they can cause adverse side effects after long term use. This can be prevented in some patients through intervention with WBRT, which can improve symptoms and allow patients to tolerate tapering of steroids (16). Nguyen et al (16) administered the dexamethasone symptom questionnaire (DSQ) to assess for steroid toxicity following WBRT (16). The study captured data for 68 patients, and at 1 month post radiation, 20% of patients were unable to be tapered off. Insomnia at week 2 post-WBRT was significantly related to a dose of ≥16mg/day, and decreased appetite loss was significantly related to longer use of steroids at baseline, but no consistent correlation between dose and QOL was determined (16).

Discussion

Factors to determine patient groups, prior to treatment, that would not benefit from WBRT is still generally inconclusive (1,8,15). It is important to continue examination into symptom outcomes and overall QOL following treatment to assess for benefit in specific patient groups. The benefit of WBRT may be diminished as patients referred to the RRRP typically have other factors disposing them to poor prognosis, such as multiple brain metastases, poor performance status, and active extracranial disease. This also contributes to the majority of our research being focused on WBRT, as more aggressive treatments in these palliative patients are rare (5). Referring physicians expectations of treatment, which are communicated to patients, may contribute to a lack of benefit seen from WBRT, as certain patients with limited survival may have been given false hope, leading to refusal of supportive care alone (5).

There is not a standardized QOL questionnaire used in brain metastases that allows for comparison across trials, decreases patient burden, and assesses symptoms related to brain metastases (1,3,11). A limitation of most of the questionnaires used in this patient population is they have been developed in a primary brain tumour population (FACT-Br, BN-20), or are general symptom assessments (ESAS).

It is unknown if assessments created for brain primary correlate correctly in brain metastases as these patients may have different experiences due to active extracranial disease (9). High attrition rate is another limitation of research studies in this population due to short life span, resulting in small sample sizes at follow-up. In our centre, we developed and are currently testing a brain metastases specific questionnaire for content and psychometric validity. This may decrease patient burden as it comprises 20 items, when compared to questionnaires used previously (FACT-Br, 53 items total). Psychometric validation is also being conducted for the FACT-Br. Our questionnaire will possibly improve data collection, and appropriately assess symptoms applicable to brain metastases patients. Additional investigation into other treatment options for brain metastases, such as SRS, should be employed at our centre to examine the symptom outcomes and QOL resulting from an emerging alternative treatment for certain subsets of patients.

Conclusion

There is a wide breadth of research done in the RRRP on brain metastases patients, and especially QOL following treatment. This has resulted in the evolution of patient assessment questionnaires to be more applicable, both in content and length, for brain metastases patients. Further upcoming research in the RRRP will focus on further validation and development of appropriate assessment tools designed specifically for this patient population. Additional investigation into alternative treatment for these advanced cancer patients is also an area of future research.

Acknowledgments

We thank the generous support of Bratty Family Fund, Michael and Karyn Goldstein Cancer Research Fund, Joseph and Silvana Melara Cancer Research Fund, and Ofelia Cancer Research Fund.

References

[1]	Wong J, Hird A, Kirou-Mauro A, Napolskikh J, Chow E. Quality of life in brain metastases radiation trials: a literature review. Curr Oncol 2008;15(5):25-45.

Review of brain metastases research in the Rapid Response Radiotherapy Program

[2]   Wong J, Hird A, Zhang L, Tsao M, Sinclair E, Barnes E, et al. Symptoms and quality of life in cancer patients with brain metastases following palliative radiotherapy. Int J Radiat Oncol Biol Phys 2009;75(4):1125-31.

[3]   Nguyen J, Sahgal A, Chow E, Danielson B. Brain metastases and quality of life. J Altern Med 2010;2(3):257-72.

[4]   Hird A, Wong J, Zhang L, Tsao M, Barnes E, Danjoux C, et al. Exploration of symptoms clusters within cancer patients with brain metastases using the Spitzer Quality of Life Index. Support Care Cancer 2010;18(3):335-42.

[5]   Barnes EA, Chow E, Tsao MN, Bradley NM, Doyle M, Li K, et al. Physician expectations of treatment outcomes for patients with brain metastases referred for whole brain radiotherapy. Int J Radiat Oncol Biol Phys 2010;76(1):187-92.

[6]   Chow E, Fan G, Hadi S, Wong J, Kirou-Mauro A, Filipczak L. Symptom clusters in cancer patients with brain metastases. Clin Oncol (R Coll Radiol) 2008;20(1):76-82.

[7]   Doyle M, Bradley NM, Li K, Sinclair E, Lam K, Chan G, et al. Quality of life in patients with brain metastases treated with a palliative course of whole-brain radiotherapy. J Palliat Med 2007;10(2): 367-74.

[8]   Chow E, Davis L, Holden L, Tsao M, Danjoux C. Prospective assessment of patient-rated symptoms following whole brain radiotherapy for brain metastases. J Pain Symptom Manage 2005;30(1):18-23.

[9]   Caissie A, Nguyen J, Chen E, Zhang L, Sahgal A, Clemons M, et al. Quality of life in patients with brain metastases using the EORTC QLQ-BN20+2 and QLQ-C15-PAL. Int J Radiat Oncol Biol Phys 2012;83(4):1238-45.

[10] Chen E, Cella D, Zeng L, Thavarajah N, Zhang L, Chang E, et al. Content validation of the FACT-Br with patients and health-care professionals to assess quality of life in patients with brain metastases. J Radiat Oncol 2012.

[11] Leung A, Lien K, Zeng L, Nguyen J, Caissie A, Culleton S, et al. The EORTC QLQ-BN20 for assessment of quality of life in patients receiving treatment or prophylaxis for brain metastases: a literature review. Expert Rev Pharmacoecon Outcomes Res 2011;11(6):693-700.

[12] Lien K, Zeng L, Nguyen J, Cramarossa G, Cella D, Chang E, et al. FACT-Br for assessment of quality of life in patients receiving treatment for brain metastases: a literature review. Expert Rev Pharmacoecon Outcomes Res 2011;11(6):701-8.

[13] Nguyen J, Zhang L, Clemons M, Vassiliou V, Danielson B, Fairchild A, et al. Content validation of the EORTC QLQ-BN20+2 with patients and health care professionals to assess quality of life in brain metastases. J Radiat Oncol 2012;1:397-409.

[14] Chen E, Nguyen J, Zhang L, Zeng L, Holden L, Lauzon N, et al. Quality of life in patients with brain metastases using the EORTC QLQ-BN20 and QLQ-C30. J Radiat Oncol 2012;1:179-86.

[15] Lock M, Chow E, Pond GR, Do V, Danjoux C, Dinniwell R, et al. Prognostic factors in brain metastases: can we determine patients who do not benefit from whole-brain radiotherapy?. Clin Oncol (R Coll Radiol) 2004;16(5):332-8.

[16] Nguyen J, Caissie A, Zhang L, Zeng L, Dennis K, Holden L, et al. Dexamethasone toxicity and quality of life in patients with brain metastases following palliative whole-brain radiotherapy. J Radiat Oncol 2012.

[17] Cramarossa G, Chow E, Zhang L, Bedard G, Zeng L, Sahgal A, et al. Predictive factors for overall quality of life in patients with advanced cancer. Support Care Cancer 2013 Jan 22.

[18] Koo K, Zeng L, Chen E, Zhang L, Culleton S, Dennis K, et al. Do elderly patients with metastatic cancer have worse quality of life scores? Support Care Cancer 2012;20(9):2121-7.

[19] Lien K, Zeng L, Zhang L, Nguyen J, Di Giovanni J, Popovic M, et al. Predictive factors for well-being in advanced cancer patients referred for palliative radiotherapy. Clin Oncol (R Coll Radiol) 2012;24(6):443-51.

SECTION THREE: SYMPTOM MANAGEMENT

In: Advanced Cancer
Editors: N. Thavarajah, N. Pulenzas, B. Lechner et al.

ISBN: 978-1-62808-239-5
© 2013 Nova Science Publishers, Inc.

Chapter 23

Review of symptom cluster research in the Rapid Response Radiotherapy Program (RRRP)

Breanne Lechner, BSc(C), Natalie Pulenzas, BSc(C),
Nemica Thavarajah, BSc(C) and Edward Chow, MBBS*
Rapid Response Radiotherapy Program, Department of Radiation Oncology,
Odette Cancer Centre, Sunnybrook Health Sciences
Centre, University of Toronto, Toronto, Ontario, Canada

Abstract

Patients with cancer often experience various concurrent symptoms which can predict changes in patient functioning, treatment outcomes and affect their quality of life. Clinical evidence of patients frequently experiencing multiple symptoms has prompted research in the identification and analysis of symptom clusters. The Rapid Response Radiotherapy Program (RRRP) provides timely radiotherapy for palliative cancer patients, focusing on quality of life (QOL) as an important endpoint. In this chapter we review the past research in the RRRP on symptom clusters in patients with advanced cancer. Research in the RRRP has addressed symptom clusters in patients with brain metastases, bone metastases and reviewed external publications concerning symptom clusters in cancer patients. Further research should aim to standardize statistical methods used for symptom cluster identification and validate symptom clusters in advanced cancer patients.

* Correspondence: Professor Edward Chow MBBS, MSc, PhD, FRCPC, Department of Radiation Oncology, Odette Cancer Centre, Sunnybrook Health Sciences Centre, 2075 Bayview Avenue, Toronto, ON Canada. Email: Edward.Chow@Sunnybrook.ca.

Introduction

Patients with cancer often experience various concurrent symptoms associated with the cancer itself, its treatment, or a combination of the two (1). These symptoms frequently predict changes in patient functioning, treatment outcomes and affect their quality of life (2). Symptoms are multidimensional concepts which can involve cognitive sensations and the biophysical functioning of the patient (2). Clinical evidence of patients frequently experiencing multiple symptoms simultaneously rather than in isolation has identified the need for further research investigating symptom clusters (2). The definition of symptom clusters by Kim et al. (3) indicates that at least two or more symptoms must be related to each other, occur together, be a stable group, and be relatively independent of other clusters. Evaluating multiple symptoms can provide information regarding the relationship between symptoms, predictors of patient outcomes and identify ideal treatment to manage specific symptom clusters (2). Thus, research in this area benefits health care providers, patients and caregivers. Symptom clusters in cancer patients can be affected by various treatments, including palliative radiotherapy (RT). Therefore, it is imperative to conduct longitudinal studies to evaluate symptom clusters in patients at baseline and at follow-up points after treatment.

Research in the Rapid Response Radiotherapy Program (RRRP) has strived to derive and analyze symptom clusters and increase the knowledge base of symptom management research. The RRRP is an outpatient clinic established in 1996 to provide timely palliative RT. Located at the Odette Cancer Centre, the RRRP provides quick access to RT to relieve symptoms and improve quality of life (QOL) in advanced cancer patients. This paper reviews previous research in the RRRP on symptom clusters in advanced cancer patients receiving RT.

Literature search

A literature search was conducted to identify studies investigating symptom clusters in cancer patients conducted by the RRRP from 2007 to present. Studies examining symptom clusters in patients with various primary cancer types and previous literature reviews regarding symptom clusters were included in the review.

The literature review identified relevant studies published between 2007 and 2013. Extensive research has been conducted regarding symptom clusters in areas including bone metastases, brain metastases, and broader literature reviews.

Symptom clusters in bone metastases

A study by Chow et al (4) explored symptom clusters in patients with bone metastases in the RRRP to determine whether bone pain was associated with any other symptoms using the Edmonton Symptom Assessment Scale (ESAS). A total of 518 patients with bone metastases provided analgesic intake information and completed the ESAS at baseline, one, two, four, eight, and twelve weeks following RT. Three clusters were identified and accounted for 66%

of the total variance at baseline. Cronbach's alpha coefficient demonstrated high internal reliability in the clusters, with a coefficient ranging from 0.61 to 0.81. It was found that pain clustered with fatigue, drowsiness, and poor sense of well-being at baseline. It was also observed that the clusters changed post-radiation in both responders and non-responders to RT and that pain clustered with different symptoms. In non-responders, three symptom clusters were consistently present, except in week eight. RT influenced the structure of symptom clusters in both responders and non-responders. This dataset of patients was reanalyzed by Khan et al (5) using different statistical methods to determine whether symptom clusters in patients with bone metastases vary when extracted using three different statistical methods. Clusters derived using Principal Component Analysis (PCA) in the previous study by Chow et al (4) were compared to symptom clusters extracted using Hierarchical Cluster Analysis (HCA) and Exploratory Factor Analysis (EFA). Clusters were derived at baseline, one, two, four, eight and twelve weeks after RT. The patient sample was further divided into responders versus non-responders to RT. A complete consensus between HCA, EFA and PCA for the number and composition of symptom clusters was not reached at any time point despite the use of an identical data set. As expected, different symptom clusters were observed in the responders and non-responders with all three statistical methods. In addition, clusters varied at each time point within each subgroup. Depression and anxiety were consistently found in the same cluster. The use of a common analytical method is necessary for consistency and comparison purposes in future symptom cluster research.

A study published in 2008, conducted in the RRRP explored symptom clusters in cancer patients with pain due to bone metastases. This study by Hadi et al (6) enrolled 348 patients with bone metastases between May 2003 and January 2007 referred for palliative RT, receiving either single or multiple fractions. The patients' worst pain at the site of treatment and seven functional interference scores were assessed using the Brief Pain Inventory (BPI) at baseline, four, eight, and twelve weeks post RT (6). PCA was performed on these items to determine interrelationships between symptoms. Principal components with an Eigenvalue higher than 0.90 and explaining more than 10% of the variance were selected. The Cronbach alpha statistic was used to estimate the internal consistency and reliability of the derived clusters. Two symptom clusters were identified. Cluster one included walking ability, general activity, normal work, enjoyment of life, and worst pain (6). Cluster two included relations with others, mood, and sleep (6). The two clusters at baseline accounted for 67% of the total variance with a Cronbach's alpha of 0.87 and 0.70 respectively (6). In patients that responded to RT, the two symptom clusters were no longer detected at four, eight, and twelve weeks post-RT. In non-responders, the same two clusters were not present at week four, re-emerged at week eight, and disappeared at week twelve (6). Hadi et al (6) concluded that the significant correlations between worst pain score and the function interference items demonstrate the importance of pain reduction as a goal for RT, as reducing pain can reduce functional interference and improve QOL.

This dataset was reanalyzed by Chen et al (7) in 2012 to determine whether symptom clusters in patients with bone metastases varied when derived using three different statistical methods. The previous BPI data was reanalyzed using HCA and EFA. Little correlation was observed in the symptom cluster findings of PCA, EFA, and HCA in the total patient sample. Absolute consensus among all three statistical methods was never reached at any assessment time point. Varying patterns of symptom cluster presentation over time were observed in the responders versus non-responders subgroups regardless of the analytical method employed. A core cluster of symptoms composed of worst pain, general activity, walking ability, normal work, and enjoyment of life frequently presented in the same cluster (7).

An additional validation study was conducted in the RRRP by Hadi and colleagues (8). This study enrolled 52 patients between February and September 2007 with bone metastases receiving either a single fraction or multiple fractions of RT (8). Again, patients provided worst pain at the site of RT and functional interference scores were assessed using the BPI at baseline, four, eight, and twelve weeks post-RT. Two symptom clusters were identified. Cluster one included worst pain, interference with general activity, normal work, and walking ability. Cluster two consisted of interference with mood, sleep, enjoyment of life, and relations with others (8). These symptom clusters were not identical to those in the previous study, therefore, the authors concluded that these differences may be an indicator of the instability of the discovered symptom clusters or may be the result of a fewer number of patients in this validation study (6, 8). Thus, further research is warranted to determine if the previously discovered symptom clusters are in fact reproducible.

Another study on symptom cluster research by Chen et al (9) was initiated identify symptom clusters at baseline in a subgroup of bone metastases patients reporting non-zero ESAS scores. A subgroup of patients reporting severity scores greater than zero for all nine ESAS symptoms at baseline was compiled from a pre-existing database of bone metastases patients identified in the RRRP. At baseline, notably different symptom clusters were identified in the non-zero subgroup compared with the total patient population regardless of the statistical method utilized. When clusters derived using different statistical methods were compared, symptom cluster results varied depending on the method employed, with a few exceptions where analogous clusters were derived using two different statistical methods at a specific time point. A complete consensus between all three methods was never observed, which emphasizes the importance of the use of standardized statistical methods in symptom cluster research (9).

Symptom clusters in brain metastases

Chow et al (10) explored the presence of symptom clusters in patients with brain metastases. Between January 1999 and January 2002, 170 patients with brain metastases referred to the RRRP completed the ESAS at baseline, one, two, four, eight, and twelve weeks after whole brain radiotherapy (WBRT). To determine interrelationships between symptoms a PCA with varimax rotation was carried out on the nine ESAS items. Three symptom clusters were found at baseline. Cluster one included fatigue, drowsiness, shortness of breath, and pain and accounted for 37%of the total variance. Cluster two included anxiety and depression, and accounted for 12% of the total variance. Cluster three included poor appetite, nausea, and a poor sense of well-being, and accounted for 13% of the total variance (10). The internal reliabilities of the three clusters using Cronbach's alpha coefficient ranged from 0.61 to 0.74 (10). This study concluded that symptom clusters appeared to exist in patients with brain metastases. Limiting factors of this study included high attrition rate due to profound deterioration in this patient population, as well as incomplete data on steroid usage, as certain symptoms can be affected by steroid usage (10).

A reanalysis of this data by Chow et al (10) was published by Chen et al (11) in 2013 to determine whether symptom clusters in patients with bone metastases varied when derived using different statistical methods. The ESAS data was reanalyzed using HCA and EFA. Symptom clusters extracted at baseline and each subsequent follow-up generally varied depending on the analytical method employed. Twelve unique clusters were found at each follow-up with each method, and at only at the eight week follow up did all three methods demonstrate the same cluster of symptoms. Symptom cluster findings using PCA and HCA correlated more strongly with each other than either did with the findings of EFA. Inconsistency in symptom cluster composition was also observed at different time intervals. While the symptom clusters differed between the three analytical methods, symptoms within determined clusters such as anxiety and depression or fatigue and drowsiness consistently clustered together over time. The authors concluded that the stability of symptoms pairs observed indicates a robust interrelationship existed between the symptoms involved (11).

An additional study by Hird et al (12) involved 129 patients with brain metastases referred to the RRRP between August 2005 to October 2007 completed the Spitzer Quality of Life Index (SQLI) and a study designed 17 item symptom questionnaire at baseline, one, two, and three months after WBRT. PCA was again used along with the Cronbach's alpha statistic. In analysis of the SQLI, the first cluster identified consisted of activity, daily living, and health (12). The second cluster consisted of support and outlook (12). Cronbach's alpha was 0.69 and 0.40 respectively, and the two clusters accounted for 64% of the variance (12). Analysis of the symptom questionnaire items revealed three clusters at baseline. Though these clusters changed slightly over time, certain symptoms remained to together despite WBRT: trouble concentrating and confusion, memory loss and decreased alertness, nausea and vomiting, dizziness and headache (12). Thus, this article concluded that symptom clusters do exist in patients with brain metastases.

A reanalysis of this compiled SQLI data was conducted by Khan et al (13) to determine whether the use of different statistical methods influenced the composition of symptom clusters derived from patients with brain metastases. Symptom clusters extracted using PCA in the previous study were compared to clusters determined using HCA and EFA at baseline, one, two, and three months following WBRT. The number and composition of symptom clusters at each time point varied based on the statistical method employed, despite the use of an identical dataset. However, some domains consistently clustered together, such as activity and daily living from the SQLI items. Additionally, memory loss, confusion, and trouble concentrating were always present in the same cluster. Nausea and vomiting also occurred in conjunction regardless of the analytical method employed. This analysis concluded that symptom clusters vary with respect to occurrence, quantity, and composition based on the statistical method utilized to extract them (9). The use of a single analytical method is essential for consistency and comparison purposes in future symptom cluster research.

Reanalysis and literature reviews

A review by Chen et al (14) was conducted to reanalyze data from the previous symptom cluster study by Fan et al. (15) using different statistical methods. The previous study by Fan et al explored symptom clusters in advanced cancer patients by applying PCA on ESAS data collected at baseline, one, two, four, eight, and twelve week follow up for 1296 patients (15). The more recent reanalysis by Chen et al (10) used this same data set and extracted symptom clusters with HCA and EFA. The symptom cluster findings of HCA and PCA correlated more frequently with each other than either did with EFA. Complete consensus of all three statistical methods was never reached (14). Thus, the authors concluded that the presence of symptom clusters in cancer patients vary depending on which statistical analysis is used (14).

A literature review published in 2011 by Chen et al (16) examined past literature on symptom clusters in lung cancer patients. Five relevant studies were identified which investigated symptom clusters in lung cancer patients. The number of symptoms in a cluster ranged from two to eleven (16). The only cluster that was consistently identified was composed of nausea and vomiting symptoms in the two studies reviewed (16). Respiratory clusters identified in two studies were also comparable, containing both dyspnea and cough, among other symptoms (16). Chen et al (16) concluded that differences in sample population characteristics, assessment tools and statistical analyses resulted in a lack of consensus in symptom clusters in patients with lung cancer.

Nguyen et al (17) published a review of research reporting symptom clusters in breast cancer patients between 2005 and 2009. Five studies relevant studies were identified that differed from each other in statistical methodology, number of symptom clusters produced, and the symptoms comprising the clusters. The number of symptom clusters extracted between the five studies varied from one to four, while the number of symptoms in a cluster ranged from two to five. One study examining symptom clusters between different patient groups and a second study examining clusters across a time trajectory had certain reproducible clusters comprising similar symptoms. There were no clusters across different studies that contained the same symptoms, though fatigue was present in at least one cluster in all five studies and depression/psychological distress was noted in four of the studies. Nausea and appetite were the only two symptoms that associated together across three of the five studies. Although there were common symptoms assessed across the five studies, no common symptom clusters could be derived from these reports. This lack of commonality may have been the result the disparities in subpopulations of patients, assessment tools, and analytical and methodological approaches (17).

In 2012, Thavarajah et al (2) reviewed empirically determined symptom clusters in patients with metastatic cancer. A total of eight relevant studies published between 2005 and 2011 were identified. The number of symptom clusters extracted varied from two to eight clusters per study, comprising of two to eight symptoms per cluster. There were no clusters consistently identified within all eight studies. Notable differences in symptoms assessed, assessment tools, statistical analysis, patient demographics were observed between the studies. The lack of consensus among the inter-study symptom clusters are likely due to the differences in patient population as well as study methodology.

A further literature review by Thavarajah et al (18) explored symptom clusters specifically in prostate cancer patients which identified two relevant studies on this topic. Both studies were longitudinal in nature and utilized cluster analysis to derive symptom clusters, though one of the studies also used three additional statistical methods. Both studies identified several symptom clusters in prostate patients, though several disparities between the two studies were determined. Differences in sample populations, assessment tools, symptoms observed and statistical methods can account for discrepancies between the two studies. Thus, the authors concluded that further research in prostate cancer symptom clusters is necessary to establish clinically relevant findings.

Discussion

Extensive research has been conducted in the RRRP regarding symptom clusters. Studies have explored symptom clusters in specific patient types with metastases to bone and brain. Symptom cluster research has also been conducted in the general population of patients with advanced cancer from various primary sites. Research identifying and analyzing symptom clusters is relevant for medical professionals in the oncology field as well as their patients. Identifying symptom clusters and their trends over time also has clinical relevance for symptom treatment and QOL improvement.

Evidently, through examination of research on symptom clusters in the RRRP, it is necessary to conduct longitudinal studies to identify symptom clusters over time. It is important for studies to determine how symptom clusters change or deteriorate over time from baseline to multiple follow up points. Longitudinal studies are also essential for examining the effect of treatment, including RT, on symptom clusters in cancer patients by assessing symptoms both at baseline and following treatment.

In addition to completing studies that are longitudinal in nature, involving large patient populations in studies is also important for symptom cluster research in order to establish findings and clusters that can be deemed significant. Conclusions from studies with smaller patient sample sizes were less definitive as discrepancies between identified symptom clusters in different studies may be the result of small patient populations (8).

For symptom cluster research, statistical analysis is also imperative. It has been identified by many of the studies conducted in the RRRP that symptom clusters can vary depending on which method of statistical analysis is used. Studies in the RRRP have used statistical methods of detecting symptom clusters including PCA, HCA, and EFA. It is important to find a standardized method of analysis for identifying symptom clusters and validate this method in the identification of symptom clusters in various patient populations (9, 14). The use of a single universal statistical method will allow various studies on symptom clusters in advanced cancer patients to be compared and analyzed together (13).

Symptom cluster investigation is a developing area of research and is promising in providing insights into symptom management for cancer patients. Symptom clusters can interfere with patients' functional status, QOL and relationships with others (3). It may be more effective to initiate interventions and assess their effects on symptom clusters rather than on single symptoms. Further research identifying underlying mechanisms of symptom clusters and impeding or manipulating these mechanisms may offer ways to treat a cluster of symptoms simultaneously (3). Research in the RRRP has shown that methodological inconsistencies between studies have resulted in a lack of consensus on symptom clusters for patient populations and have thus impeded the determination of clinically relevant findings (16).

Conclusion

Although there is still debate in the literature on what defines a symptom cluster and which statistical method should be used to identify symptom clusters, it is evident that research in the area is significant. The efforts of the RRRP have aimed to broaden the available information on symptom clusters in patients with advanced cancer and how these clusters are impacted by RT. There are still inconsistencies in research methodologies and results for patients with various primary cancers and sites of metastases. Thus, continued research in the RRRP is warranted to further determine the clinical implications of symptom clusters and validate the methods used to identify them.

Acknowledgments

We thank the generous support of Bratty Family Fund, Michael and Karyn Goldstein Cancer Research Fund, Joseph and Silvana Melara Cancer Research Fund, and Ofelia Cancer Research Fund.

References

[1]   Bedi H, Hird A, Campos S, Chow E. Symptom clusters in metastatic cancer: A critical appraisal. J Pain Manage 2010;3(1):17-29.

[2]   Thavarajah N, Chen E, Zeng L, Bedard G, Di Giovanni J, Lemke M, et al. Symptom clusters in patients with metastatic cancer: A literature review. Expert Review of Pharmacoecon Outcomes Res 2012;12(5):597-604.

[3]   Kim HJ, McGuire DB, Tulman L, Barsevick AM. Symptom clusters: Concept analysis and clinical implications for cancer nursing. Cancer Nurs 2005;28:270-82.

[4]   Chow E, Fan G, Hadi S, Filipczak L. Symptom clusters in cancer patients with bone metastases. Support Care Cancer 2007;15(9):1035-43.

[5]   Khan L, Cramarossa G, Chen E, Nguyen J, Zhang L, Tsao M, et al. Symptom clusters using the edmonton symptom assessment system in patients with bone metastases: A reanalysis comparing different statistical methods. World J Oncol 2012;3(1):23-32.

[6]   Hadi S, Fan G, Kirou-Mauro A, Hird A, Filipczak L. Symptom clusters in cancer patients with metastatic bone pain. J Palliat Med 2008;11(4):591-600.

[7]   Chen E, Khan L, Zhang L, Nguyen J, Cramarossa G, Tsao M, et al. Symptom clusters in patients with bone metastases - A reanalysis comparing different statistical methods. Supportive Care Cancer 2012;20(11):2811-20.

[8]   Hadi S, Zhang L, Hird A, de Sa E, Chow E. Validation of symptom clusters in patients with metastatic bone pain. Curr Oncol 2008;15(5):211-8.

[9]   Chen E, Nguyen J, Cramarossa G, Khan L, Zhang L, Tsao M, et al. Symptom clusters in patients with advanced cancer: Sub-analysis of patients reporting exclusively non-zero ESAS scores. J Palliat Med 2012;26(6):826-33.

[10]   Chow E, Fan G, Hadi S, Wong J, Kirou-Mauro A, Filipczak L. Symptom clusters in cancer patients with brain metastases. Clin Oncol (R Coll Radiol) 2008;20(1):76-82.

[11]   Chen E, Khan L, Zhang L, Nguyen J, Zeng L, Bedard G, et al. Symptom clusters in patients with brain metastases-a reanalysis comparing different statistical methods. J Radiat Oncol 2013;2(1):95-102.

[12]   Hird A, Wong J, Zhang L, Tsao M, Barnes E, Danjoux C, et al. Exploration of symptoms clusters within cancer patients with brain metastases using the spitzer quality of life index. Support Care Cancer 2010;18(3):335-42.

[13]   Khan L, Cramarossa G, Lemke M, Nguyen J, Zhang L, Chen E, et al. Symptom clusters using the spitzer quality of life index in patients with brain metastases--a reanalysis comparing different statistical methods. Support Care Cancer 2013;21(2):467-73.

[14] Chen E, Nguyen J, Khan L, Zhang L, Cramarossa G, Tsao M, et al. Symptom clusters in patients with advanced cancer: A reanalysis comparing different statistical methods. J Pain Symptom Manage 2012;44(1):23-32.

[15] Fan G, Hadi S, Chow E. Symptom clusters in patients with advanced-stage cancer referred for palliative radiation therapy in an outpatient setting. Support Cancer Ther 2007;4(3):157-62.

[16] Chen E, Nguyen J, Cramarossa G, Khan L, Leung A, Lutz S, et al. Symptom clusters in patients with lung cancer: A literature review. Expert Rev Pharmacoecon Outcomes Res 2011;11(4):433-9.

[17] Nguyen J, Cramarossa G, Bruner D, Chen E, Khan L, Leung A, et al. A literature review of symptom clusters in patients with breast cancer. Expert Rev Pharmacoecon Outcomes Res 2011;11(5):533-9.

[18] Thavarajah N, Chen E, Bedard G, Lauzon N, Zhou M, Chu D, Chow E. Symptom clusters in patients with prostate cancer: a literature review. J Pain Manage 2012;5(4): 303-10.

In: Advanced Cancer
Editors: N. Thavarajah, N. Pulenzas, B. Lechner et al.

ISBN: 978-1-62808-239-5
© 2013 Nova Science Publishers, Inc.

Chapter 24

Symptom clusters in metastatic cancer: A critical appraisal

Harleen Bedi, BSc(C), Amanda Hird, BSc(C),
*Sarah Campos, BSc(C) and Edward Chow, MBBS, PhD, FRCPC**

Rapid Response Radiotherapy Program, Department of Radiation Oncology,
Odette Cancer Centre, Sunnybrook Health Sciences Centre,
University of Toronto, Toronto, Ontario, Canada

Abstract

Advanced cancer patients often present with multiple concurrent symptoms that may have synergistic effect on patient morbidity. Previous research in oncology has suggested that certain symptoms tend to occur together, stay relatively stable over time, and remain relatively independent of other symptoms, with or without a shared etiology. Research on the co-management of symptoms through the analysis of symptom clusters can improve palliative care in oncology. This literature review analyzes symptom cluster studies in metastatic cancer. Common advanced cancer symptoms are discussed to explore their relationship within a cluster. Methods: A literature search was conducted to identify studies on symptom clusters in advanced cancer. Additionally, studies analyzing conceptual issues, statistical modelling and physiological mechanisms of symptoms common to advance cancer were examined. Results: The literature review identified 11 relevant studies published between 1997 and 2008. Eight studies focussed on metastatic cancer while three studies investigated symptom clusters in oncology patients representing various disease stages. Discussion: Investigation of symptom clusters is complicated and is influenced by several conceptual, methodological and patient related factors. Studies reviewed differed in their definitions of symptom clusters, types of assessment questionnaires and statistical analyses. Further research to explore the

* Correspondence: Edward Chow MBBS, PhD, FRCPC, Department of Radiation Oncology, Odette Cancer Centre, Sunnybrook Health Sciences Centre, 2075 Bayview Avenue, Toronto, ON, Canada M4N 3M5. Tel: 416-480-4998; Fax: 416-480-6002; E-mail: Edward.Chow@sunnybrook.ca.

mechanisms underlying symptom clusters and the stability of clusters over time will validate research on this concept.

Introduction

Oncology patients often present with multiple symptoms that co-occur and may be caused by the cancer itself, its treatment, or a combination of the two (1). A symptom is defined as a "subjective experience reflecting the biopyschosocial functioning, sensations, or cognition of an individual" (2, pg 669). Symptoms are multidimensional and can include a patient's perceptions of prevalence, intensity and distress (3).

Past research in cancer symptom management has followed a reductionist approach by investigating a few clinically significant symptoms individually (4). Though this approach reveals extensive information about certain symptoms, it does not determine particular groups of symptoms that are commonly observed to co-occur and correlate in cancer patients. Dodd et al (5) pioneered the concept of "symptom clusters" to research on the concurrence and co-management of symptoms commonly observed in cancer. A symptom cluster was proposed to be constructed of symptoms that were related without necessarily sharing a common etiology (5).

Exploration of symptom clusters has revealed new avenues in symptom management and palliative care of cancer patients. Research on the influence of groups of symptoms on patient outcomes has led to increased awareness of symptom clusters, and was recently supported by the National Institutes of Health (NIH) at the State-of-the-Science Conference on "Symptom Management in Cancer: Pain, Depression and Fatigue" (6).

Successive studies of symptom clusters have refined the definition of what should qualify as a symptom cluster. Kim et al (7) defined a symptom cluster as a group of two or more related symptoms that co-occur and form a stable group independent of other clusters. Additionally, Miaskowski et al (4) suggested symptoms should share a common etiology, have common variance and produce outcomes different from individual symptoms to be considered related. Nevertheless considerable debate exists around determining a common, working definition of symptom clusters (4,8-10).

Contemporary research in symptom clusters has either followed the deterministic model or the heuristic model. The deterministic model investigates the validity and reliability of pre-defined symptom clusters (10). In contrast, the heuristic model statistically examines relationship between list of symptoms to derive clusters (10). Generally symptom clusters studies have employed a cross-sectional design to examine the concurrence of symptoms at any given time (10). Nonetheless, analysis of symptom clusters in chronic diseases such as cancer can benefit from longitudinal studies that investigate symptom profiles over time.

Common statistical approaches employed for derivation of symptom clusters include correlation and related measures of association, graphical modelling, factor analysis and cluster analysis. Correlation and related measures of association provide concrete mathematical evidence for the concurrence of two or more symptoms (10). On the other hand, graphical modelling is an effective tool for visual representation of conditional relationships in multivariate random observations (10). Alternatively, factor analysis can identify groups of symptoms that share an underlying mechanism (10). Furthermore, cluster analysis can identify clinical subgroups that present common symptom patterns (10).

Despite the variance among previous studies in terms of definition, methodological approaches to derivation and statistical analyses, symptom clusters are a major issue in metastatic cancer. The investigation of symptom clusters has the potential to greatly contribute to the symptom management and palliative care of this population. The present study delved into the origin of symptom cluster research in metastatic cancer populations. An exhaustive review of literature on symptom clusters in advanced cancer was conducted to understand the current state of knowledge on this concept. Additionally, symptoms commonly observed in advanced cancer are summarized and the physiological or psychological mechanisms underlying a cluster of symptoms are explored. Moreover, limitations in concept definition, methodology and application of research findings are critically analyzed. Recommendations for future research on symptom clusters in advanced cancer population are proposed.

Literature search

A literature search was conducted in the following databases to identify studies investigating symptom clusters in advanced cancer patients: Medline (1950 to October 2008), PubMed, Embase (1980 to 2008), Embase reviews (including Cochrane Central Register of Controlled Trials (CCTR), National Health Service Economic Evaluation, Cochrane Database of Systematic Reviews (COCH), Cochrane Methodology Register Database (CMR), Database of Abstracts of Reviews of Effects (DARE), Health Technology Assessment Database (DTA) and ACP Journal Club. The search was restricted to publications in English and studies conducted in humans. The keywords used for search included "symptom cluster", "symptom constellation", "co-occurrence of symptoms". The results were combined with "metastases" and "advanced cancer". Studies on conceptual issues in symptom clusters and statistical modelling were analyzed. Additionally, studies examining physiological mechanisms underlying symptoms common to advanced cancer were reviewed to investigate the reasons for occurrence of symptom clusters.

Results

The literature review identified 11 relevant studies published between 1997 and 2008. Eight studies focussed on metastatic cancer while three studies investigated symptom clusters in oncology patients representing various disease stages. A summary of clinical population, symptom clusters, statistical analyses and assessment tool in each study is presented in tables 1 and 2.

Dodd et al (5) pioneered symptom cluster research in 2001. The study attempted to validate a symptom cluster including pain, fatigue and sleep insufficiency in cancer patients receiving chemotherapy. Information on symptom distress was collected by the 33-item Quality of Life- Cancer (QoL-CA) questionnaire. The deterministic model was analyzed by two-stage hierarchical multiple regression.

Table 1. Review of symptom clusters in advanced cancer patients

Reference	Cancer site	Sample Size	Symptom cluster	Statistical Analysis	Assessment Tools
Chow et al (11)	Bone metastases	518	Cluster 1: fatigue, pain, drowsiness, poor sense of well-being Cluster 2: anxiety, depression Cluster 3: shortness of breath, nausea, poor appetite	Principal component analysis with varimax rotation	Edmonton Symptom Assessment System
Hadi et al (12)	Bone metastases	348	Cluster 1: walking ability, general activity, normal work, enjoyment of life, worst pain Cluster 2 : relations with others, mood, sleep	Principal component analysis with varimax rotation	Brief Pain Inventory
Chow et al (13)	Brain metastases	170	Cluster 1: fatigue, pain, drowsiness, shortness of breath Cluster 2: anxiety, depression Cluster 3: shortness of breath, nausea, poor appetite	Principal component analysis with varimax rotation	Edmonton Symptom Assessment System
Sarna and Brecht (15)	Advanced lung cancer (women)	60	Cluster 1: Emotional/Physical Suffering- pain frequency, pain severity, bowel, appearance, outlook Cluster 2: Gastrointestinal- nausea frequency, nausea severity, appetite Cluster 3: Respiratory Distress- cough, breathing, insomnia, Cluster 4: Malaise- fatigue, concentration	Principal component analysis with varimax rotation	13-item Symptom Distress Scale
Chan et al (14)	Advanced lung cancer (undergoing radiation treatment)	27	Cluster 1: breathlessness, anxiety, fatigue	Multivariate analysis of variance	100 mm horizontal visual analog scale
Fan et al (9)	Metastases to miscellaneous sites (common primary: lung, breast, prostrate)	1296	Cluster 1: Nausea, appetite loss, poor sense of well-being, pain Cluster 2: fatigue, drowsiness, shortness of breath Cluster 3: anxiety, depression	Principal component analysis with varimax rotation	Edmonton Symptom Assessment System
Teunissen et al (17)	Metastases to miscellaneous sites (common primary: GI, breast, gynaecological, head and neck)	181	Cluster 1: nausea, dysphagia, dyspnea, confusion, depressed mood	Multivariate analysis	49-symptom checklist (derived by the Dutch Centres for Development of Palliative Care)

Reference	Cancer site	Sample Size	Symptom cluster	Statistical Analysis	Assessment Tools
Walsh and Rybicki (18)	Metastases to miscellaneous sites (common primary: lung, breast, colorectal, prostrate)	922	Cluster 1: Fatigue: anorexia-cachexia (fatigue, weakness, lack of energy, anorexia, early satiety, weight loss, taste change, dry mouth) Cluster 2: neuropsychological (sleep, depression, anxiety) Cluster 3: upper gastrointestinal (dizziness, dyspepsia, belching, bloating) Cluster 4: nausea-vomiting Cluster 5: aerodigestive (dyspnea, cough, hoarseness, dysphagia) Cluster 6: debility (edema, confusion) Cluster 7: pain (pain, constipation)	Cluster analysis (agglomerative hierarchical with average linkage)	38-item Eastern Cooperative Oncology Group performance status and severity checklist

Table 2. Review of symptom clusters in cancer patients combined across different stages

Reference	Cancer site	Sample Size	Symptom cluster	Statistical Analysis	Assessment Tools
Fox and Lyon (19)	Ovarian cancer survivors (mostly stage III advanced)	76	Cluster 1: depression, fatigue	Hierarchical multiple regression analysis	Short Form- 36 Health Status Survey subscales, Fox Simple Quality of Life Scale
Bender et al (20)	Breast cancer	154 (40 Early Sage, 88 Sage I/II/III, 26 Stage IV)	Cluster 1 : Fatigue- fatigue, weakness, lacking energy Cluster 2 : Cognitive impairment- memory problems, concentration loss Cluster 3 : mood problems- anxiety, depression	Hierarchical cluster analysis	Profile of Mood States, Symptom Checklist, Daily symptom diary, Kupperman Index, Menopausal Quality of Life Scale, Functional Assessment of Cancer Therapy: Anemia/ Fatigue Scale
Glaus et al (21)	Breast cancer (receiving hormone therapy)	373 (301 Early Stage, 72 Late Stage)	Cluster 1 : menopausal- hot flashes/sweats, weight tiredness/ fatigue, weight gain, vaginal dryness, decreased sexual interest	Cluster Analysis (agglomerative hierarchical method)	Checklist for Patients with Endocrine Therapy, International Breast Cancer Study Group Linear Snalogue Scale for patients with endocrine treatment

Inter-correlations among fatigue, pain and sleep insufficiency were observed to be small and the hierarchical regression model explained only 48.4% of the total variance in functional status (5). Thus, the study was unable to confirm the symptom cluster of pain, fatigue and sleep insufficiency in the cancer population. However, the initial work stimulated further research in symptom clusters to improve quality of life in cancer patients.

Symptom clusters in bone metastases

Two studies have investigated symptom clusters in bone metastases patients. Chow et al (11) examined if bone pain clustered with other advanced cancer symptoms in 518 patients. Principal component analysis (PCA) with varimax rotation on the symptoms assessed by the Edmonton Symptom Assessment System (ESAS) questionnaire yielded a three cluster solution that accounted for 66% of the total variance. Cluster 1 included fatigue, pain, drowsiness, poor sense of well-being while anxiety and depression comprised cluster 2. Lastly, cluster 3 consisted of shortness of breath, nausea, and poor appetite. Cronbach's alpha coefficient ranged from 0.61 to 0.81, demonstrating high internal reliability. The clusters were found to disintegrate during the follow-ups conducted 1, 2, 4, 8 and 12 weeks post radiation treatment in both responders and non-responders to radiotherapy (RT) (11). Nevertheless some symptoms often appeared in the same cluster, for instance fatigue and drowsiness, and anxiety and depression remained together at each assessment.

Following a similar design, Hadi et al (12) attempted to validate symptom clusters in bone metastases. The Brief Pain Inventory (BPI) was used to assess symptom distress in 348 patients with bone metastases. In contrast to Chow et al (11), PCA with varimax rotation yielded a two factor solution that accounted for 67% of the total variance. Cluster 1 included walking ability, general activity, normal work, enjoyment of life and worst pain while cluster 2 included relations with others, mood and sleep. The two symptom clusters disintegrated at 4, 8, and 12 weeks post RT in the responder group and followed an inconsistent pattern in the non-responders. The disintegration of symptom clusters in responders following RT alluded to the effectiveness of palliative RT in alleviating symptomatic bone pain and reducing functional interference over time (12).

Symptom clusters in brain metastases

Only one study investigating symptom clusters in brain metastases was identified in the literature search. Chow et al (13) utilized a design similar to their previous study on bone metastases (11) to explore symptom clusters in 170 brain metastases patients referred to an outpatient palliative RT clinic. The most common primary cancer sites were lung, breast and gastrointestinal. Principal component analysis with varimax rotation on the ESAS questionnaire revealed three clusters; cluster 1 contained fatigue, drowsiness, shortness of breath, and pain; cluster 2 consisted of anxiety and depression; and cluster 3 included poor appetite, nausea and poor sense of well-being. Similar to preceding longitudinal studies (11, 12), the symptom clusters were observed to change in follow-up weeks, alluding to their dynamic nature.

Symptom clusters in advanced lung cancer

Two studies focussed on symptom clusters in advanced lung cancer patients. Chan et al (14) investigated the existence of a symptom cluster consisting of breathlessness, fatigue, and anxiety in patients undergoing palliative RT. Data was collected from 27 patients at three time points: 1 day prior to RT (Baseline, T0), week 3 (T1) and week 6 (T2) after commencement of RT using 100 mm horizontal visual analog scales (VAS). The three symptoms shared moderate to strong relationships (Spearman coefficient= 0.49-0.66) and the cluster had a high internal consistency (Cronbach a = 0.69 to 0.82) at the three time points.

Another study by Sarna and Brecht (15) applied factor analysis with varimax orthogonal rotation to the 13-item Symptom Distress Scale. The study sampled 60 women with advanced lung cancer and generated four symptom clusters explaining 63.3% of the total variance. The four clusters identified were emotional or physical suffering, gastrointestinal distress, respiratory distress and malaise. Nevertheless, reliability and validity of these findings is questionable due to the small sample size and lack of male representation in the studied population (16).

Symptom clusters in patients with metastases to miscellaneous sites

Three studies investigated symptom clusters in patients with any site of metastases. Fan et al (9) analyzed 1296 metastatic patients, primarily with metastases to the bone (64%) from primary lung, breast, and prostate cancer. Principal component analysis with varimax rotation was employed on the 9-symptom ESAS scale. Based on Kim et al's (7) definition, three clusters were identified, which accounted for 62% of the total variance. Cluster 1 was composed of nausea, lack of appetite, poor sense of well-being and pain. Cluster 2 included fatigue, drowsiness and shortness of breath, while cluster 3 was comprised of anxiety and depression.

Teunissen et al (17) conducted a prospective analysis on 181 advanced metastases patients. Gastrointestinal, breast, gynaecological or head and neck were the most common primary cancer sites in this cohort, and bone, lymph node, liver, lung and viscera were the most common sites of metastasis. A 49-symptom checklist derived by the Dutch Centres for Development of Palliative Care was utilized. Multivariate analysis of 20 symptoms, which occurred in more than 10% of the patient sample, yielded a symptom cluster composed of nausea, dysphagia, dyspnea, confusion and depressed mood. The obtained symptom cluster was later validated to accurately predict survival in hospitalized cancer patients.

In contrast, Walsh and Rybicki (18) utilized the 38-item Eastern Cooperative Oncology Group (ECOG) performance status and symptom severity checklist to measure symptom distress in 922 patients with metastatic cancer. The ECOG checklist graded each symptom on a four point scale as present/absent, mild, moderate or severe. The most common primary cancer sites were lung, breast, colorectal and prostate. Twenty five symptoms with greater than 15% prevalence were statistically analyzed. Cluster analysis using agglomerative hierarchical method with average linkage yielded seven symptom clusters (fatigue, anorexia-cachexia, neuropsychological, upper gastrointestinal, nausea-vomiting, aerodigestive, debility, and pain) when a cut-off of correlation > 0.68 was employed. The symptoms within each cluster are listed in Table 1.

Symptom clusters in cancer patients combined across different stages

Fox and Lyon (19) explored symptom clusters in survivors of ovarian cancer. The multipurpose Short Form- 36 (SF-36) Health Status Survey subscales for general health status and the Fox Simple Quality of Life Scale (FSQOLS) for quality of life assessment were employed. Following Kim et al's (2005) definition, hierarchical multiple regression analysis identified a symptom cluster of depression and fatigue, which explained 41% of total variance.

Bender et al (20) analyzed symptom data from three independent studies to identify symptom clusters common across three phases of breast cancer. The study population consisted of 40 women in early stage (received primary surgery but not yet initiated adjuvant therapy); 88 in stage I, II, or III (completed surgery and adjuvant chemotherapy, may have been receiving hormonal therapy); and 26 in stage IV (metastatic cancer). Information on symptom distress was extracted from a variety of self-report questionnaires such as Profile of Mood States (POMS), symptom checklist, daily symptom diary, Kupperman Index, Menopausal Quality of Life Scale, and Functional Assessment of Cancer Therapy (FACT): Anaemia/Fatigue Scale. Hierarchical cluster analysis identified symptom clusters related to fatigue, cognitive impairment and mood problems common in each of the three different phases of breast cancer.

Glaus et al (21) explored a menopausal symptom cluster and its relationship with fatigue in 373 breast cancer patients undergoing hormonal treatment (301 with early stage cancer and 72 with late stage cancer). The Checklist for Patients with Endocrine Therapy (C-PET) and the International Breast Cancer Study Group (IBCSG) Linear Analogue Scale for patients with endocrine treatment were used for symptom assessment. Agglomerative hierarchical cluster analysis confirmed a menopausal symptom cluster, composed of hot flashes, weight tiredness, weight gain, vaginal dryness, and decreased sexual interest.

Discussion

The field of symptom clusters is complicated due to the presence of several confounding factors. The symptom cluster studies conducted in advanced cancer populations differed in the type of symptom assessment questionnaires employed and methods of statistical analyses.

Mularski et al (22) noted that the use of different assessment tools of uncertain quality had made it difficult to compare results across studies on symptom clusters. Additionally, the necessity of uniformity in assessment tools utilized by quality of life studies has been emphasized by the National Institutes of Health, State-of-the-Science Conference Statement on "Improving End-of-Life Care" (23). The differences in symptom clusters identified by two studies on bone metastases (11,12) (see table 1) can be attributed to the different assessment questionnaires employed. A lack of consensus on a symptom assessment tool and statistical methodology is a limitation in the extrapolation of findings and generalization of symptom clusters from various studies (9, 14, 15, 17, 18, 20, 21) (see tables 1 and 2).

Most common assessment tools utilized in symptom cluster studies include the ESAS, M.D. Anderson Symptom Inventory, Symptom Distress Scale and BPI. These self-report, multi-symptom assessment questionnaires are widely used to measure the presence, severity and frequency of symptoms such as pain, fatigue, nausea, depression, lack of appetite, dyspnea in general cancer patients (24). Nevertheless, symptom clusters in advanced cancer may be specific to the type of cancer, treatment, or a combination of both factors (24). A comparison of symptom clusters identified by Chow et al (11) in bone metastases patients and brain metastases patients (13) exemplifies the disadvantage of using a general questionnaire. Both studies utilized the ESAS to assess symptom distress. Consequently, the symptom clusters derived included symptoms common to both cancer types and do not allow an effective diagnosis or clinical management of the particular cancer populations examined. Thus, assessment tools specifically designed and validated for a particular cancer population are preferred over a general questionnaire (22) to ensure the extraction of symptom clusters that are relevant to the specific symptomatology of that cancer.

Additionally, several symptom cluster studies were conducted in patients with different cancer types (9,17,18) and disease stages (19-21). It is necessary to recognize that patients with different stages and types of cancer have different symptom experiences. In their analysis of ovarian cancer survivors with different stages of the disease, Fox and Lyon (19) identified a cluster that correlated depression with fatigue. The study did not explore more specific quality of life items affecting ovarian cancer-specific disease and treatment-related symptoms. Moreover, symptom distress can be confounded by the use of symptom management strategies, such as opioids used to relieve pain, RT and chemotherapy (1). For instance, Sarna and Brecht (15) observed that symptom distress was significantly related to treatment (chemotherapy was associated with fewer serious problems with insomnia). Hence, symptom management efforts must be considered when assessing symptom distress.

There is much variability in how symptoms within a cluster may be correlated. The "partial mediation model" (25) alludes to the complexity in understanding dynamics of symptom concurrence in advanced cancer. The model explains how two symptoms can influence each other indirectly through effect on a common symptom, for instance, pain could affect sleep and indirectly influence subjective reports of fatigue (25). Thus, the validity of symptom clusters must be confirmed by investigating the underlying pathophysiology behind observed symptom groups, or by reviewing previous literature and conducting further research. Owing to the complications in statistical analysis of symptom clusters, Kim et al (10) have proposed the use of a multimodal strategy for further investigations. Their study suggested using a graphical modelling of multiple symptoms to gain insight into the type and direction of relationship between symptoms, followed by structural equation modelling to test the viability of the model.

Several studies have correlated psychological distress (anxiety, depression, psychological distress or sadness) with physical burden (fatigue, weakness or decreased physical activity) in advanced cancer patients (10, 15,19). For instance, Chen and Chang (26) observed an increased occurrence of insomnia, pain, anorexia, fatigue, and wound or pressure sores in depressed patients. Similarly, Lloyd-Williams et al (27) have affirmed a significant correlation between a patient's subjective feeling of physical symptoms, such as pain and fatigue, and psychological distress.

Subsequent research by Teunissen et al (28) investigated the effect of anxiety and depression on presence and severity of physical symptoms in hospitalized advanced cancer patients. Anxiety and depression were measured by the Hospital Anxiety and Depression Scale (HADS) and the ESAS. Conversely, this study did not find a relationship between anxiety or depressed mood and symptom presence or symptom intensity. In a review of research by Chen and Chang (26), Teunissen et al (28) noted that the relationship between depression and physical symptom distress could be confounded owing to a high Karnofsky score (KPS) (Table 3) (29) in the cancer population analyzed (mean KPS of study sample was 81%) and the chemotherapy treatment being administered.

Table 3. The Karnofsky Performance Status Scale (KPS) (29)

Score	Description
100	Normal, no complaints, no evidence of disease.
90	Able to carry on normal activity; minor signs or symptoms of disease.
80	Normal activity with effort; some signs or symptoms of disease.
70	Cares for self, unable to carry on normal activity or do active work.
60	Requires occasional assistance, but is able to care for most of his/her needs.
50	Requires considerable assistance and frequent medical care.
40	Disabled, requires special care and assistance.
30	Severely disabled, hospitalization indicated. Death not imminent.
20	Very sick, hospitalization indicated. Death not imminent.
10	Moribund, fatal processes progressing rapidly.
0	Dead

The KPS is used to measure the functional status, daily mobility and degree of dependence on medical care of cancer patients. The scale has intervals of 10% and measures performance on a range of 0% (dead) to 100% (normal, no complaints, no evidence of disease). Higher scores on the KPS indicate better physical mobility and functioning while lower scores signify greater symptom burden (40).

When Teunissen et al (28) applied the DSM-criteria (Diagnostic and Statistical Manual of Mental Disorders) to analyze depression in patients observed by Lloyd-Williams et al (27), no significant differences in symptom rating could be found between depressed and non-depressed patients. Therefore, contrary to the assumption made in palliative medicine, presence and intensity of physical symptom distress may not be a reliable predictor of anxiety or depression in the advanced cancer population or vice-versa (28).

A significant volume of research has been conducted to advance knowledge on the occurrence of symptom clusters in advanced cancer. However, research on mechanisms underlying the manifestation of symptom clusters specific to advanced cancer has not been discussed extensively in the palliative literature.

Several studies investigating symptom clusters in oncology populations have referred to the "sickness behaviour" described in animal models to explain symptom clusters observed. For instance, the sickness symptom cluster observed by Chen and Tseng (16) in the general cancer population was composed of fatigue, pain, sleep disturbance, lack of appetite and drowsiness. This cluster was found to be remarkably similar to the "sickness behaviour" described for animals (16). The sickness behaviour in animals is characterized by pyrexia, fatigue, somnolence, psychomotor retardation, anhedonia and impaired cognitive functioning (16,30). This behaviour is thought to be mediated by proinflammatory cytokines (such as interleukin-1, interleukin-6, interferon-a and tumour necrosis factor-a) and the study questioned the existence of a similar underlying mechanism in humans (31).

Analyses of causal factors underlying commonly observed symptoms in advanced cancer can provide the theoretical framework for correlations between symptoms in a cluster. Few symptoms commonly observed in advanced cancer include anorexia, cachexia, dyspnea, delirium, nausea, vomiting and fatigue.

Anorexia and cachexia are major causes of morbidity and mortality in advanced cancer (32). While both anorexia and cachexia can result in weight loss and reduced tolerance to RT, chemotherapy and surgery, mechanisms underlying their expression are different (32,33). Anorexia occurs when appetite signals, normally derived from neuropeptide Y within the hypothalamus, are diminished while satiety signals generated by melacortins are amplified (32). In contrast, cachexia is a systemic inflammatory response caused by cytokines (tumour or host generated) such as leukemia-inhibiting factor and tumour necrosis factor, or specific cachexins that detrimentally alter carbohydrate, lipid and protein metabolism (32). Management of cachexia also depends upon correction of several secondary causes, such as emotional distress, pain, dyspnea, and several reversible gastrointestinal disorders (33).

Dyspnea is a subjective sense of difficulty in breathing which is associated with a multidimensional physical, social and emotional component (32,34). While the occurrence of dyspnea has been related to weakness of respiratory muscles (34,35), no tests exist yet to indicate its severity. Hence, reports on symptom distress due to dyspnea vary with a patient's subjective experience.

Under metastatic conditions, dyspnea can result from complications of therapy or comorbidities (such as cachexia and anemia) (32). Additionally, Dudgeon et al (35) observed a significant correlation between intensity of dyspnea and the intensity of anxiety. The cluster composed of breathlessness, anxiety and fatigue, identified by Chan et al (14), exemplifies the need to investigate common mechanisms underlying the presentation of these symptoms in advanced lung cancer populations.

Advanced cancer patients that present with delirium can be challenging to manage under palliative settings (36). Delirium can be manifested as disturbance in consciousness, reduced concentration, impaired memory or language disturbance (32). It can be precipitated due to several factors such as medication, infection, central nervous system malignancies, pain, and surgery (32,36). Several patient related factors such as age, pre-existing cognitive dysfunction, nutritional deficits, hearing or visual dysfunction and unfamiliar surroundings may predispose the development of delirium (32). A few symptom cluster studies have correlated cognitive impairment with depression (17) and fatigue (15). Additionally, Bender et al (20) identified a cognitive impairment cluster that was common to breast cancer patients across different stages of the disease. Notably, above studies did not utilize validated tools, such as the Delirium Rating Scale, the Confusion Assessment Method, or the Mini-Mental Status Examination (32), to screen for delirium. Rather the assessments were made from single-item screening question or general symptom distress checklists (28). Thus the correlations observed must be confirmed by further investigations of the causal mechanisms.

Furthermore, nausea and vomiting are frequently observed in advanced cancer. While nausea is an unpleasant, subjective feeling of wanting to vomit, vomiting is the forceful expulsion of gastric contents (32, 37). Metabolic abnormalities, brain metastases, chemotherapy, RT, constipation and certain medications (opioids, antibiotics, non-steroidal anti-inflammatory drugs, and vitamin / mineral supplements) can dispose a patient to develop nausea and vomiting (32,37). Emotional distress (for instance, anxiety, and fear) and pain can also stimulate the development of nausea (32,37). Nausea and vomiting centres in the medulla have been hypothesized to share common afferent neural pathways (32), which may explain their concurrence in advanced cancer patients (18).

Advanced cancer patients often report fatigue as a distressing symptom. Cancer-related fatigue is defined "as an unusual, persistent, subjective sense of tiredness, related to cancer or cancer treatment that interferes with usual functioning" (38, pg 152). Though the exact pathways for fatigue are unknown, it is speculated that multiple factors such as cancer treatment (chemotherapy/radiotherapy), co-morbid illnesses, cachexia, anaemia, sleep disorders, psychological factors (anxiety/depression), pain, nausea, dyspnea, medications may predispose the development of fatigue (32). Therefore, the clustering of fatigue with symptoms such as anorexia (18), pain (11,13), anxiety (14) and depression (19) can be explained. Further investigations of pathophysiology of symptoms common in advanced cancer would validate the symptom clusters observed in this population.

Symptom clusters research in advanced cancer is complicated due to several variables that can confound the symptom experience. Subjective reports of symptom distress can be confounded by long-term experience with the disease, presence of multiple symptoms, duration of disease experience or any other perceptual disorders (3).

Additionally, factors such as education level, language skills, and ethnicity can affect a patient's reports of symptom distress (3,9). In an investigation of symptom clusters in women with advanced lung cancer, Sarna and Brecht (15) confirmed that personal and subjective factors can affect the symptom experience. For instance, higher education levels were significantly associated with poorer outlook and associated distress, and lower income was correlated with serious disruptions in sleeping (15). Therefore, adoption of objective measures of symptom presence and severity, administered by trained nurses or physicians, could eliminate problems associated with a subjective, self-report questionnaire.

It is important to monitor how symptom clusters observed in advance cancer population change over time to establish a definite relationship between symptoms within a cluster. Longitudinal studies can provide information on the effectiveness of management strategies commonly employed to treat or contain the cancer. Only a few studies have delved into the longitudinal patterns in symptom clusters observed in advanced cancer patients (11-14). These studies confirmed the effectiveness of palliative RT in alleviating symptomatic bone pain and reducing symptom burden and functional interference over time. Additionally, Chan et al (14) confirmed the concurrence of breathlessness, fatigue, and anxiety in advanced lung cancer patients by observing a strong correlation between the three symptoms 3 weeks and 6 weeks after palliative radiotherapy. Further investigations on the stability of symptom clusters over time, would validate the concept of symptom clusters and improve quality of life in advanced cancer populations by allowing a co-management of various symptoms that form a cluster.

Importantly, prioritization of certain symptoms by patients can increase the possibility of those symptoms being relieved through clinical intervention (39). This hypothesis was confirmed for some physical symptoms, such as pain and constipation (39). However symptom prioritization had little influence over the alleviation of subjective symptoms such as nausea, fatigue, physical function, role function and activity (39).

In view of the fact that patients who prioritize certain symptoms report higher initial scores for those symptoms and describe a significantly better treatment outcome than those who do not do so, palliative care could be focussed on relieving the most prioritized symptoms to optimize patient care and increase cost effectiveness in palliative oncology.

Acknowledgments

This study was supported by the Michael and Karyn Goldstein Cancer Research Fund. We would like to thank Rene E. Harrison, PhD, Department of Biological Sciences, University of Toronto for her comments.

References

[1]   Barsevick AM, Whitmer K, Nail LM, Beck SL, Dudley WN. Symptom cluster research: Conceptual, design, measurement, and analysis issues. J Pain Symptom Manage 2006;31(1):85-95.

[2]   Dodd M, Janson S, Facione N, Faucett J, Froelicher ES, Humphreys J, et al. Advancing the science of symptom management. J Adv Nurs 2001;33(5):668-76.

[3]   Lenz ER, Pugh LC, Milligan RA, Gift A, Suppe F. The middle-range theory of unpleasant symptoms: An update.(middle-range nursing theory). Adv Nurs Sci 1997;19(3):14-27.

[4]   Miaskowski C, Dodd M, Lee K. Symptom clusters: The new frontier in symptom management research. J Natl Cancer Inst Monogr 2004(32):17-21.

[5]   Dodd MJ, Miaskowski C, Paul SM. Symptom clusters and their effect on the functional status of patients with cancer. Oncol Nurs Forum 2001;28(3):465-70.

[6]   National Institutes of Health Consensus State-of-the-Science Statements. Symptom Management in cancer: pain, depression, and fatigue 2002;19(4):1-29. Accessed 2008 Nov 12. URL: http://consensus.nih.gov

[7]   Kim HJ, McGuire DB, Tulman L, Barsevick AM. Symptom clusters - concept analysis and clinical implications for cancer nursing. Cancer Nurs 2005;28(4):270-82.

[8]   Armstrong TS. Symptoms experience: A concept analysis. Oncol Nurs Forum 2003;30(4):601-6.

[9]   Fan G, Hadi S, Chow E. Symptom clusters in patients with advanced-stage cancer referred for palliative radiation therapy in an outpatient setting. Support Cancer Ther 2007;4(3):157-62.

[10]   Kim HJ, Abraham IL. Statistical approaches to modeling symptom clusters in cancer patients. Cancer Nurs 2008;31(5):E1-E10.

[11]   Chow E, Fan G, Hadi S, Filipczak L. Symptom clusters in cancer patients with bone metastases. Support Care Cancer 2007;15(9):1035-43.

[12]   Hadi S, Fan G, Hird AE, Kirou-Mauro A, Filipczak LA, Chow E. Symptom clusters in patients with cancer with metastatic bone pain. J Palliat Med 2008;11(4):591-600.

[13]   Chow E, Fan G, Hadi S, Wong J, Kirou-Mauro A, Filipczak L. Symptom clusters in cancer patients with brain metastases. Clin Oncol (R Coll Radiol) 2008;20(1):76-82.

[14]   Chan CW, Richardson A, Richardson J. A study to assess the existence of the symptom cluster of breathlessness, fatigue and anxiety in patients with advanced lung cancer. Eur J Oncol Nurs 2005;9(4):325-33.

[15]   Sarna L, Brecht M. Dimensions of symptom distress in women with advanced lung cancer: A factor analysis, Heart and Lung: The Journal of Acute and Critical Care, 1997;26(1):23-30.

[16]   Chen ML, Tseng HC. Symptom clusters in cancer patients. Support Care Cancer 2006;14(8):825-30.

[17]   Teunissen SC, de Graeff A, de Haes HC, Voest EE. Prognostic significance of symptoms of hospitalised advanced cancer patients. Eur J Cancer 2006;42(15):2510-6.

[18]   Walsh D, Rybicki L. Symptom clustering in advanced cancer. Support Care Cancer 2006;14(8):831-6.

[19]   Fox SW, Lyon D. Symptom clusters and quality of life in survivors of ovarian cancer. Cancer Nurs 2007;30(5):354-61.

[20]   Bender CM, Ergun FS, Rosenzweig MQ, Cohen SM, Sereika SM. Symptom clusters in breast cancer across 3 phases of the disease. Cancer Nurs 2005;28(3):219-25.

[21]   Glaus A, Boehme C, Thurlimann B, Ruhstaller T, Hsu Schmitz SF, Morant R, et al. Fatigue and menopausal symptoms in women with breast cancer undergoing hormonal cancer treatment. Ann Oncol 2006;17(5):801-6.

[22]   Mularski RA, Dy SM, Shugarman LR, Wilkinson AM, Lynn J, Shekelle PG et al. A systematic review of measures of end-of-life care and its outcomes. Health Serv Res 2007;42(5):1848-70.

[23]   National Institutes of Health State-of-the-Science Conference Statement. "Improving End-of-Life Care and Outcomes" 2004 Dec 6-8;21(3):1-28. Accessed 2008 Oct 21. URL: http://consensus.nih.gov/2004/2004EndOfLifeCareSOS024PDF.pdf

[24]   Lacasse C, Beck SL. Clinical assessment of symptom clusters. Seminars in Oncology Nursing 2007;23(2):106-12.

[25]   Beck SL, Dudley WN, Barsevick A. Pain, sleep disturbance, and fatigue in patients with cancer: Using a mediation model to test a symptom cluster. Oncol Nurs Forum 2005;32(3):542.

[26]   Chen ML, Chang HK. Physical symptom profiles of depressed and nondepressed patients with cancer. Palliat Med 2004;18(8):712-8.

[27]   Lloyd-Williams M, Dennis M, Taylor F. A prospective study to determine the association between physical symptoms and depression in patients with advanced cancer. Palliat Med 2004;18(6):558-63.

[28]   Teunissen SC, de Graeff A, Voest EE, de Haes JC. Are anxiety and depressed mood related to physical symptom burden? A study in hospitalized advanced cancer patients. Palliat Med 2007;21(4):341-6.

[29]   Karnofsky DA, Abelmann WH, Craver LF, Burchenal JH. The use of the nitrogen mustards in the palliative treatment of carcinoma. With particular reference to bronchogenic carcinoma. Cancer 1948; 1(4):634-656.

[30]   Kent S, Bluthe RM, Kelly KW, Dantzer R. Sickness behaviour as a new target for drug development. Trends Pharmacol Sci 1992;13:24-9.

[31]   Cleeland CS, Bennett GJ, Dantzer R, Dougherty PM, Dunn AJ, Meyers CA, et al. Are the symptoms of cancer and cancer treatment due to a shared biologic mechanism? A cytokine-immunologic model of cancer symptoms. Cancer 2003;97(11):2919-25.

[32]   Lagman RL, Davis MP, LeGrand SB, Walsh D. Common symptoms in advanced cancer. Surg Clin North Am 2005;85(2):237-55.

[33]   MacDonald N. Cancer cachexia and targeting chronic inflammation: A unified approach to cancer treatment and palliative/supportive care. J Support Oncol 2007;5(4):157-62.

[34]   Dudgeon DJ, Lertzman M. Dyspnea in the advanced cancer patient. J Pain Symptom Manage 1998;16(4):212-9.

[35]   Dudgeon DJ, Lertzman M, Askew GR. Physiological changes and clinical correlations of dyspnea in cancer outpatients. J Pain Symptom Manage 2001;21(5):373-9.

[36]   Lawlor PG, Gagnon B, Mancini IL, Pereira JL, Hanson J, Suarez-Almazor ME, et al. Occurrence, causes, and outcome of delirium in patients with advanced cancer: A prospective study. Arch Intern Med 2000;160(6):786-94.

[37]   Twycross R, Back I. Nausea and vomiting in advanced cancer. Eur J Palliat Care 1998;5(2):39-45.

[38]   Mock V, Atkinson A, Barsevick A, Cella D, Cimprich B, Cleeland C, et al. National Comprehensive Cancer N. NCCN practice guidelines for cancer-related fatigue. Oncology (Williston) 2000;14(11A):151-61.

[39]   Stromgren AS, Goldschmidt D, Groenvold M, Petersen MA, Jensen PT, Pedersen L, et al. Self-assessment in cancer patients referred to palliative care: A study of feasibility and symptom epidemiology. Cancer 2002;94(2):512-7.

[40]   Chen ML, Lin CC. Cancer symptom clusters: a validation study. J Pain Symptom Manage 2007;34(6):590-9.

In: Advanced Cancer
Editors: N. Thavarajah, N. Pulenzas, B. Lechner et al.

ISBN: 978-1-62808-239-5
© 2013 Nova Science Publishers, Inc.

Chapter 25

Symptom clusters in patients with prostate cancer: A literature review

Nemica Thavarajah, BSc(C), Emily Chen, BSc(C),
Gillian Bedard, BSc(C), Natalie Lauzon, BSc MRT(T),
Michelle Zhou, BSc(C), Dominic Chu, MBBCh BAO(C)
and Edward Chow, MBBS[*]

Rapid Response Radiotherapy Program, Odette Cancer Centre,
Sunnybrook Health Sciences Centre, University of Toronto,
Toronto, Canada

Abstract

This chapter presents a review of the literature reporting empirically determined symptom clusters in prostate cancer patients. Methods: We conducted a literature search on symptom clusters in prostate cancer patients using EMBASE, MEDLINE, and CINAHL. Studies examining the presence of predetermined clusters were excluded. Two relevant studies published in 2008 were identified. Results: Both studies were longitudinal in nature and utilized cluster analysis to derive symptom clusters, while the first study, conducted by Maliski et al, used this in combination with three other statistical methods. Several clusters were identified in each study ranging from two to six symptoms per cluster. Maliski et al observed a combination of psychosocial and physical symptoms in patients receiving different types of prostate cancer treatments while the second study, conducted by Capp et al solely analyzed radiation-induced rectal symptoms across a time trajectory. Pain and bowel dysfunction were two symptoms commonly observed in both studies despite the lack of similar symptom clusters derived between the two studies. Differences in sample populations, assessment tools, symptoms observed, and analytical methods can account for discrepancies between the studies. Conclusion:

---

[*] Correspondence: Professor Edward Chow, MBBS, MSc, PhD, FRCPC, Department of Radiation Oncology, Odette Cancer Centre, Sunnybrook Health Sciences Centre, 2075 Bayview Avenue, Toronto, ON M4N 3M5, Canada. E-mail: Edward.Chow@sunnybrook.ca.

Further exploration in prostate cancer symptom cluster research will ideally facilitate efficient and effective symptom management in future clinical practice by improving patient outcomes and quality of life.

Introduction

Patients with cancer often experience an assortment of concurrent symptoms associated with their disease or treatment (1,2). These symptoms frequently predict changes in patient functioning, failures of treatment, post-therapeutic outcomes, and affect their overall quality of life (2). Symptoms can reflect cognitive sensations or biopsychosocial functioning of the patient and are a major component of morbidity in cancer care (3,4). Clinical evidence of patients frequently experiencing multiple symptoms simultaneously rather than in isolation has fostered the need for further research in symptom clusters (5,6).

Although there is no general consensus in the literature pertaining to what defines a symptom cluster, it is commonly described as two or more concurrent symptoms experienced by a patient. For instance, a symptom cluster may constitute of symptoms such as fatigue and pain. These symptoms, however, do not necessarily need to share the same etiology to be considered a cluster. Pain may arise from the progression of the disease itself whereas fatigue may arise as a side effect of systemic treatment (3,7).

Most research in the past has focused on single symptoms in isolation rather than focusing on concurrent symptoms and its deleterious effects on patient outcomes such as mood, physical functioning, and overall quality of life (3,7-9). Consequently, it is imperative that symptom clusters are continually derived and analyzed in symptom management research through longitudinal and cross-sectional study designs. Evaluating multiple symptoms can benefit health care practitioners, patients, and caregivers, as it provides information pertaining to the relationship between these symptoms, predictors of patient outcomes, and ideal interventions to manage specific symptom clusters (9).

Two different conceptual approaches are used in symptom cluster research to identify symptom clusters and evaluate the effect of multiple symptoms on patients. The first is an empirical approach that involves identifying symptom clusters by administering a symptom assessment tool. After collecting patients' ratings of the presence or absence and severity of symptoms, the results are analyzed using statistical procedures such as cluster or factor analysis. The second approach involves grouping cancer patients based on experiences of specific symptom clusters which are identified through a common underlying mechanism. Patients complete a questionnaire pertaining to these symptoms and are sorted into subgroups based on the severity of their experience with the symptom cluster (10).

Previous studies in symptom cluster research have focused largely on heterogeneous cancer populations. Focusing symptom cluster research in specific cancer populations may prove to be more beneficial in identifying common symptom clusters experienced by patients undergoing similar treatment modalities and disease progression. Identifying symptom clusters in homogeneous cancer populations may also aid in developing characterized treatment plans and forecasting potential symptoms experienced by patients (11, 12).

Prostate cancer is one of the most common cancers diagnosed among men and the incidence of prostate cancer has significantly increased in the past 20 years (13). Common symptoms experienced by prostate cancer patients include sexual dysfunction, urinary incontinence, and increased bowel symptoms (14). Typical treatments for prostate cancer can include one or a combination of treatments such as radiation therapy, brachytherapy, androgen-ablation therapy, cytotoxic chemotherapy, or a radical prostatectomy (15). As more men are being diagnosed with prostate cancer and survival rates are increasing, it is becoming progressively important to place a greater emphasis on improving the quality of life of prostate cancer patients. The main objective of this article is to provide a literature review of empirically determined symptom clusters in prostate cancer patients.

Literature review

A literature review was conducted using the EMBASE (1947 to week 46 of 2011), Ovid MEDLINE (1948 to November 2011), and CINAHL (1981 to November 2011) databases to examine studies reporting symptom clusters in prostate cancer patients at different stages of their disease. Search terms 'prostate cancer', 'prostate carcinoma', 'prostate neoplasm' or 'prostate tumor' were coupled with 'symptom cluster', 'concurrent symptoms', 'symptom constellations', co-occurring symptoms', symptom combinations', or 'multiple symptoms' to elicit relevant literature. Reference lists retrieved for these publications were also cross-referenced for further relevant articles.

The literature search revealed a total of 34 different articles from all three databases. Two reviewers screened abstracts of identified articles fitting the eligibility criteria in both an independent and duplicate manner. Only peer-reviewed articles statistically determining prostate cancer symptom clusters were included in this review. Studies examining predetermined symptom clusters, non-English studies, and studies involving a heterogeneous patient population were excluded.

Our findings

Two studies published in 2008 were identified, both of which empirically determined symptom clusters among prostate cancer patients (see table 1). (16-17). The primary endpoint of both studies was to determine symptom clusters in men treated for their prostate cancer; however, one study specifically examined longitudinal radiation-induced rectal symptoms among locally advanced prostate cancer patients (17).

Maliski et al explored symptom clusters among 402 men treated for prostate cancer at a large teaching medical center in the United States (16). Health-related quality of life surveys were administered at baseline as well as 1, 2, 4, 8, 12, 18, and 24 months after receiving a single or combination of treatments including external beam radiation therapy, surgery, and brachytherapy. The PCI-SF is a 15-item assessment tool utilized in this study which focuses on six domains: bowel function, sexual function, urinary function, bowel bother, sexual bother, and urinary bother. The second assessment tool used to assist in gathering symptom-related data experienced by prostate cancer patients was the Medical Outcomes Study Short Form, version 2 (SF-36). The SF-36 focuses on both physical and mental scores across eight multi-item subscales: social functioning, vitality, general health perceptions, pain, emotional well-being, physical functioning, role limitations related to emotional issues, and role limitations related to physical issues.

Maliski et al conducted four different symptom and patient-based analyses to derive symptom clusters as outlined in table 1 (16). Frequency and co-occurrence is a symptom-based analysis that involves distributing the PCI-SF and SF-36 into quartiles and identifying the frequency of specific symptoms in comparison to the remaining symptoms. Definite symptom clusters were not identified using this method as the researchers focused on a comparison of the frequency of specific symptoms with others individually. Correlations analysis is another symptom-based analysis which identifies symptoms that are highly correlated with others. Five symptom clusters were identified using this method, as outlined in table 1, in which fatigue commonly clustered with other symptoms in four out of five clusters. Factor analysis is also a symptom-based analysis which involves determining groups of highly correlated variables through the use of a covariance matrix and developing a factor solution.

This analysis revealed two significant clusters (cluster 1: fatigue, emotional distress; cluster 2: sexual dysfunction, bowel dysfunction, pain). Cluster analysis was the only patient-based analysis employed, and resulted in four distinct clusters, as outlined in Table 1. Sexual dysfunction was a key component of all four clusters derived through cluster analysis. The results of the four analyses concluded that fatigue and emotional distress were two symptoms that commonly clustered together. Furthermore, a strong correlation between sexual dysfunction and urinary dysfunction were expected as both symptoms are characteristic of prostate cancer treatment-related side effects.

Capp et al took on a unique approach by examining longitudinal radiation-induced rectal symptoms amongst 802 men with locally advanced prostate cancer at 18 different centers across Australia and New Zealand (17). Modified Litwin self-assessment questionnaires were distributed and Gastro-intestinal CTC scores (version 2) were collected from patients at baseline, end of radiotherapy, four monthly intervals for the first two years, and at six monthly intervals afterwards. The data collected specifically pertained to rectal symptoms including diarrhea, bowel frequency, mucus loss, bleeding, abdominal cramps, pain, looseness, and urgency.

The researchers utilized the cluster analysis approach when deriving symptom clusters for each time interval of data. Both pain and urgency were identified as key focal points of cluster composition. At immediate completion of radiotherapy, six prominent symptom clusters emerged and were characterized based on rectal symptoms experienced in patients, as illustrated in table 1. Pain dominated four out of the six symptom clusters identified (cluster 1: urgency, pain; cluster 2: cramps, pain, urgency; cluster 3: diarrhea, pain, bowel frequency, looseness; cluster 4: looseness, bowel frequency, mucus loss, blood; cluster 5: frequency, urgency, pain, mucus loss; cluster 6: urgency, mucus loss).

Due to the longitudinal nature of this study, symptoms were also categorized based on the severity as to which these symptom were expressed at each time interval. Four prominent symptom clusters were identified after one to three years of receiving radiation treatment (cluster 1: minimal occult bleeding, diarrhea, mucus loss; cluster 2: urgency, bowel frequency, looseness, bleeding; cluster 3: urgency, diarrhea, pain, mucus loss; cluster 4: urgency, bleeding, mucus loss).

Table 1. Studies identifying symptom clusters in prostate cancer patients

Study (year)	Design	Sample size (n)	Diagnosis	Analytical method	Symptom cluster	Associated symptoms
Maliski *et al.* (2008)	Longitudinal	402	Prostate cancer	Frequency and co-occurrence (symptom-based), correlations (symptom-based), factor analysis (symptom-based), cluster analysis (patient-based)	Correlations: Cluster 1 Cluster 2 Cluster 3 Cluster 4 Cluster 5 ------------------ Factor Analysis: Cluster 1 Cluster 2 ------------------ Cluster Analysis: Cluster 1 Cluster 2 Cluster 3 Cluster 4	Correlations: 1) sexual dysfunction, urinary dysfunction 2) sexual dysfunction, bowel dysfunction, emotional distress, fatigue, pain 3) urinary dysfunction, emotional distress, fatigue 4) fatigue, emotional distress 5) fatigue, pain ------------------------------------ Factor Analysis: 1) fatigue, emotional distress 2) sexual dysfunction, bowel dysfunction, pain ------------------------------------ Cluster Analysis: 1) pain, fatigue, sexual dysfunction 2) urinary dysfunction, sexual dysfunction 3) fatigue, emotional distress, sexual dysfunction 4) bowel dysfunction, sexual dysfunction

Table 1. (Continued)

Study (year)	Design	Sample size (n)	Diagnosis	Analytical method	Symptom cluster	Associated symptoms
Capp *et al.* (2008)	Longitudinal	802	Localized T2b,c, T3, T4, and N0M0 prostate cancer	Cluster analysis	End of Radiotherapy:	End of Radiotherapy:
					Cluster 1	1) urgency, pain
					Cluster 2	2) cramps, pain, urgency
					Cluster 3	3) diarrhea, pain, bowel frequency, looseness
					Cluster 4	4) looseness, bowel frequency, mucus loss, blood
					Cluster 5	5) frequency, urgency, pain, mucus loss
					Cluster 6	6) urgency, mucus loss
					------------------	------------------------------------
					1 to 3 Years After Radiotherapy	1 to 3 Years After Radiotherapy:
					Cluster 1	1) minimal occult bleeding, diarrhea, mucus loss
					Cluster 2	2) urgency, bowel frequency, looseness, bleeding
					Cluster 3	3) urgency, diarrhea, pain, mucus loss
					Cluster 4	4) urgency, bleeding, mucus

Urgency dominated three out of four of the symptom clusters derived. The results also revealed that patients exhibiting minimal symptoms at baseline also reported minimal symptoms at the end of radiotherapy treatment as well as three years following radiation. Capp et al. effectively demonstrated the multidimensional nature of radiation-induced rectal symptoms experienced by prostate cancer patients by incorporating the severity and dynamic pattern of symptoms expressed by patients over time.

Discussion

Symptom cluster research is a field of study of increasing importance, particularly within homogeneous patient populations. Limited information pertaining to the relationships between multiple concurrent symptoms associated with patient outcomes (including quality of life, functional status, and emotional wellbeing) are known to date (18). This is evident in prostate cancer symptom cluster research as only two studies, to our knowledge, exist concerning this particular patient population (16,17). Several disparities in symptom clusters derived in both studies are evident, making it difficult to formulate a general consensus of standard symptom clusters exhibited by prostate cancer patients. Varying definitions of symptom clusters, types of symptoms, analytical methods, assessment tools, and patient demographics can account for such discrepancies amongst the two studies.

Maliski et al identified symptom clusters based on two different methods: patient-based and symptom-based (16). A symptom-based approach typically yields symptom clusters based on symptoms that occur together most frequently whereas a patient-based approach group patients by their probability of experiencing certain symptoms. Maliski et al. analyzed a combination of psychosocial (i.e. emotional well-being, social functioning, health perceptions, etc.) and physical symptoms (i.e. sexual function, urinary function, bowel function, etc.) when formulating symptom clusters. Capp et al. adopted a more unconventional approach by incorporating the severity of each symptom experienced, as well as the symptoms that cluster together at specific time points (prior to treatment, at completion of treatment, and after one, two, and three years of completion) (17). The researchers for this study solely focused on rectal toxicities (i.e. diarrhea, urgency, abdominal cramps, etc.) when developing clusters, rather than psychosocial symptoms. This creates a large discrepancy in the clusters derived from each study as Maliski et al incorporated a combination of different quality of life issues whereas Capp et al solely focused on physical symptoms affecting quality of life, but in greater detail. Despite the lack of similar symptom clusters derived between the two studies, pain and bowel dysfunction were two symptoms commonly observed in both studies.

Population samples also varied amongst the two studies, which may alter the types of clusters that arise in patients. Maliski et al. included prostate cancer patients receiving a large range of different treatments such as brachytherapy, external beam radiation therapy, or surgery, and excluded patients receiving hormone ablation therapy (16). Capp et al (17) however focused on patients receiving radiotherapy treatment exclusively. Including a diverse population of prostate cancer patients undergoing any type of treatment may be beneficial in deriving prostate cancer symptom clusters for future studies as side effects and symptoms can vary depending on the type of treatment (i.e. surgery versus radiation).

Both studies were longitudinal in nature, as both involved collecting data from prostate cancer patients at several time intervals after receiving treatment (16,17). Longitudinal studies can be beneficial in symptom cluster research as it can account for varying symptom presentations over time. Capp et al acknowledged that the extent to which patients experience particular symptoms changes over time as they adapt and become sensitized to certain symptoms (17). Sensitization to symptoms could potentially lead to a different combination of symptoms expressed over time, resulting in the emergence of new symptom clusters.

Other studies focus solely on individual symptoms expressed by prostate cancer patients, rather than on multiple concurrent symptoms (19,20). Talcott et al identified bowel and bladder symptoms commonly occurring in men shortly after receiving radiotherapy, which eventually subsided after a year (19). Hanlon et al (20) also quantified both bladder and bowel quality of life symptoms in prostate cancer patients receiving radiotherapy. The results revealed that rectal urgency and bowel incontinence often resulted in a decreased quality of life in patients. These studies both demonstrated the dynamic nature of symptoms experienced by prostate cancer patients and its effect on overall quality of life. Despite the relevant findings of these types of studies, it is ideally beneficial to identify symptom clusters in this patient population for further practicality. Identifying prostate cancer symptom will aid in the development of characterized treatment plans and forecasting potential symptoms experienced by patients based on the nature of specific symptoms having the tendency to cluster together.

Further exploration in prostate cancer symptom cluster research is necessary to confidently establish clinically relevant findings. Based on the findings of the two reviewed literature, it would be recommended that future studies incorporate a diverse sample population of prostate cancer patients receiving a single or combination of different treatments including brachytherapy, external beam radiation, surgery, hormone therapy, chemotherapy, etc (16,17). Studies longitudinal in nature incorporating the observation of both psychosocial and physical symptoms will also aid in accounting for the dynamic presentation of concurrent symptoms in prostate cancer patients. Empirically determined prostate cancer symptom clusters will ideally facilitate more efficient and effective symptom management in future clinical practice and in turn improve patient outcomes and quality of life.

Acknowledgment

We thank the generous support of Bratty Family Fund, Michael and Karyn Goldstein Cancer Research Fund, Joseph and Silvana Melara Cancer Research Fund, and Ofelia Cancer Research Fund. We also thank Mr Henry Lam from Sunnybrook Library service in the literature search. The authors have no conflicts of interest to disclose.

References

[1] Chen ML, Tseng HC. Symptom clusters in cancer patients. Support Care Cancer 2006;8(14):825-30.

[2] Fan G, Filipczak L, Chow E. Symptom clusters in cancer patients: A review of the literature. Curr Oncol 2007;5(14):173-9.

[3] Dodd MJ, Miaskowski C, Paul SM. Symptom clusters and their effect on the functional status of patients with cancer. Semin Oncol Nurs 2010;26(3):168-74.

[4] Wang XS, Fairlough DL, Liao Z, Komaki R, Chang JY, Mobley GM, Cleeland CS. Longitudinal study of the relationship between chemoradiation therapy for non-small cell lung cancer and patient symptoms. J Clin Oncol 2006;24(27):4485-91.

[5] Miaskowski C. Symptom clusters: establishing the link between clinical practice and symptom management research. Support Care Cancer 2006;14:792-4.

[6] Kim E, Jahan T, Aouizerat BE, et al. Differences in symptom clusters identified using occurrence rates versus symptom severity ratings in patients at the end of radiation therapy. Cancer Nurs 2009;32(6):429-36.

[7] Dodd MJ, Miaskowski C, Lee KA. Occurrence of symptom clusters. J Natl Cancer Inst Monogr 2004;32:76-8.

[8] Glover J, Miaskowski C, Dibble S, Dodd MJ. Mood states of oncology outpatients: does pain make a difference? J Pain Symptom Manage 1995;10(2):120-8.

[9] Miaskowski C, Dodd MJ, Lee KA. Symptom clusters: the new frontier in symptom management research. J Natl Cancer Inst Monogr 2004;32:17-21.

[10] Miaskowski C, Aouizerat BE, Dodd MJ, Coope B. Conceptual issues in symptom clusters research and their implications for quality-of-life assessment in patients with cancer. J Natl Cancer Inst Monogr 2007;37:39-46.

[11] Gift AG. Symptom clusters related to specific cancers. Semin Oncol Nurs 2007;23(2):136-41.

[12] Bender CM, Ergyn FS, Rosenzweig MQ, et al. Symptom clusters in breast cancer across 3 phases of the disease. Cancer Nurs 2005;28:219-25.

[13] Yin M, Bastacky S, Chandran U, Becich MJ, Dhir R. Prevalence of incidental prostate cancer in the general population: a study of healthy organ donors. J Urol 2008;179(3):892-5.

[14] Talcott JA, Manola J, Clark JA, et al. Time course and predictors of symptoms after primary prostate cancer therapy. J Clin Oncol 2003;21(21):3979-86.

[15] Denmeade SR, Isaacs JT. A history of prostate cancer treatment. Nat Rev Cancer 2002;2(5):389-96.

[16] Maliski SL, Kwan L, Elashoff D, Litwin MS. Symptom clusters related to treatment for prostate cancer. Oncol Nurs Forum 2008;35(5):786-93.

[17] Capp A, Inostroza-Ponta M, Bill D, et al. Is there more than one proctitis syndrome? A revisitation using data from the TROG 96.01 trial. Radiother Oncol 2009;90(3):400-7.

[18] Gilbertson-White S, Aouizerat BE, Miaskowski C. A review of the literature on multiple symptoms, their predictors, and associated outcomes in patients with advanced cancer. Palliat Support Care 2011;9(1):81-102.

[19] Talcott JA, Rieker P, Clark JA, et al. Patient-reported symptoms after primary therapy for early prostate cancer: results of a prospective cohort study. J Clin Oncol 1998;16(1):275-83.

[20] Hanlon AL, Bruner DW, Peter R, Hanks GE. Quality of life study in prostate cancer patients treated with three-dimensional conformal radiation therapy: comparing late bowel and bladder quality of life symptoms to that of the normal population. Int J Radiat Oncol Biol Phys 2001;49(1):51-9.

In: Advanced Cancer
Editors: N. Thavarajah, N. Pulenzas, B. Lechner et al.

ISBN: 978-1-62808-239-5
© 2013 Nova Science Publishers, Inc.

Chapter 26

Dedicated out-patient palliative radiation treatment clinics for patients with advanced cancer

Justin Kwong, BSc(C), Florencia Jon, MRTT*, Lori Holden, MRTT, Liang Zeng, BSc(C), Shaelyn Culleton, BSc(C), Cyril Danjoux, MD, May Tsao, MD, Elizabeth Barnes, MD, Arjun Sahgal, MD, Kristopher Dennis, MD and Edward Chow, MBBS

Rapid Response Radiotherapy Program, Department of Radiation Oncology,
Odette Cancer Centre, Sunnybrook Health Sciences Centre,
University of Toronto, Toronto, Canada

Abstract

Quality of life for advanced cancer patients is of utmost importance. To address this concern, eight cancer centres across Canada have established palliative radiotherapy clinics dedicated to providing rapid access to radiotherapy for patients suffering from debilitating symptoms. The first of such clinics was the Rapid Response Radiotherapy Program (RRRP), established in 1996 at Toronto Sunnybrook Odette Cancer Centre. Since then, there has been much progress in initiating similar programs elsewhere across Canada, but a current detailed summary of their status is lacking. This report reviews and summarizes the emergence and current status of rapid access palliative radiotherapy programs in Canada and a similar specialized clinic in Australia since the time of their inception.

---

* Correspondence: Florencia Jon, BSc, MRT(T), Department of Radiation Therapy, Sunnybrook Odette Cancer Centre, 2075 Bayview Ave, Toronto, Ontario, M4N 3M5 Canada. Tel: 416-480-6100 ext.7543; Fax: 416-480-6002; E-mail: Florencia.Jon@sunnybrook.ca.

Introduction

In patients with advanced cancer, palliative radiotherapy is a useful modality for improving quality of life. It plays a significant role in alleviating symptoms such as dyspnea, bleeding, hemoptysis, neurologic deficits, and most commonly, pain. In Europe and North America, approximately 50% of prescribed radiotherapy treatments for cancer patients are palliative in nature (1).

Typically in Canada, the interval between referral and initiation of treatment may be several weeks (2). For potentially curative cases, Canadian Association of Radiation Oncology (CARO) has established a policy that consultation with a radiation oncologist should take place no more than 2 weeks after referral and treatment should start within 10 working days after consultation, therefore a wait of up to 4 weeks is generally acceptable (3,4). However, for terminally-ill patients, such an extended wait is unacceptable as these patients have limited life expectancy and are usually suffering from debilitating symptoms; most commonly bone pain.

From 1986 to 1995, only one quarter of patients who died of cancer in Ontario had ever received palliative radiotherapy (4). This suggests that the significance and potential role of palliative radiation for patients with advanced cancer had been underappreciated or that resources limited efforts to provide appropriate radiotherapy in this setting.

In Canada, with an increased demand for radiotherapy and inadequate radiotherapy resources waitlists for patients became inevitable and rapid access to palliative radiotherapy was a problem (3). Patients with limited life expectancy who require urgent radiation were expected to wait alongside patients with curative cancers. At the 1996 Canadian symposium on palliative radiotherapy, it was concluded that the establishment of a separate radiotherapy clinic devoted to rapidly assessing, planning and treating symptomatic patients in the same day was an excellent method of managing the needs of palliative patients.

This article details the emergence and status of rapid response radiotherapy clinics in Canada with some selected information published by their groups for context.

Our search

We conducted a Medline search for reports related to palliative radiotherapy programs throughout Canada. Search terms included "radiotherapy", "irradiation", "radiation treatment", "palliative", "care", "clinic", "program", "rapid", "fast", "track", "response", "access" and "symptom". Secondary search terms included "brain metastases" and "bone metastases", "pain" and "waiting time".

The search results were manually reviewed. Information regarding history and current status of each palliative radiotherapy clinic was extracted. Research results that had indications for the progress and awareness of rapid access palliative radiotherapy were also extracted. Abstracts from articles returned in the search were reviewed and those with rapid access palliative radiotherapy clinics were selected for full article review.

Our findings

The Sunnybrook Odette Cancer Centre Rapid Response Radiotherapy Program (RRRP)

Soon after the aforementioned 1996 Canadian symposium on palliative radiotherapy, Canada's first rapid response radiotherapy program (RRRP) was established in Toronto at the Sunnybrook Odette Cancer Centre. The goal of this clinic was to provide timely palliative radiotherapy within a week of referral and to decrease the number of clinic visits needed for patients (1).

Upon initiation of the RRRP in June 1996, the clinic ran for 2 half-days and was staffed by 2 radiation oncologists, 1 nurse and 1 radiation therapist. By July 1998, the Sunnybrook RRRP expanded to include a total of 4 radiation oncologists, 1 nurse and 1 radiation therapist. The number of clinics was increased to 3.5 per week. Today, the RRRP clinic runs 5 times per week and is staffed by 5 radiation oncologists, 5 nurses, 1 advanced practice radiation therapist, 1 palliative radiation therapist and 1 research assistant. The nurses and radiation therapists coordinate to maintain the efficient booking of patients and timely transition for patients from consultation to radiation planning to treatment delivery (2). The research assistant is responsible for maintaining the overall flow of the clinic and accruing patients to clinical trials.

As part of the referral screening procedure, patients referred to the RRRP were to have an estimated survival of less than 12 months and were scheduled to be seen within 3 working days of referral. All relevant imaging and information were to accompany the patient at consultation. Patients could expect to be assessed and treated on the same day if indicated. Following an appointment with a patient, the radiation oncologist would fax an assessment and management note to the referring physician detailing the case disposition to avoid delays in communication due to transcription (1). Since its inception, the RRRP has helped streamline patient referrals and treatment for patients suffering from end-stage symptoms (5).

In July 1998, the RRRP completed a study in which a referring physician satisfaction survey was mailed out to all physicians who had referred at least one patient to the RRRP between January 1996 and June 1998 (1). Of the 126 referring physicians, most of which were in community practice in the Greater Toronto and neighbouring catchment areas, 64 completed the questionnaire. This corresponded to a response rate of 51%. There was a higher response rate for physicians who referred 10 or more patients compared to physicians who referred less than 5 patients. 33% of responding physicians reported having referred more patients for palliative radiotherapy since the establishment of the RRRP. Most of the referring physicians (75%) reported being "very" or "extremely satisfied" with the service provided by the RRRP. Reasons for referral reported by physicians included: quick access to treatment (70%), satisfaction with services provided (59%), generally refer to Toronto Sunnybrook Regional Cancer Centre (48%), proximity to patient's residence (47%) and patient's preference (27%). The survey also indicated some areas of potential improvement for the program. Referring physicians mentioned weaknesses of the program, including poor accessibility to palliative-care service in general, difficulty in contacting radiation oncologists, poor communication of case dispositions to the referring physician and the extended delay for a dictated consult note to reach the referring physician (1).

The RRRP team took steps to enhance awareness of palliative radiotherapy by coordinating outreach educational sessions at local hospitals and community facilities. As well, information packages, which included indications for palliative radiotherapy, directions to Sunnybrook, and RRRP referral forms, were distributed to family physicians and community health care providers. To ensure that referring physicians and palliative care specialists were well-informed regarding RRRP activity and research, a quarterly newsletter entitled "Hot Spot" was distributed to referring physicians, family practitioners, palliative health-care workers and local health-care institutions (2).

A previous retrospective review by Danjoux et al (5) summarized the RRRP clinic activity from 1996-2003. A total of 3290 patients were referred to the RRRP within the study period. There was an increase in number of cases from 200 cases annually from 1996 to 1997 to over 500 cases annually from 2000 to 2002. There was a slight dip in the number of cases seen in 2003, at 480 cases due to SARS. It was found that the overall median interval from referral to consultation was 8 days, with a range from 5 to 11 days. Sixty percent of patients seen were consulted, planned and treated on the same day of initial consultation. The most common reason for referral was painful bone metastases which was present in 70% of patients (5).

To update previous research, a retrospective review of the RRRP between 2004 to 2008 was conducted by De Sa et al (6). The RRRP had 3267 referrals within the study period. It was found that the overall median interval from referral to consultation was 4 days, confirming an improved referral system from the 1996 to 2003 review (8 days). Over eighty percent of patients were simulated and treated within 7 days of initial consultation. The most common reason for referral was painful bone metastases in 52.4% of patients (6).

The success of the RRRP has instigated the inception of the Bone Metastases Clinic at the Sunnybrook Odette Cancer Centre (7). In January 1999, the RRRP along with the Division of Orthopedics at Sunnybrook Health Sciences Centre initiated this clinic to provide a multidisciplinary approach to the care of advanced cancer patients with bone metastases. The staff for this clinic include radiation oncologists, orthopaedic surgeons, nurses, radiation therapists, pharmacists and interventional radiologists. Similar to the RRRP, the goals of this clinic are to improve efficiency in consulting and treating symptomatic patients (7).

Ongoing research at the RRRP

The RRRP acts as a hub for researchers to collect patient data and accrue patients to clinical trials. Since its inception, the number of studies conducted has continuously increased. Currently, every patient in the RRRP is assessed for eligibility into a clinical trial. There are currently 10 open clinical trials accruing patients from the RRRP. As well, baseline data and case disposition for every patient consulted in the clinic is recorded into a prospective database by a research assistant. This database has acted as a rich resource for publications.

Other cancer centers across Canada have since developed programs similar to the RRRP. Although each centre has adopted its own unique model, the central theme remains to provide rapid access radiotherapy for palliative patients. In Canada, there are currently 8 established rapid response radiotherapy clinics distributed in the provinces of Alberta, Ontario, British Columbia and Quebec.

Ottawa Hospital Rapid Palliative Radiotherapy Program (RPRP) (Ottawa, Ontario)

The RPRP was established at the Ottawa Regional Cancer Centre in 1999 to provide palliative radiotherapy for symptomatic patients with advanced cancer. A retrospective audit revealed that from 1999 to 2001, painful bone metastases were present in 81% of all patients referred to the program and they were the most common reason for referral. The audit also revealed that by 2001, only 19 out of 148 patients treated by the RPRP were referred by family physicians (8). Subsequently, a study was conducted to assess the awareness of the RPRP and the perceptions of the efficacy of palliative radiotherapy amongst family practitioners in Eastern Ontario (8). A 30-item survey was distributed to 400 randomly selected family physicians in Eastern Ontario. Only 31 responders (18%) were aware of the RPRP and only 15 responders (9%) had previously referred patients to the RPRP

However, 96 responders (56%) reported having referred patients for palliative radiotherapy outside of the RPRP. Of the 172 responders, 149 (87%) reported having been involved with the care of patients with advanced cancer and 138 responders (80%) reported providing palliative care for their patients on a regular basis (8). The survey also identified that family physicians were significantly more likely to refer to the RPRP were those who had previously sought advice from a radiation oncologist and physicians who had provided palliative care for patients (8).

The results from the survey suggested that the underutilization of the RPRP by family physicians in Eastern Ontario was partially due to a lack of awareness of the program itself, uncertainty of the benefits of radiotherapy (55%) and perceptions of extended wait times for cons ultation and treatment (55%). More than 30% of responders were unaware of the efficacy of radiotherapy in patients with malignant spinal cord compression, hematuria or hemoptysis. This may indicate that previous awareness programs had been unsuccessful and investigation into new methods of informing family practitioners may be necessary. The survey revealed that 86% of responders were interested in attending education tutorials on radiation oncology (8).

Princess Margaret Hospital Palliative Radiation Oncology Program (PROP) (Toronto, ON)

The PROP at the Princess Margaret hospital is dedicated to providing palliative radiotherapy to symptomatic advanced cancer patients, with a specific focus on bone and brain metastases and incurable lung tumours. Approximately 450 patients per year are served by the program and about 50% of the patients are referred for painful bone metastases (9). Patients are seen within 2 weeks of referral, unless the request is marked urgent in which case the patient is seen in less than a week. Each clinic is staffed by a radiation oncologist and advanced practice nurse (RN) case manager; specialists are involved as necessary (10).

The sequence in which the patient is consulted is highly structured; first, the RN assesses the patient, taking notes of the patient's current medication. As well, the RN gives the patient the Edmonton Symptom Assessment System (ESAS) which is a questionnaire that assesses the severity of 9 symptoms the patient may be experiencing; 6 of which are physical and 3 psychological (11). Afterwards, the radiation oncologist, together with the RN, assesses the patient and reviews the patient's chart and medical and psychosocial history. Appropriate recommendations for palliative treatment, education, counselling and necessary referrals are provided to the patient. A complete note is dictated by the Radiation Oncologist and is faxed to the patient's family physician and oncologist (10).

Tom Baker Cancer Centre Fast Track Clinic (Calgary, Alberta)

In 2002, the Fast Track Clinic was established at the Tom Baker Cancer Centre in Calgary, Alberta to provide rapid access radiotherapy to advanced cancer patients with painful bone metastases. A patterns-of-practice audit was later performed to evaluate the impact of the rapid access clinic. The retrospective review consisted of a cohort of patients who had radiographic confirmation of bone metastases and were first-time users of palliative radiotherapy. From 2003 to 2005, 275 patients initially received palliative RT at the rapid access clinic (12). Results of the study demonstrated that elderly (>80 years old) and out of area patients (>50 km from cancer centre) were at a disadvantage to accessing radiotherapy, which was consistent with other studies (12). The most significant result found was that patients initially treated through the Fast Track clinic returned for more courses of palliative radiotherapy at a significantly higher rate than patients assessed and treated through a routine clinical care pathway (12).

Cross Cancer Institute Rapid Access Palliative Radiotherapy Program (RAPRP) (Edmonton, Alberta)

In July 2006, the RAPRP was established to provide palliative radiotherapy to advanced cancer patients with painful bone metastases. Patients are referred not only from Alberta, but also from British Columbia, Saskatchewan and the Northwest Territories. As such, the RAPRP is considered to have one of the largest catchment areas amongst all palliative radiotherapy clinics in Canada (13).

The RAPRP staffs include a radiation oncologist, a registered nurse (RN), nurse practitioner, clinical pharmacist, radiation therapist, occupational therapist, social worker and registered dietician. For each patient, a clinic day would last approximately 4 to 6 hours. Initially, the RN would orient the patient to the clinic. Either the registered nurse, pharmacist or radiation therapist would administer screening tools. The pharmacist would then investigate the patient's medication history. The nurse practitioner along with the radiation oncologist would assess the patient for suitability for radiotherapy. Multidisciplinary consultation with an occupational therapist, social worker or registered dietician would be conducted if necessary. Simulation of radiotherapy would then be conducted by the radiation oncologist and radiation therapist. Lastly, meal break for patients while radiotherapy is planned, radiotherapy delivery, survey completion and telephone follow-up after radiation treatment would be supervised by the radiation therapist (14). Currently, the program runs 1 day a week and may accommodate up to 4 patients per day but has been averaging 2 or 3 patients (13).

A 25-week pilot phase from January 2007 to June 2007 was conducted in which patients eligible for single-fraction radiotherapy were consulted and treated on the same day. There were 86 patients referred to the RAPRP over the pilot period and 58 of them were considered for radiotherapy and assessed in clinic. The median duration from referral to clinic visit was 5 days, although it ranged from 0 to 20 days (14).

The average reported patient-rated pain improved from 6.1/10 to 2.6/10 (10 being the worst pain) from baseline to 4 weeks post radiotherapy, respectively. As well, patients describing severe pain decreased from 34% to 3% from baseline to 4 weeks post radiotherapy, respectively. After the 4 week period, the average number of symptoms, as measured by ESAS, decreased from 6.2 to 5.2 and more than 75% of patients reported that all their symptoms were stabilized or improved (14). All patients reported being satisfied with their experience and recommended the RAPRP clinic to other patients who had a similar condition (14).

Mater Centre Rapid Response Palliative Radiotherapy Clinic (RRPRC) (South Brisbane, Queensland, Australia)

According to guidelines from the Royal Australian and New Zealand College of Radiologists, the ideal wait time for palliative patients is no more than 2 days. With this in mind, the RRPRC was established in 2005 at the Mater Centre of Princess Alexandra Hospital in South Brisbane, Queensland, Australia.

The clinic was established based on the Canadian model of a specialized palliative radiotherapy clinic. Goals of the clinic include providing efficient palliative radiotherapy to patients with a prognosis of less than 18 months, reducing suffering and number of clinic visits for patients, delivering same-day consultation and treatment, providing community palliative support, and developing an academic basis for research in palliative radiotherapy (15).

Before initiating the clinic, a 6-month pilot study was conducted to compare 2 palliative patient groups; those seen in RRPRC and those seen in non-RRPRC at the Mater Centre. Data, including patient, referral and treatment details, was collected from 292 patients, 78 of which were seen in the RRPRC (15). Results showed that that RRPRC patients were more likely to be treated within 24 hours (74% RRPRC, 27% Non-RRPRC) and receive a single fraction of treatment (65% RRPRC, 42.6% Non-RRPRC). With these findings, it was confirmed that this clinic successfully provided timely and efficient radiotherapy for palliative patients (15).

Today, the clinic is functional every Thursday for 5 hours. The staff consists of a radiation oncologist, radiation oncology nurse, occupational therapist, radiation therapist and clinical trial coordinator. When feasible, patients are consulted, planned and treated on the same day.

Telephone follow-up is conducted 2 weeks post-treatment by the clinic nurse. A 4-week clinic follow-up is also offered. For research purposes, a prospective database is updated with patient information and patients are continuously accrued to clinical trials (15). The RRPRC continues to act as a model for other palliative radiotherapy clinics in Australia.

Discussion

Since the establishment of the first dedicated rapid response palliative radiotherapy clinic in 1996 in Canada, there has been a limited amount of published literature on the collective progress of such clinics across Canada. Within the research published, there have been many indications which suggest an increased need for palliative radiotherapy in the future. The establishment of dedicated palliative radiotherapy clinics has been shown to reduce wait times and achieve considerable satisfaction from both patients and physicians (1,14,16). Despite these findings, the use of palliative radiotherapy in Canada is generally underutilized (4,17). According to a study conducted by Fitzgibbon et al (16), this may be explained by a knowledge gap which may exist between potential referring physicians and radiation oncologists. As demonstrated by the survey of family physicians in Eastern Ontario, family physicians may be unaware of palliative radiotherapy programs, uncertain of palliative radiotherapy benefits and may have perceptions of extended wait times for consultation and treatment (18).

As 86% of responders were interested in attending radiation oncology tutorials, educational seminars may be an effective way to reduce this knowledge gap and dispel misconceptions on palliative radiotherapy, ultimately increasing utilisation (8). The Sunnybrook RRRP actively promotes its program by offering outreach educational sessions and half-day educational elective courses and distributing an information package and a quarterly newsletter "Hotspot" to palliative care workers and physicians. The RRRP is also listed in the directory of Palliative Information Services of the Metropolitan Toronto Palliative Care Council (2). This focus on awareness may have contributed to the RRRP's success in being able to consult on average, over 500 patients per year from 2004 to 2008 (6).

Despite the considerable benefits of palliative radiotherapy clinics as outlined above, there are some limitations of these programs as well as potential conflicts they create with other oncology services that warrant comment here. The establishment of rapid response palliative radiotherapy clinics, while reducing radiation treatment wait time for symptomatic patients with advanced cancer, may in fact increase radiation treatment wait times for patients seeking potentially curative radiation. Because of the finite amount of radiation oncologists, associated staff, clinic rooms, treatment machines and computed tomography (CT) simulation machines, allocating resources to patients with terminal cancers then takes away from patients who could be receiving curative therapy. With this dilemma, cancer programs are faced with the challenge to strike a balance between improving the quality of life for terminal cancer patients and increasing the probability of curing cancer patients. Increasing the radiation treatment waiting time for curable cancer patients increases the probability for the cancer to metastasize to other areas of the body, which may deem the patient incurable.

Allocating resources to palliative radiotherapy may also put a strain on overall resources in the long run. With curative patients having to wait a longer time for treatment, their disease may progress which in turn creates an even greater demand for treatment. This unnecessary demand for treatment could have been prevented if the cancer had been treated at an earlier stage. Also, as indicated by a study by Wu et al., patients who attended a rapid access palliative radiotherapy clinic returned for retreatment more often than those who followed a regular care pathway (12). This finding may indicate that providing short term, less complicated doses of radiation may in fact have an impact on resource utilization.

The establishment of rapid access palliative radiotherapy clinics also may not necessarily increase the overall number of patients receiving palliative radiotherapy because patients may also receive this service through a primary tumour-site specific clinical care pathway (12). The nature of the rapid access palliative radiotherapy clinic may also not be cost effective. Because patients may have a CT simulation performed immediately after consultation, some clinics, such as the RRRP, have a dedicated CT simulation machine reserved for urgent palliative radiotherapy patients. In having a reserved CT simulation machine, it is possible for there to be a lag in flow in between consultation and CT scanning in which the CT simulation machine is left unused for extended periods of time in between patient consultations. There is also the challenge of coordinating the same day treatment in treatment units that are already overbooked.

Our current review is also limited by the information available in the literature. The setting of the rapid access clinics may have changed since the publication of the experience. Readers are cautioned to check the latest update from the corresponding clinics.

Conclusion

Since the establishment of urgent palliative radiotherapy at Sunnybrook Hospital, 7 other specialised rapid access radiotherapy clinics have been developed in Canada and one in Australia from our literature search. Although each clinic varies slightly in their focus and structure, they all have the same goal of providing timely palliative radiotherapy for symptomatic patients with advanced cancer. With the substantial success seen at Toronto Sunnybrook's RRRP, other cancer programs across Canada have modeled their palliative radiotherapy clinics in a similar fashion. Outside of Canada, clinics such as the RRPRC in Australia have followed suit (15). Referral to urgent palliative radiotherapy clinics has been documented to successfully decrease wait times and provide prompt treatment for terminal-phase advanced cancer patients. This has achieved satisfaction from both patients and physicians (1,14,16). To maximize the potential for providing urgent palliative radiotherapy in Canada, further steps are required to improve the awareness of urgent palliative radiotherapy amongst potential referring physicians.

Acknowledgments

We thank Dr. Jackson Wu and Mrs. Stacy Yuen for assistance. This study was supported by the Michael and Karyn Goldstein Cancer Research Fund.

References

[1]   Chow E, Wong R, Vachon M, Connolly R, Andersson L, Szumacher E et al. Referring physicians' satisfaction with the rapid response radiotherapy program. Support Care Cancer 2000;8:405-9.

[2]   Danjoux C, Szumacher E, Andersson L, Franssen E, Wong R, Chow E et al. Palliative radiotherapy at Toronto-Sunnybrook Regional Cancer Centre: The Rapid Response Radiotherapy Program. Curr Oncol 2000;7:52-6.

[3]   Wait time alliance member assessments of 10 – year plan to strengthen health care. Wait time alliance for timely access to health care Spring 2008;pp1-15. Accessed 2010 Oct18. URL:http://www. waititmealliance.ca/images/Spring2008/WTA-Assessment-Report-EN.pdf.

[4]   MacKillop WJ, Zhou Y, Quirt CF. A comparison of delays in the treatment of cancer with radiation in Canada and the United States. Int J Radiat Oncol Biol Phys 1995;32:531-9.

[5]   Danjoux C, Chow E, Drossos A, Holden L, Hayter C, Tsao M et al. An innovative rapid response radiotherapy program to reduce waiting time for palliative radiotherapy. Support Care Cancer 2006; 14:38-43.

[6]   De Sa E, Sinclair E, Mitera G, Wong J, Danjoux C, Hird A et al. Continued success of the rapid response radiotherapy program: a review of 2004-2008. Support Care Cancer 2009;7:757-62.

[7]   Chow E, Finkelstein J, Connolly R, Andersson L, Pope J, Axelrod T et al. New combined bone metastases clinic: the ultimate one-stop for cancer patients with bone metastases. Curr Oncol 2000;7:205-8.

[8]   Huang J, Zhou S, Groome P, Tyldesley S, Zhang-Solomans J, Mackillop WJ. Factors affecting the use of palliative radiotherapy in Ontario. J Clin Oncol 2001;19:137-44.

[9]   Haddad P, Wong RKS, Pond GR, Soban F, Williams D, McLean M et al. Factors influencing the use of single vs multiple fractions of palliative radiotherapy for bone metastases: a 5-year review. Clin Oncol 2005;1716:430-4.

[10]   Zimmerman C, Seccareccia D, Clarke A, Warr D, Rodin G. Bringing palliative care to a Canadian cancer center: the palliative care program at Princess Margaret Hospital. Support Care Cancer 2006;14:982-7.

[11]   Bruera E, Kuehn N, Miller MJ, Selmser P, Macmillan K. The Edmonton Symptom Assessment System (ESAS): a simple method of assessment of palliative care patients. J Pall Care 1991;7:6-9.

[12]   Wu J, Kerba M, Wong R, McKimmon E, Eigl B, Hagen NA. Patterns of practice in palliative radiotherapy for painful bone metastases: impact of a regional rapid access clinic on access to care. Int J Radiat Oncol Biol Phys 2010;78(2):533-8.

[13]   New radiotherapy streamlines access for bone metastases patients. Accessed 2010 Aug18. URL:.http://ww.cancerboard.ab.ca/Research/OurResearchers/ResearchStories /Bone%20Metastases

[14]   Fairchild A, Pituskin E, Rose B, Ghosh S, Dutka J, Driga A et al. The rapid access palliative radiotherapy program: blueprint for initiation of a one-stop multidisciplinary bone metastases clinic. Support Care Cancer 2009;17:163-70.

[15]   Holt TR, Yau VKY. Innovative program for palliative radiotherapy in Australia. J Med Imaging Radiat Oncol 2010;54:76-81.

[16]   Fitzgibbon EJ, Samant R, Meng J, Graham ID. Awareness and use of the Rapid Palliative Radiotherapy Program by family physicians in Eastern Ontario: a survey. Curr Oncol 2006;13:27-32.

[17]   Samant R. How should we describe the benefits of palliative radiotherapy? Curr Oncol 2006;13:230-4.

[18]   Barnes EA, Hanson J, Neumann CM, Nekoliachuk L, Bruera E. Communication between primary care physician and radiation oncologists regarding patients with cancer treated with palliative radiotherapy. J Clin Oncol 2000;18(15):2902-7.

In: Advanced Cancer ISBN: 978-1-62808-239-5
Editors: N. Thavarajah, N. Pulenzas, B. Lechner et al. © 2013 Nova Science Publishers, Inc.

Chapter 27

Needs assessment of patients and their caregivers

Luluel Khan, MD, Sarah Hugh, Shah Ansari, Andrew Chiang, MD, Liang Zeng, BSc, Roseanna Presutti, BSc , Gunita Mitera, PhD, Liying Zhang, PhD, Elizabeth Barnes, MD, Cyril Danjoux, MD, Arjun Sahgal, MD, Edward Chow, MBBS and May Tsao*, MD

Rapid Response Radiotherapy Program, Department of Radiation Oncology, Odette Cancer Centre, Sunnybrook Health Sciences Centre, University of Toronto, Toronto, Ontario, Canada

The purpose of this chapter was to perform a needs assessment within a palliative radiotherapy clinic in patients and their caregivers. Specifically, the study sought to answer the following questions: 1) what were the met and unmet needs of patients with bone and brain metastases undergoing palliative radiotherapy as perceived by patients and their caregivers; 2) was there good inter rater reliability between the two groups. Methods: Twenty patients and 20 caregivers participated in the study by completing a questionnaire based on the Problems and Needs in Palliative Care – short version (PNPC-sv) tool. Quantitative statistical analysis was performed on the data to determine the most frequent identified and unmet patient needs of patients and caregivers. Percent agreement and Kappa Cohen statistics were calculated to assess concordance. Results: Patients identified fatigue and pain as the most pressing concerns whilst care givers identified loss of autonomy and psychosocial concerns as their primary concerns. There was very good to moderate agreement for the 10 most commonly identified problems between patients and care givers. Conclusion: Identification of patient and care giver met and unmet needs can facilitate appropriate timely referral to specialized palliative care and psychosocial oncology which can minimize patient distress and improve quality of life.

---

* Correspondence: May Tsao, MD, Department of Radiation Oncology, Odette Cancer Centre, Sunnybrook Health Sciences Centre, 2075 Bayview Avenue, Toronto, ON M4N 3M5, Canada. Tel: 416-480-4806; Fax: 416-480-6002; E-mail: may.tsao@sunnybrook.ca.

Introduction

Physical distress in patients with advanced disease is one of the most consistent predictors of depression and other manifestations of psychological distress (1). Apart from the physical ramifications of advanced disease the significant social, economic and psychological impact of such disease has been exhaustively studied and made clear. Palliative care aims to positively impact quality of life (QOL) for patients with incurable illnesses through management of pain, physical and psychosocial distress (2). Many of these distressing symptoms are not reported by patients with advanced disease unless specific enquiry is made (3). By identifying the met and unmet needs of palliative care patients, and anticipating future needs of these patients, better quality of care is achievable.

Identifying these states can often be difficult during oncology clinic visits due to oncologists' time constraints, discomfort and frequent lack of experience in responding to emotional reactions. Further, some patients minimize distress or are reluctant to disclose psychological symptoms because they fear being judged as weak or inadequate or because they are unaware of the availability of treatment for them. Recent observations highlight that humans are fundamentally relational in nature and that social relatedness is an essential dimension of physical and psychological well-being (4). There is also abundant evidence that the perception of social support protects the emotional well-being of individuals facing cancer or other stressful life circumstances (5). In the palliative care setting in particular, patient perceptions of end of life QOL are greatly influenced by their relationships with their caregivers, families and close friends. As a result the identification of the met and unmet needs of patients from the perspective of patients and their caregivers is crucial to the needs assessment of a palliative clinic. As aforementioned the time constraints of a traditional oncologic practice to elucidate these needs is frequently not present in the palliative clinic.

The purpose of this paper was to perform a needs assessment within a palliative radiotherapy clinic, among palliative radiotherapy patients and their caregivers. Specifically, the study sought to answer the following questions: 1) what were the met and unmet needs of patients with bone and brain metastases undergoing palliative radiotherapy as perceived by patients and their caregivers; 2) was there good inter rater reliability between the two groups?

Our study

The Rapid Response Radiotherapy Program (RRRP) within Department of Radiation Oncology at the Odette Cancer Centre at the Sunnybrook Health Sciences Centre was established in 1996. The RRRP is an outpatient clinic that provides timely access to palliative radiation for cancer patients. Between 2003 and 2006, the median time from referral to treatment at RRRP was 6 days down from 49 days in 1996. Most patients are simulated and treated on the day of their initial consultation to help provide quick symptom relief and improve patient quality of life.

Study population

The study population consisted of 20 patients who had advanced cancer, who were referred to RRRP for the treatment of symptomatic bone and brain metastases as well as their caregivers. "Caregivers" was defined as those who accompanied the patient to clinic and met at least one of the following criteria: (1) lived with the patient, (2) first degree relative of the patient or (3) identified themselves as being knowledgeable of the patient's daily activities and care. Research subjects were recruited in patient caregiver pairs where possible. Inclusion criteria included fluency in English. Patients were not excluded due to poor performance status or unable to physically complete surveys. The study obtained ethics approval from Sunnybrook Health Sciences Centre.

Data collection

Participants were recruited upon presentation to the RRRP clinic, following consultation with the RRRP team but prior to receiving radiation therapy, which would often be on the same day as consultation. Patients who presented without a caregiver were not asked to participate in the study. Patients and caregivers who agreed to participate were then given the Adapted Problems and Needs in Palliative Care – short version (PNPC-sv) questionnaire (Appendix 1). This tool is divided into eight categories of patient needs: daily activities, physical symptoms, autonomy, social issues, psychological issues, spiritual issues, financial problems, and informational needs. Patients and caregivers were asked to identify which of the 33 potential needs, spanning the eight categories, were problems (yes, somewhat, or no) and for which issues they would like professional attention. At the end of the questionnaire patients were asked to list relevant issues that were missing as well as questions and comments.

Statistical analysis

Descriptive statistics was expressed as means and standard deviations for quantitative variables and as proportions for qualitative variables. The percentage (%) of agreement was calculated between patients and caregivers on each item of the aPNPC. The weighted Kappa Cohen statistic (k) was also calculated after adjusting for weighting information to test for the percent agreement between the two groups at the 95% confidence interval. Some weighted kappa values were not calculated due to the lower number of cells in the cross-table. A kappa value of 1 implies perfect agreement and values less than 1 imply less perfect agreement. The following agreement categories were used in the study: <0.20 indicates poor agreement, 0.20-0.40 indicates fair agreement, 0.41-0.60 indicates moderate agreement, 0.61-0.80 indicates good agreement, and 0.81-1.00 indicates very good agreement (11). All statistical analysis was conducted using Statistical Analysis Software version 9.2 for Windows.

Our findings

Table 1. Top Rankings of identified problems from 20 patients' responses

Ranking	Item of Identified Problems	Patients (n = 20)
1	PHS2: Fatigue	19 (95.0%)
2	PHS1: Pain	17 (85.0%)
3	AUT1: Difficulties in continuing the usual activities	15 (78.9%)
4	ADL2: Personal transportation	14 (73.7%)
5	AUT3: Being dependent on others	14 (73.7%)
6	PSY3: Fear of metastases	13 (68.4%)
7	AUT4: Experiencing loss of control over one's life	12 (63.2%)
8	PSY1: Depressed mood	12 (63.2%)
9	PHS3: Sleeping problems	11 (57.9%)
10	PSY4: Difficulty coping with the unpredictability of future	11 (57.9%)

Table 2. Top Rankings of identified problems from 20 caregivers' responses

Ranking	Item of Identified Problems	Caregiver (n = 20)
1	AUT1: Difficulties in continuing the usual activities	20 (100.0%)
2	PHS2: Fatigue	18 (90.0%)
3	PSY4: Difficulty coping with the unpredictability of future	16 (84.2%)
4	ADL2: Personal transportation	14 (70.0%)
5	PHS1: Pain	14 (70.0%)
6	PSY2: Fear of physical suffering	13 (68.4%)
7	SPI4: Difficulties to accept the disease	13 (68.4%)
8	PHS3: Sleeping problems	13 (65.0%)
9	AUT3: Being dependent on others	13 (65.0%)
10	AUT4: Experiencing loss of control over one's life	11 (57.9%)

Table 3. Top Rankings of unmet needs from 20 patients' responses

Ranking	Item of Unmet Needs	Patients (n = 20)
1	ADL3: Doing light housework	5 (25.0%)
2	PHS1: Pain	5 (25.0%)
3	PHS2: Fatigue	5 (25.0%)
4	ADL2: Personal transportation	4 (22.2%)
5	PHS3: Sleeping problems	4 (21.1%)
6	ADL1: Body care, washing, dressing, or toilet	4 (20.0%)
7	PSY3: Fear of metastases	3 (17.6%)
8	PHS8: Prickling or numb sensation	3 (16.7%)
9	AUT4: Experiencing loss of control over one's life	3 (16.7%)
10	PSY2: Fear of physical suffering	3 (16.7%)

The needs identified by patients and their care givers are highlighted in table 1 and 2 respectively. Patients identified fatigue and pain as the most pressing concerns while care givers identified loss of autonomy and psychosocial concerns as their primary concerns. The unmet needs identified by patients were increasing dependency on others for day to day functioning along with physical symptoms such as pain and fatigue. It is interesting to note, that most of unmet concerns for caregivers were in the psychosocial/ spiritual categories (table 3 and 4 respectively). Concordance between the two groups are illustrated through percent agreement in table 5 and weighted Cohen's kappa in table 6. There is very good to moderate agreement for the ten most commonly identified problems.

Table 4. Top Rankings of unmet needs from 20 caregivers' responses

Ranking	Item of Unmet Needs	Caregiver (n = 20)
1	PHS7: Sexual dysfunction	19 (100.0%)
2	SOC1: Problems in relationship with life companion	19 (100.0%)
3	SOC4: Finding others not receptive to talking about the disease	18 (100.0%)
4	PSY5: Difficulties to show emotions	17 (100.0%)
5	SPI2: Difficulties to be of avail for others	18 (100.0%)
6	SPI4: Difficulties to accept the disease	18 (100.0%)
7	FIN1: Extra expenditures because of the disease	19 (100.0%)
8	FIN2: Loss of income because of the disease	19 (100.0%)
9	PHS1: Pain	7 (35.0%)
10	PSY2: Fear of physical suffering	5 (29.4%)

Table 5. Percentage of agreement (ranking) on the problems from patients and their caregivers

Ranking	Item of Problems	Agreement between 20 Patients and their Caregivers n (% agreement)
1	SPI3: Difficulties concerning meaning of death	14 (100.0%)
2	SOC1: Problems in relationship with life companion	14 (87.5%)
3	INF1: Insufficient information	15 (78.9%)
4	SOC2: Difficulties in talking about the disease with life companion	15 (78.9%)
5	SOC4: Finding others not receptive to talking about the disease	14 (77.8%)
6	SPI1: Difficulties to be engaged usefully	14 (72.2%)
7	PHS7: Sexual dysfunction	13 (72.2%)
8	PHS9: (Nightly) sweating or hot flushes	13 (72.2%)
9	PHS6: Itch	13 (72.2%)
10	PHS1: Pain	14 (70.0%)

Table 6. The weighted Kappa statistics (with 95% confidence intervals) among two observers on each problem item

Ranking	Item of Problems	Weighted Kappa	95% Confidence Interval	Strength
1	SPI3: Difficulties concerning meaning of death	1.0000	1.0000, 1.0000	Very Good
2	INF1: Insufficient information	0.6025	0.2174, 0.9876	Good
3	PHS3: Sleeping problems	0.5476	0.2889, 0.8063	Moderate
4	PHS1: Pain	0.5349	0.2045, 0.8653	Moderate
5	ADL2: Personal transportation	0.5280	0.2319, 0.8240	Moderate
6	FIN1: Extra expenditures because of the disease	0.5097	0.1878, 0.8316	Moderate
7	SOC4: Finding others not receptive to talking about the disease	0.5000	0.0757, 0.9243	Moderate
8	PHS7: Sexual dysfunction	0.5000	0.1328, 0.8672	Moderate
9	SPI1: Difficulties to be engaged usefully	0.4375	0.0372, 0.8378	Moderate
10	SOC1: Problems in relationship with life companion	0.4286	-0.2299, 1.0000	Moderate

Discussion

In a recent review, Teunissesn et al (6) reported thirty seven symptoms almost always occurring in greater than 10 percent of patients. Overall, fatigue, pain, lack of energy, weakness and loss of appetite were the most frequent symptoms occurring in greater than 50% of patients. Not surprisingly, the patients in this study also reported fatigue and pain as the most commonly identified problems. Patients identified lack of autonomy, physical symptoms and psychosocial concerns as the needs most often not met. This is of significance as main reason for referral for palliative radiotherapy is for pain control. The combination of physical and psychosocial factors strongly predicts depression in patients with advanced disease (7). Thus, identification of physical symptoms and timely referral to specialized palliative care may ultimately help to prevent the emergence of psychological distress (8).

Caregivers were more likely to report that psychosocial/ spiritual needs were unmet rather than physical needs. While it is important to note that some literature has shown discordance between patient needs as stated by patients and those stated by caregivers (9).This does not completely discount caregiver-reported patient needs. Caregivers become more responsible for making proxy decisions for palliative patients and communicating patient needs to healthcare providers as the disease process progresses (10). Therefore, addressing the patient needs identified by caregiver priorities is important in providing appropriate patient-centred care despite the possibility that caregivers may actually overestimate palliative patient needs.

Looking at the agreement between patients and caregivers we see that in our palliative radiotherapy setting we are not addressing the spiritual, psychosocial at times even the physical symptoms for some of our patients. The analysis of agreement does illustrate that most of the problems are in the psychosocial/ spiritual domain. While the pressure of clinical and other demands may interfere with the extent to which physicians are able to address these concerns, attention to the process of communication may allow patients to feel understood and supported, even when time is brief. The use of multidisciplinary teams including volunteers (who can clarify information, allow emotional expression, and reinforce themes that have already been introduced by the oncologist), may also be of value.

Our study is a first step in identifying the palliative care needs of the patient population seen at the RRRP. We were able to obtain intra-comparator ratings to show that both groups had similar problem lists. Although further studies are necessary, it is encouraging to note the possibility of future goal oriented palliative therapy as being beneficial even when the patient is unable to fully communicate his or her desires.

Significant limitations of this study include a small sample size, and the possible inability to generalize this data to other palliative populations as only radiotherapy patients were considered. Other limitations include self selection of study participants.

Acknowledgments

We thank the support of Mrs. Stacy Yuen and Ms Kristina Facchini.

References

(1)   Rodin G, Lo C, Mikulincer M et al. Pathways to distress: the multiple determinants of depression, hopelessness, and the desire for hastened death in metastatic cancer patients. Soc Sci Med 2009;68(3):562-9.

(2)   Osse BH, Vernooij-Dassen MJ, de Vree BP et al. Assessment of the need for palliative care as perceived by individual cancer patients and their families: a review of instruments for improving patient participation in palliative care. Cancer 2000;88(4):900-11.

(3)   Homsi J, Walsh D, Rivera N et al. Symptom evaluation in palliative medicine: patient report vs systematic assessment. Support Care Cancer 2006;14(5):444-53.

(4)   Lo C, Walsh A, Mikulincer M, et al. Measuring attachment security in patients with advanced cancer: psychometric properties of a modified and brief Experience in Close Relationships scale. Psychooncology 2009;18:490-9.

(5)   Bloom JR, Stewart SL, Johnston M, et al. Sources of support and the physical and mental well-being of young women with breast cancer. Soc Sci Med 2001;53:1513-24.

(6)   Teunissen SC, Wesker W, Kruitwagen C, et al. Symptom prevalence in patients with incurable cancer: a systematic review. J Pain Symptom Manage 2007;34:94-104.

(7)   Lo C, Zimmermann C, Rydall AC, et al. Longitudinal study of depressive symptoms in patients with metastatic gastrointestinal and lung cancer. J Clin Oncol 2010;28:3084-9.

(8)   Holland, JC, Andersen B, Breitbart WS, et al. Distress management. J Natl Compr Cancer Netw 2010;8:448-85.

(9)   Doyle M, Bradley M, Li K et al. Quality of life in patients with brain metastases treated with a palliative course of whole-brain radiotherapy. J Pall Med 2007;10(2):367-74.

(10)   Fleming DA, Sheppard VB, Mangan PA, Taylor KL et al. Caregiving at the end of life: perceptions of health care quality and quality of life among patients and caregivers. J Pain Symptom Manage 2006;31(5):407-420.

Appendix 1

DAILY ACTIVITIES

Is this a problem?			Your problems and needs for care	Do you want professional attention for this?		
Yes	Some what	No		Yes	As is	No
☐☐	☐☐	☐☐	Body care, washing, dressing, or toilet	☐☐	☐☐	☐☐
			Personal transportation			
			(cycling, driving a car, using public transportation, etc.)			
☐☐	☐☐	☐☐	Doing light housework (tidying up, etc.)	☐☐	☐☐	☐☐
☐	☐	☐	_____	☐	☐	☐

If you would like any of these problems and needs addressed, how would you like them addressed?

Why is this area of problems and needs important to you?

PHYSICAL SYMPTOMS

Is this a problem?			Your problems and needs for care	Do you want professional attention for this?		
Yes	Some what	No		Yes	As is	No
☐	☐	☐	Pain	☐	☐	☐
☐	☐	☐	Fatigue	☐	☐	☐
☐	☐	☐	Sleeping problems	☐	☐	☐
☐	☐	☐	Shortness of breath	☐	☐	☐
☐	☐	☐	Cough	☐	☐	☐
☐	☐	☐	Itch	☐	☐	☐
☐	☐	☐	Sexual dysfunction	☐	☐	☐
☐	☐	☐	Prickling or numb sensation	☐	☐	☐
☐	☐	☐	(Nightly) sweating or hot flushes	☐	☐	☐
			_____			
☐	☐	☐	_____	☐	☐	☐

If you would like any of these problems and needs addressed, how would you like them addressed?

Why is this area of problems and needs important to you?

PATIENT VERSION

Problems and needs in palliative care radiation therapy questionnaire

AUTONOMY

Is this a problem?			Your problems and needs for care	Do you want professional attention for this?		
Yes	Some what	No		Yes	As is	No
☐	☐	☐	Difficulties in continuing the usual activities	☐	☐	☐
☐	☐	☐	Difficulty in handing over tasks to another person	☐	☐	☐
☐	☐	☐	Being dependant on others	☐	☐	☐
☐	☐	☐	Experiencing loss of control over one's life	☐	☐	☐
☐	☐	☐	_____	☐	☐	☐

If you would like any of these problems and needs addressed, how would you like them addressed?

Why is this area of problems and needs important to you?

SOCIAL ISSUES

Is this a problem?			Your problems and needs for care	Do you want professional attention for this?		
Yes	Some what	No		Yes	As is	No
☐	☐	☐	Problems in the relationship with life companion	☐	☐	☐
☐	☐	☐	Difficulties in talking about the disease with life companion	☐	☐	☐
☐	☐	☐	Finding it difficult to talk about the disease, because of not wanting to burden others	☐	☐	☐
☐	☐	☐	Finding others not receptive to talking about the disease	☐	☐	☐
☐	☐	☐	Difficulties in finding someone to talk to (confidante)	☐	☐	☐
☐	☐	☐	_____	☐	☐	☐

If you would like any of these problems and needs addressed, how would you like them addressed?

Why is this area of problems and needs important to you?

PATIENT VERSION

Problems and needs in palliative care radiation therapy questionnaire

PSYCHOLOGICAL ISSUES

Is this a problem?				Do you want professional attention for this?		
Yes	Some what	No	*Your problems and needs for care*	Yes	As is	No
☐	☐	☐	Depressed mood	☐	☐	☐
☐	☐	☐	Fear of physical suffering	☐	☐	☐
☐	☐	☐	Fear of metastases	☐	☐	☐
☐	☐	☐	Difficulty coping with the unpredictability of the future	☐	☐	☐
☐	☐	☐	Difficulties to show emotions	☐	☐	☐
☐	☐	☐	_____	☐	☐	☐
☐	☐	☐	_____	☐	☐	☐

If you would like any of these problems and needs addressed, how would you like them addressed?

Why is this area of problems and needs important to you?

SPIRITUAL ISSUES

Is this a problem?				Do you want professional attention for this?		
Yes	Some what	No	*Your problems and needs for care*	Yes	As is	No
☐	☐	☐	Difficulties to be engaged usefully	☐	☐	☐
☐	☐	☐	Difficulties to be of avail for others	☐	☐	☐
☐	☐	☐	Difficulties concerning the meaning of death	☐	☐	☐
☐	☐	☐	Difficulties to accept the disease	☐	☐	☐
☐	☐	☐	_____	☐	☐	☐
☐	☐	☐	_____	☐	☐	☐

If you would like any of these problems and needs addressed, how would you like them addressed?

Why is this area of problems and needs important to you?

PATIENT VERSION
Problems and needs in palliative care radiation therapy questionnaire

FINANCIAL PROBLEMS

Is this a problem?				Do you want professional attention for this?		
Yes	Some what	No	*Your problems and needs for care*	Yes	As is	No
☐	☐	☐	Extra expenditures because of the disease	☐	☐	☐
☐	☐	☐	Loss of income because of the disease	☐	☐	☐
☐	☐	☐	_____	☐	☐	☐
☐	☐	☐	_____	☐	☐	☐

If you would like any of these problems and needs addressed, how would you like them addressed?

Why is this area of problems and needs important to you?

NEED FOR INFORMATION

Is this a problem?				Do you want professional attention for this?		
Yes	Some what	No	*Your problems and needs for care*	Yes	As is	No
☐	☐	☐	Insufficient information (about the disease and its treatment, aids and agencies that can provide help, alternative healing methods, etc.)	☐	☐	☐

For what topics would you like more information?

If you would like any of these problems and needs addressed, how would you like them addressed?

Why is this area of problems and needs important to you?

Do you have anything else to add about your problems and needs?

In: Advanced Cancer ISBN: 978-1-62808-239-5
Editors: N. Thavarajah, N. Pulenzas, B. Lechner et al. © 2013 Nova Science Publishers, Inc.

Chapter 28

Determining the accuracy of health care professionals in predicting the survival of patients with advanced metastatic cancer

*Edward Chow[*], MBBS, George Hruby, MBChB,
Kristin Harris, BSc, Katherine Enright, MD,
Emily Sinclair, MRT (T) and Grace Chan, RN*
Rapid Response Radiotherapy Program, Odette Cancer Centre,
Sunnybrook Health Sciences Centre, Toronto, Canada

In this chapter we compare the clinician predicted survival (CPS) with the actual survival (AS) of patients with advanced cancer. Methods: Participants were asked to estimate the median survival as well as the upper and lower range of expected survival in whole months from the time of referral to the outpatient radiotherapy clinic for five real cases presented in the survey. Secondly, the participants were asked to rank the five most important prognostic factors they considered in answering the previous questions. Finally they were asked to provide some basic information concerning time spent in their field of expertise so one could compare and contrast the survival estimates according to different disciplines, and according to their years of experience. Results: The response rates to the survey from physicians, nurses and radiation therapists were 50%, 53% and 59% respectively. In general, the survival prediction from all disciplines was not accurate. The predictions tended to be optimistic in patients with short-lived survival (= 6 months) and pessimistic in patients with longer survival (= 9 months). There did not appear to be significant differences in the direction of survival prediction among the three disciplines. The accuracy of survival prediction did not depend on the experience of the health care professionals. Conclusions: Survival predictions are important, but, given the poor predictions of the clinicians, it is necessary to develop better predictive models for

[*] Correspondence: Edward Chow, MBBS, PhD, FRCPC, Department of Radiation Oncology, Odette Cancer Centre, Sunnybrook Health Sciences Centre, 2075 Bayview Avenue, Toronto, ON M4N 3M5 Canada. E-mail: Edward.Chow@sunnybrook.ca

survival using clinical parameters rather than relying on intuition and clinical judgment alone.

Introduction

Patients with advanced cancer and their families often request an estimate of the life expectancy to plan end-of-life issues and remaining time together. Medical professionals also rely on such estimates to guide appropriate clinical decisions, plan supportive care, and allocate resource use (1).

Clinicians tend to be overly optimistic in the survival prediction of terminally ill cancer patients (2-4). This may result in delaying referral to hospice and other end-of-life care (5,6). The choice of dose fractionation in palliative radiotherapy or the use of chemotherapy may also depend on the survival prediction.

The primary purpose of this study was to compare the clinician predicted survival (CPS) with the actual survival (AS) of patients with advanced cancer. The secondary objectives were to examine whether the CPS improved with clinician experience and the impending death of the patient.

A survey was conducted to determine the ability to predict survival in patients with advanced metastatic cancer among health care professionals including nursing staff, oncologists, palliative care physicians and radiation therapists. The objectives were to enhance our understanding of health care professionals' (HCP) predictions of survival in patients with metastatic cancer; to compare and contrast the survival estimates among the various disciplines; and to examine the impact of prognostic factors which are readily available in the out-patient/ hospice setting on the HCPs' quantitative assessment of survival for each patient.

Our study

The Rapid Response Radiotherapy Program at Odette Cancer Centre provides quick access to radiotherapy to relieve suffering and improve the quality of life of patients with advanced cancer. Patients referred have a pathologic diagnosis of cancer and documentation of metastatic disease by pathologic confirmation, clinical examination, or imaging studies. Five real cases were presented in the survey (see appendix 1). The time to death from any cause was the outcome. The survival time was measured from the date of the first consultation at the Rapid Response Radiotherapy Program. Participants were asked to estimate the median survival as well as the upper and lower range of expected survival in whole months from the time of referral to the outpatient radiotherapy clinic. A summary of the Karnofsky Performance Status (KPS) was supplied in appendix 2.

Whole month of remaining life span was chosen in order to quantify any differences between the estimated and observed survival in each of the 5 cases. Secondly, the participants were asked to rank the five most important prognostic factors they considered in answering each of the cases. Finally they were asked to provide some basic information concerning time spent in their particular field of expertise so one can compare and contrast the survival estimates according to different disciplines, and to their years of experience. This project was approved by the research ethics board at Odette Cancer Centre.

Our findings

The response rates to the survey from physicians, nurses and radiation therapists were 50%, 53% and 59% respectively (see table 1). Their years of licensure are listed in table 2.

Table 1. Return rates of the survey

Discipline	Surveys Sent	Surveys Completed	Return Rate
Physicians	48	24	50%
Oncology Nurses	62	33	53%
Radiation Therapists	98	58	59%

Table 2. The year of licensure

Disciplines	Before 1970	1970-1979	1980-1989	1990-1999	After 1999
Physicians (n=24)	0	2 (8%)	4 (17%)	9 (38%)	9 (38%)
Oncology Nurses (n=33)	7 (21%)	11 (33%)	7 (21%)	6 (18%)	2 (6%)
Radiation Therapists [a] (n=58)	0	6 (10%)	16 (28%)	22 (38%)	13 (22%)

[a] 1 missing

Table 3. Survival prediction

Case No.	Actual Survival (in months)	Survival Prediction	Disciplines (median and range in months)		
			Physicians	Nurses	Radiation Therapists
1	< 1	ES	4 $(2-8)$	6 $(2-36)$	6 $(2-24)$
		LR	2 $(0-4)$	3 $(1-12)$	3 $(0-18)$
		UR	8 $(3-12)$	9 $(2-24)$	9 $(3-36)$
2	6	ES	12 $(1-48)$	12 $(2-60)$	10 $(1-48)$
		LR	6 $(0-12)$	6 $(0-24)$	6 $(1-36)$
		UR	24 $(4-120)$	15 $(3-84)$	14 $(5-60)$
3	9	ES	6 $(1-24)$	8 $(1-24)$	5 $(1-36)$
		LR	3 $(0-12)$	4 $(0-14)$	2 $(0-24)$
		UR	12 $(3-60)$	12 $(2-36)$	8 $(2-48)$
4	16	ES	12 $(6-72)$	12 $(2-60)$	16 $(3-118)$
		LR	6 $(0-36)$	10 $(1-48)$	10 $(1-36)$
		UR	24 $(8-108)$	24 $(3-54)$	24 $(6-60)$
5	12	ES	6 $(1-12)$	9 $(2-120)$	6 $(1-48)$
		LR	2 $(0-6)$	5 $(1-60)$	4 $(0-24)$
		UR	12 $(5-24)$	12 $(3-100)$	11 $(2-72)$

Note: ES = Estimated survival
LR = Lower range of expected survival
UR = Upper range of expected survival

The estimated survival with the lower and upper ranges of expected survival of the five cases from the health care professionals is detailed in table 3. In general, the survival prediction from the disciplines was not accurate. The prediction tended to be optimistic in patients with short-lived survival (= six months) and pessimistic in patients with longer survival (= nine months). There did not appear to be a significant difference in the direction of survival prediction among the three disciplines. The accuracy of survival prediction did not depend on the experience of the health care professionals either.

When asked to rank the most important factors (in descending order of importance) in estimating the patient's survival, physicians listed Karnofsky Performance Status (KPS), primary cancer site, site of metastases, weight loss and age of the patients. The responses from nurses were primary cancer site, histologic grade of the tumor, site of metastases, time of onset of metastases and KPS whereas those from the radiation therapists were site of metastases, histological grade of tumor, time of onset of metastases, primary cancer site and KPS.

Discussion

Accurate prediction of survival is very important in advanced cancer and the management and especially in the pain management of these cases in final stages. Patients and families can set appropriate goals and plan end-of-life issues. It enables clinicians to make appropriate treatment decisions and recommendations, researchers to select relevant patient groups for clinical trials, and health care administrators to allocate resources in end-of-life care.

It has been observed that clinicians consistently overestimate survival (2,7). A systematic review of physicians' survival predictors in terminally ill cancer patients suggested that survival of patients was typically 30% shorter than predicted (8). The authors emphasized that doctors need to be aware of their tendency to overestimate prognosis in cancer patients who are approaching death. This optimism may have serious implications for the patients in terms of inappropriate application of disease controlling treatment and delay referral to a hospice, and or supportive or palliative care. The steering Committee of the European Association for Palliative Care has recently published evidence based clinical recommendations on prognostic factors in advanced cancer patients. They caution that clinical prediction of survival should not be based on experience alone, but in conjunction with other prognostic factors (9). Our survey revealed the prediction tended to be optimistic in patients with short-lived survival and pessimistic in patients with longer survival. We cannot be confident of this observation whether this may be due to the small sample size or the use of the survey. However the range provided by the clinicians included the actual survival time. This supports what often occurs in clinical practice that clinicians feel more comfortable and are more accurate when providing ranges. The various disciplines reported using primary cancer site, site of metastases and KPS when formulating survival. These factors are known to be predictive of survival. Future studies may try to develop a predictive model based on these factors and we are trying to do so in our centre.

Some studies have concluded that, toward the end of the patient's life, physicians became better at anticipating the timing of death (10,11). This is analogous to what meteorologists call the "horizon effect" in that short-term forecasts are usually more accurate than long-term

Determining the accuracy of health care professionals in predicting the survival ... 231

forecasts (12). However, this effect was not apparent in our study nor in others reported in the literature (13-15). Other studies have observed that doctors in the upper quartile of practice experience were the most accurate in their prediction of patient survival (16,17). We also did not observe such a trend in our study. However, our study was limited to a single institution and compliance was < 60% for all disciplines. Furthermore, the number of cases may have been too small to demonstrate small differences within the disciplines and between the disciplines. Our study employed a survey to assess clinician predicted survival which may not be a valid method of measuring the accuracy of health care professionals in predicting the survival of patients with advanced metastatic cancer. They were not provided of the opportunity of face to face contact with the patients.

Life expectancy is an important factor in decision-making. It may play a role when radiation oncologists decide on radiation dose fractionation schemes, transition from prolonging life to controlling symptoms and improving quality of life, and hospice referral. Excessive optimism may have a negative impact on all of these decisions. Parkes, in his recent commentary, aired his disappointment that doctors are still no better at predicting the length of survival of our terminally ill patients than they were 27 years ago. He also stated that if all predictions had been divided by 2, they would have been marginally more accurate (18).

Survival predictions are important, but, given the poor predictions of the clinicians, it is necessary to develop good predictive models for survival using clinical parameters rather than relying on intuition and clinical judgment alone. Research instruments such as Morita's palliative prognostic index (19-21) and Maltoni's palliative prognostic score (22,23) have had recent success, both of which were shown to predict short-term survival reasonably well. We employed ESAS as the instrument tool in our survey. There are also limitations in the prognostic models that they tend to do better when predicting survival in populations rather than individuals and they may not be much better and accurate than clinical judgment alone. Some of the models such as palliative prognostic score also include clinical predicted survival as one of the indices. Furthermore, our study was intended to be exploratory. Hopefully, with further research, we can fine-tune these models, including the one developed at our clinic (24) and make more reliable clinical predictions. Until that time, we would do better to stop guessing and, when predictions are needed, to make use of the available predictive instruments. Prognoses should be based on proven indexes and not intuition (18).

In practice, if asked to provide survival estimates, we need to inform patients and their families that, in general, clinicians' estimates are far from accurate. It may also be more useful to provide a range rather than discuss median survival figures. If discussing median survival, patients and their families need to understand the limitations of this statistical construct.

In a study from Sydney, 11 medical oncologists were asked to estimate survival in 86 cases. The survival predictions were well calibrated but imprecise. Almost two-thirds (61%) of patients had actual survivals that fell between half and double that of their predicted survivals. Therefore ranges based on simple multiples of the predicted survival time convey both prognosis and its uncertainty (25).

Finally, it may be important to switch patient and family focus on the quality, rather than the quantity, of their remaining time.

Acknowledgments

We thank Ms Stacy Lue for the secretarial support, Michael and Karyn Goldstein Cancer Research Fund and all participants in completing the survey. We declare no conflicts of interest.

References

(1)   Maher EJ. How long have I got doctor? Eur J Cancer 1994;3:283-4.

(2)   Chow E, Harth T, Hruby G, et al. How accurate are physicians' clinical predictions of survival and the available prognostic tools in estimating survival times in terminally ill cancer patients? A systematic review. Clin Oncol 2001;13:209-18.

(3)   Heyse-Moore LH, Johnson-Bell VE. Can doctors accurately predict the life expectancy of patients with terminal cancer? Palliat Med 1987;1:165-6.

(4)   Parkes CM. Accuracy of predictions of survival in later stages of cancer. BMJ 1972;2:29-31.

(5)   Demer C, Johnston-Anderson AV, Tobin R, et al. Cost of hospice care: Late versus early entry [Abstract]. Proc ASCO 1992;11:392.

(6)   National Hospice Organization (NHO) Newsline, 1992. Stats show continued growth in programs and patients. NHO Newsline 1993; 3:1–2.

(7)   Vigano A, Dorgan M, Buckingham J, et al. Survival prediction in terminal cancer patients: A systemic review of the medical literature. Palliat Med 2000;14:363-374.

(8)   Glare P, Virik K, Jones M, et al. A systemic review of physicians' survival predictions in terminally ill cancer patients. BMJ 2003;327 (7422):1048-9.

(9)   Maltoni M, Caraceni A, Brunelli C, et al. Prognostic factors in advanced cancer patients: evidence-based clinical recommendations – a study by the steering committee of the European Association for Palliative Care. J Clin Oncol 2005;23(25):6240-8.

(10)   Mackillop WJ, Quirt CF. Measuring the accuracy of prognostic judgments in oncology. J Clin Epidemiol 1997;50:21-9.

(11)   Oxenham D, Cornbleet MA. Accuracy of prediction of survival by different professional groups in a hospice, Palliat Med 1998;12:117-8.

(12)   Stanski HR, Wilson LJ, Burrows WR. Survey of common verification methods in meteorology. Downsview, ON: Environment Canada Atmospheric Environment Service Research Report (MSRB) 1989:89-95.

(13)   Bruera E, Miller MJ, Kuehn N, et al. Estimate of survival of patients admitted to a palliative care unit: A prospective study. J Pain Symptom Manage 1992;7:82–86.

(14)   Evans C, McCarthy M. Prognostic uncertainty in terminal care: Can the Karnofsky index help? Lancet 1985;1:1204-6.

(15)   Vigano A, Dorgan M, et al. The relative accuracy of the clinical estimation of the duration of life for patients with end of life cancer. Cancer 1999;86:170-6.

(16)   Christakis NA, Lamont EB. Extent and determinants of error in doctors' prognoses in terminally ill patients: Prospective cohort study. BMJ 2000;320:469-73.

(17)   Maltoni M, Nanni O, Derni S et al. Clinical prediction of survival is more accurate than the Karnofsky performance status in estimating life span of terminally ill cancer patients. Eur J Cancer 1994;6: 761-6.

(18)   Parkes CM. Commentary: Prognoses should be based on proved indices not intuition. BMJ 2000;19:473.

(19)   Morita T, Tsunoda J and Inoue S et al. Prediction of survival of terminally ill cancer patients. A prospective study. Jap J Cancer Chemother 1998; 25:1203-11.

(20)   Morita T, Tsunoda J, Inoue S, et al. Survival prediction of terminally ill cancer patients by clinical symptoms: Development of a simple indicator. Jap J Clin Oncol 1999;29:156-9.

(21) Morita T, Tsunoda J, Inoue S, et al. The palliative prognostic index: A scoring system for survival prediction of terminally ill cancer patients. Support Care Cancer 1999;7:128-33.

(22) Maltoni M, Nanni O, Pirovano M, et al. Successful validation of the palliative prognostic score in terminally ill cancer patients. Italian Multicenter Study Group on Palliative Care. J Pain Symptom Manage 1999;7:240-7.

(23) Pirovano M, Maltoni M, Nanni O, et al. A new palliative prognostic score: A first step for the staging of terminally ill cancer patients. J Pain Symptom Manage 1999;17:231-9.

(24) Chow E, Fung KW, Panzarella T, et al. A predictive model for survival in metastatic cancer patients attending an out-patient palliative radiotherapy clinic. Int J Radiat Oncol Biol Phys 2000;53: 1291-1302.

(25) Stockler MR, Tattersall MH, Boyer MJ et al. Disarming the guarded prognosis: predicting survival in newly referred patients with incurable cancer. Br J Cancer 2006:94:208-12.

Appendix 1

Case 1

Small cell lung cancer, extensive disease at diagnosis with bilateral intra-pulmonary nodules and multiple bone metastases. Reason for referral to the Outpatient Radiotherapy Clinic: post surgical decompression of spinal cord C7-T2.

Clinical Status at time of referral to the Outpatient Radiotherapy Clinic

- 67 year old male
- No liver, brain, adrenal or lymph node involvement.
- Small intra-pulmonary nodules on chest radiograph, no pleural effusion

Significant symptoms: (0 = absence of symptom, 10 = worst possible symptom)

- Pain   5/10
- Fatigue   5/10
- Dyspnoea   3/10
- Loss of appetite   9/10
- Sensation of well being   7/10

KPS:	40
Weight Loss (>10% in last 6/12):	Yes
Analgesia:	Tylenol as required
Date of initial cancer diagnosis:	8 months previously
Chemotherapy:	cis-platinum + etoposide
	4 cycles completed 4 months ago

Please provide your survival estimates in whole months (0,1,2,3…) from the time of referral to the Outpatient Radiotherapy Clinic.

My estimated survival for this patient is [   ] months

His lower range of expected survival is [   ] months

His upper range of expected survival is [   ] months.

Case 2

Metastatic ductal breast cancer

Reason for referral to the Outpatient Radiotherapy Clinic: post-surgical fixation of pathological fracture of the left hip.

Clinical status at time of referral to the Outpatient Radiotherapy Clinic

- 67 year old female
- Sites of metastases: lung nodules, mediastinal lymphadenopathy, multiple bony sites including pelvis, femurs, ribs, cervical and thoracic spine. No liver or brain metastases.

Significant symptoms: (0 = absence of symptom, 10 = worst possible symptom)

- Pain   0/10
- Fatigue   8/10
- Loss of appetite   9/10
- Dyspnoea   0/10
- Sensation of well being   8/10

KPS:	50
Weight Loss (>10% in last 6/12):	No
Analgesia:	Morphine 90 mg daily
	Amitryptiline 75 mg daily
Date of initial cancer diagnosis:	35 months previously
	Estrogen receptor positive (ER+) at diagnosis.
Treatment	1. modified radical mastectomy then adjuvant cyclophosphamide, methotrexate and fluorouracil (CMF x 6) 34-27 months ago
	2. adjuvant tamoxifen, commenced 27 months ago
Date metastases first diagnosed	2 weeks ago (fractured hip).

Please provide your survival estimates in whole months (0,1,2,3…) from the time of referral to the Outpatient Radiotherapy Clinic.

My estimated survival for this patient is [   ] months

Her lower range of expected survival is [   ] months

Her upper range of expected survival is [   ] months

Case 3

Metastatic Lobular Breast Cancer
Reason for referral to the Outpatient Radiotherapy Clinic: tender lytic sacral metastasis

Clinical status at time of referral to the Outpatient Radiotherapy Clinic

– 78 year old female
– Sites of metastases: multiple bony sites, diffuse metastases to stomach, right colon, para-aortic lymph nodes and ileum (the bulky metastases were excised)

Significant symptoms: (0 = absence of symptom, 10 = worst possible symptom)

- Pain   5/10
- Fatigue   8/10
- Dyspnoea   5/10
- Loss of appetite   10/10
- Sensation of well being   8/10

KPS: 60
Weight Loss (>10% in last 6/12): Yes
Analgesia: Tylenol 3, 6 tablets daily
Date of initial cancer diagnosis: 4 months previously
                                                   Presented with metastatic disease
                                                   ER (+) at diagnosis.
Treatment   1. Surgical excision of abdominal metastases 4 months ago.
                                                   2. Tamoxifen, commenced after surgery
                                                   3. Clodronate, commenced 1 month ago.

Please provide your survival estimates in whole months (0,1,2,3…) from the time of referral to the Outpatient Radiotherapy Clinic.

My estimated survival for this patient is [   ] months

Her lower range of expected survival is [   ] months

Her upper range of expected survival is [   ] months

Case 4

Prostate cancer with bone metastases
Reason for referral to the Outpatient Radiotherapy Clinic: painful cervical spine and left hip

Clinical Status at time of referral to the Outpatient Radiotherapy Clinic

- – 69 year old male
- – Sites of metastases: Cervical spine, skull, pelvis and femurs

Significant symptoms: (0 = absence of symptom, 10 = worst possible symptom)
- Pain   3/10
- Fatigue   0/10
- Dyspnoea   0/10
- Loss of appetite   1/10
- Sensation of well being   1/10

KPS:	80
Weight Loss (>10% in last 6/12):	Yes
Analgesia:	100 mg of morphine equivalent per day
Date of initial cancer diagnosis:	16 months previously (PSA 54 ng/dL). Prostatic biopsy confirmed Gleason Score 8 prostatic carcinoma.
Treatment	1. Orchiectomy and casodex 11 months ago 2. PSA dropped to 34 ng/dL(7 months ago) but has risen steadily to 3. 107ng/dL at time of referral for XRT
Date metastatic disease diagnosed	12 months ago Bone scan revealed increased uptake in the lumbar spine and pelvis, not present at diagnosis.

Please provide your survival estimates in whole months (0,1,2,3…) from the time of referral to the Outpatient Radiotherapy Clinic.

My estimated survival for this patient is [＿＿＿＿] months

Her lower range of expected survival is [＿＿＿＿] months

Her upper range of expected survival is [＿＿＿＿] months

Case 5

Breast cancer with brain metastases
Reason for referral to the Outpatient Radiotherapy Clinic: 2 brain metastases.

Clinical status at time of referral to the Outpatient Radiotherapy Clinic

- 62 year old female
- Sites of metastases: brain and lung.

Significant symptoms: (0 = absence of symptom, 10 = worst possible symptom)

- Pain   2/10
- Fatigue   3/10
- Dyspnoea   4/10
- Loss of appetite   4/10
- Sensation of well being   4/10

KPS:	90
Weight Loss (>10% in last 6/12):	No
Analgesia:	450 mg daily morphine equivalent
Date of initial cancer diagnosis:	33 months previously
	T2N1, ER+, high grade

Treatment
1. Left modified radical mastectomy, 33 months ago
2. CMF x 6 completed 27 months ago
3. Tamoxifen started 27 months ago

Date metastatic disease diagnosed 18 months previously (lung metastases)
Treated with:
4. Arimidex (from 18 to 9 months ago),
5. Megace, commenced 9 months ago due to further progression of the 3 lung nodules

---

Please provide your survival estimates in whole months (0,1,2,3…) from the time of referral to the Outpatient Radiotherapy Clinic.

My estimated survival for this patient is [   ] months

Her lower range of expected survival is [   ] months

Her upper range of expected survival is [   ] months

Questionnaire

A. In which year did you gain your fellowship/ certification   _____
                                                                                                    date

Specialty (please put X on one of the followings)

Medical Oncology   _____
Radiation Oncology   _____
Surgical Oncology   _____
Palliative Care Physician   _____
Other, please specify   _____

B   In which year did you gain your Nursing diploma / degree   _____

date

In which year did you begin working in oncology   _____

date

C.   In which year did you gain your Radiation Therapy diploma / degree_____

date

Of the following 9 items, please rank the 5 you consider the most important (in descending order of importance) in helping you estimate the patient's survival
1.   Age of patient
2.   Primary Cancer Site
3.   Histologic grade of disease
4.   Time from initial cancer diagnosis to onset of metastatic disease (the disease free interval)
5.   Site of metastases
6.   Karnofsky Performance Status (KPS)
7.   Weight loss >/= 10% over the last 6 months
8.   Symptom Distress e.g. pain, appetite, dyspnoea, sense of "well being"
9.   Analgesic intake

Please place the corresponding number (1-9) in the space provided below:

The most important factor is _____

The second most important factor is _____

The third most important factor is _____

The fourth most important factor is _____

The fifth most important factor is _____

Appendix 2

Karnofsky Performance Status Index	
100	Normal, no complaints, no evidence of disease
90	Able to carry on normal activity, minor signs of symptoms of disease
80	Normal activity with effort, some signs or symptoms of disease
70	Cares for self, unable to carry on normal activity or to do work

60	Requires occasional assistance from others but able to care for most needs
50	Requires considerable assistance from others and Frequent medical care
40	Disabled, requires special care and assistance
30	Severely disabled, hospitalization indicated, death not imminent
20	Very sick, hospitalization necessary, active supportive treatment necessary
10	Moribund
0	Dead

In: Advanced Cancer
ISBN: 978-1-62808-239-5
Editors: N. Thavarajah, N. Pulenzas, B. Lechner et al. © 2013 Nova Science Publishers, Inc.

Chapter 29

Rapid Response Radiotherapy Program and multidisciplinary bone metastases clinic

Janet Nguyen, BSc(C), Arjun Sahgal, MD, Emily Sinclair, MRTT,
Gunita Mitera, MRTT, Macey Farhadian, RN, Cyril Danjoux, MD,
Joel Finkelstein, MD, Albert Yee, MD, Michael Ford, MD,
Robyn Pugash, MD, Urban Emmenegger, MD,
Anita Chakraborty, MD and Edward Chow*, MBBS
Rapid Response Radiotherapy Program and Bone Metastases Site Group,
Odette Cancer Centre, Sunnybrook Health Sciences Centre, University of Toronto,
Toronto, Ontario, Canada

Waiting for radiotherapy (RT) in Ontario has been a major problem for the past decade. In 1996, the Sunnybrook Odette Cancer Centre (OCC) initiated a Rapid Response Radiotherapy Program (RRRP) to provide timely palliative RT for symptom relief of patients with advanced cancer. Nearly all patients were simulated for radiation treatment on the same day of consultation, with the majority starting treatment on the same day as simulation. The Bone Metastases Clinic (BMC) was initiated in 1999 to provide a coordinated multidisciplinary approach to the care of cancer patients with bone metastases. This dedicated care approach saves time, effort and human resources that both patients and health care providers would otherwise expend during separate, sequential visits to various specialists for consultation. The Prostate Bone Metastases Clinic (PBMC) was also initiated in conjunction with the BMC, as prostate cancer is the most common cancer in Canada among men. Research is an integral part of the RRRP and the BMC/PBMC. At these clinics, the majority of patients are eligible for at least one ongoing study and all patients are registered on a prospective database, which is

---

* Correspondence: Edward Chow, MBBS, PhD, FRCPC, Department of Radiation Oncology, Odette Cancer Centre, Sunnybrook Health Sciences Centre, 2075 Bayview Avenue, Toronto, ON M4N 3M5, Canada. E-mail: Edward.Chow@sunnybrook.ca

important in order to obtain prospective outcome data. These innovative research programs at the OCC have been recognized in the medical community as a model for other centres to emulate.

Introduction

The Rapid Response Radiotherapy Program (RRRP) was initiated in 1996 with the goal of providing timely palliative RT within a week of referral for patients with metastatic disease requiring radiotherapy. The RRRP is a service that community physicians and oncologists, within the city of Toronto, can directly refer patients to. The aim is to expedite palliative radiotherapy referrals rather than the patient requiring a referral to their primary oncologist first, and then to a radiation oncology service. For the patient with symptomatic metastases, long wait times are unacceptable and negatively impact their quality of life. The RRRP team is structured to ensure a streamlined approach to both the referral process and delivery of radiation.

As patients were often referred to orthopedics from the RRRP for consideration of surgical procedures for bone metastases, in 1999, a dedicated bone metastases clinic (BMC) was initiated (1). The idea was to staff this clinic with radiation oncologists, medical oncologists, orthopaedic surgeons, interventional radiologists, radiation therapists, pain specialists and a nurse co-ordinator. The BMC provides an innovative approach to the care of cancer patients with bone metastases allowing patients to see multiple health care professionals in a single visit.

Given that prostate cancer is the fourth most common cancer worldwide, and the most common cancer in Canada among men (2,3), many patients with advanced disease will develop metastases to the bone (4). As such, the Prostate Bone Metastases Clinic (PBMC) was initiated and operates jointly with the BMC, specializing in treating patients with prostate cancer. In addition to the above-mentioned staff operating the BMC, specialists in prostate cancer are also present to provide therapy and advise specifically for these patients (5).

Apart from the innovative approach to streamline care for palliative patients, research is an integral part of these programs. Studies are constantly ongoing at the RRRP and the BMC/PBMC. The majority of patients seen are usually eligible and accrued to studies, giving the patient an opportunity to contribute to research. This clinic has been successful in research and contributed to many advances in the care of palliative patients. This chapter will focus on these innovative palliative care programs initiated at the OCC, which now serve as a model for other cancer centers to emulate.

Rapid Response Radiotherapy Program (RRRP)

Waiting times for radiation therapy (RT) in Ontario have been a major problem for the past decade in spite of an increase in resources. The median waiting time from referral to start of RT treatment deteriorated from 5.1 weeks in 1993 to 7 weeks in 2002 (6). The majority of Ontario patients waited longer for RT than is recommended by the consensus-based targets established by the Canadian Association of Radiation Oncologists (2 weeks from referral to consultation; two weeks from consultation to treatment) (6,7). The situation is not unique to Ontario, as other Canadian provinces, Australia, New Zealand and the UK have experienced similar problems (8-11).

The number of new cancer cases in Ontario is projected to increase by more than 60% by 2020 and to double by 2028 (6). Demand may be greater than indicated since RT is underutilized in Ontario (6,12,13). According to most referral systems, patients for whom palliative RT is prescribed must wait for treatment along with patients requiring curative irradiation. The tendency to prioritize cases, which means in practice that patients waiting for curative RT are offered treatment as soon as possible in order to preclude progression of their disease to an incurable stage, has led to a situation in which palliative patients are given low priority on waiting lists. Inevitably under this system, patients with terminal cancer continue to suffer while waiting their turn for irradiation. The fiscal and psychological cost of caring for these patients, either at home or in healthcare facilities, with nonradiotherapeutic measures is also substantial. There needs to be a fine balance between resource allocation for curative and palliative RT, since ideally, no patient should be denied access to effective treatment.

An aging population and a greater awareness of the effectiveness of RT have led to an increased demand for RT services. Radiation therapy can be used for cure, as adjuvant treatment or palliation of symptoms of advanced disease. Palliative RT should not be discounted as it may account for nearly 50% of the workload of an RT department (14). Symptomatic patients with limited life expectancy often find it difficult to make separate visits for consultation, radiotherapy simulation and planning before starting treatment. Furthermore, a long waiting time with multiple visits before starting treatment may discourage referral for palliative RT.

An innovative approach

In a symposium on palliative RT in 1996, our palliative care physician suggested that "a separate palliative RT clinic, where access is rapid and patients can be assessed, planned and treated on the same day, is an excellent way of handling the special needs of those patients" (15).

To meet the challenge of providing palliative RT within a week of referral, we initiated the RRRP and reorganized the referral process to minimize the number of clinic visits (16,17). When appropriate, consultation, simulation, treatment planning and initiation of treatment occurr on the same day. In order to simultaneously coordinate these activities on the day of consultation, it is necessary for all relevant information and imaging studies to accompany the patient. This is clearly communicated to the referring physician and patient when they are given their appointment date. The RRRP team is resource intensive consisting of radiation oncologists, nurses, radiation therapists and research assistants.

For patients with symptomatic metastases and limited life expectancy, waiting lists prolong suffering with the potential for the patient to die before being treated. Strategies to reduce waiting times have focused on managing demand and increasing resources. Previous reports from Ontario showed that when resources were limited, workload shifted from palliative to curative RT. When RT resources expanded in the early 1990s, the use of curative RT rapidly increased, but the use of palliative RT did not (18). Therefore, increasing resources alone may not improve the waiting list for palliative RT patients unless the RT delivery process is optimized.

The RRRP was initiated in 1996 as two half-day clinics per week staffed by two radiation oncologists, a nurse and a radiation therapist. To meet the increase in referrals, we added another three weekly half-day clinics. Since 2000, five radiation oncologists have a weekly half-day RRRP clinic. The number of cases seen increased from 200 to 500 annually; however, in 2003, we observed a 13% drop in the number of new cases, which was partly due to the impact of severe acute respiratory syndrome (SARS) on access to health care facilities (see figure 1) (19).

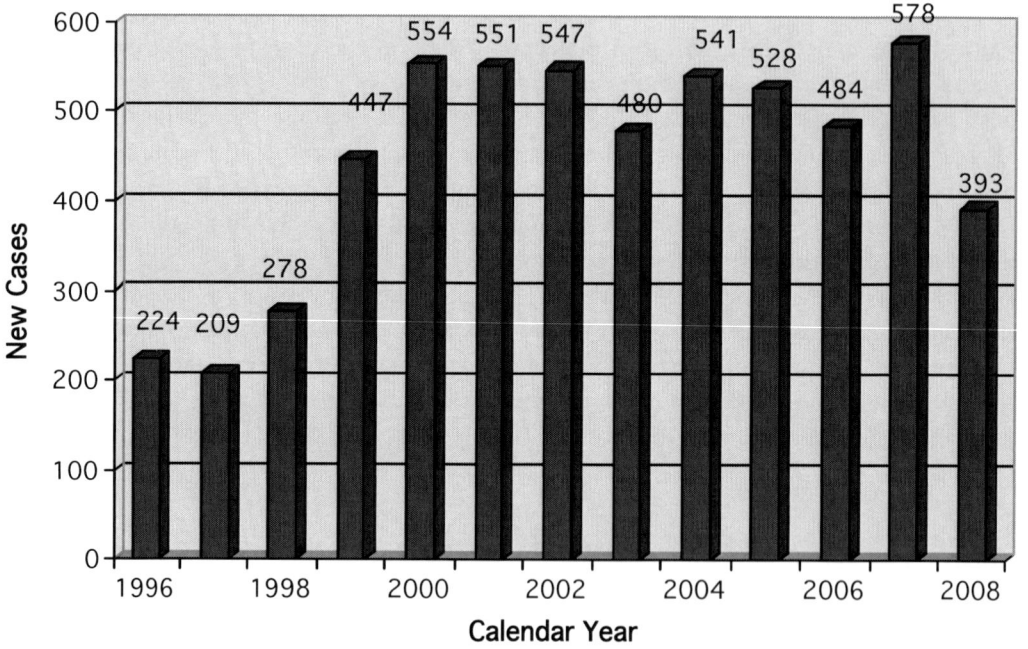

*Data collected for the calendar year 2008 consists of cases referred to RRRP clinic between January 1 – July 31 inclusive
*Source: reference 2 and 23

Figure 1. Number of new RRRP cases by calendar year*.

What is an approprate waiting time for palliative RT?

When Canadian and American radiation oncologists were asked how long they thought it was acceptable to wait for RT for different case scenarios, for palliation of painful bone metastases the Canadian response was 17 days and the American response was 5 days (11). The RRRP overall median time from referral to treatment was eight days, which is closer to the expectation of American than Canadian radiation oncologists. It was much shorter than the median time of 5 to 7 weeks for all patients seen at OCC, or in other Ontario RT facilities over the same period (6). In other words, patients were seen in the RRRP within 8 days of referral during a period when the median provincial wait time increased from 5 to 7 weeks.

The 500 new palliative RT cases seen by the RRRP annually represent about 10% of all new cases referred to OCC for radiation consultation. Patients who require emergency palliative RT, such as for spinal cord compression, are usually seen and treated on the day of their referral either in the RRRP or by the radiation oncologist on call when the referral is made outside of the RRRP clinic times. About 5% of all patients seen in the RRRP are referred for emergency RT.

Our program is faced with some challenges. First, a previous study showed that 25% of RRRP patients are either hospital or hospice in-patients at the time of initial consultation, and travel by ambulance (20). An accompanying nurse from the in-patient ward looks after those patients during their day-stay at the OCC. The need for a comfortable ambulance waiting area, their medications and other medical needs for that day pose an additional challenge to our program. Second, RRRP patients are not routinely followed up at our centre but referred back to their palliative care physician for ongoing care. To compensate for the lack of outcome information, which is usually obtained from routine follow-up, we phone the patient to assess their response to treatment if the patient has been accrued to a study. Since a significant number of our patients are frail and find it difficult to travel, they prefer the convenience of a phone assessment. We are exploring the possibility of involving other health care providers who routinely see the patient at home, or in the referring institution, to collect and provide us with relevant outcome information. Third, the RRRP may be criticized for diverting radiotherapy resources and further lengthening the waiting time for curative RT. We therefore need to strike a balance between competing demands and resource allocation, to optimize the care we provide for all patients whether for cure or palliation. Finally, our next challenge is to provide the same support and fast track process for all palliative patients within the OCC. When a decision is made in a busy clinic that a patient requires palliative RT, it is very difficult for the radiation oncologist to leave their clinic and arrange for radiotherapy simulation and initiate treatment on that day. A possible solution for OCC radiation oncologists who are not involved with the RRRP, is to delegate the coordination and overview of the simulation and initiation of palliative RT treatment to an advanced-practice RRRP radiation therapist. The development of an advanced-practice independent radiation therapist is another innovation in palliative RT.

Review of the program

Since its inception in 1996, there have been two reviews measuring the continued success of the RRRP (21,22). Between 1996 and 2003, there were 3,290 cases referred to the RRRP for palliative RT consultation. Over 200 cases were seen annually in the first 2 years and this increased to over 500 in the years 2000 to 2002 (Figure 1). The majority of patients (76%) seen in the RRRP were new patients to the OCC (Table 1), with the main reason for referral to the RRRP for bone pain (70%) (Table 2). The 3,290 cases made a total of 4,570 visits to the centre, and received 4,272 courses of irradiation. The average number of visits for consultation and treatment was 1.38 for each new case. The majority of patients received palliative RT following consultation (84%) (Table 2). The most common RT dose fractionation for patients with bone metastases was a single 8-Gy fraction (45%), while the majority of patients with brain metastases were treated using 20 Gy in five daily fractions (88%) (Table 3).

Table 1. Descriptive Statistics for Patients Seen at the RRRP, January 1999 – July, 2008 inclusive (n = 6,557)

	1999 – 2003 Cases (%)	2004 – 2008 Cases (%)
Source of referral		
New patients to OCC	2499 (76%)	1494 (46%)
Old cases registered at OCC	791 (24%)	1773 (54%)
Total	3290	3267
Age (years)		
Median (Range)	69 (21 – 95)	68 (21 – 101)
Gender		
Male	1792 (54%)	1719 (53%)
Female	1498 (46%)	1584 (47%)
Total	3290	3267
Primary Cancer Site		
Lung	1078 (32%)	1117 (34%)
Genitourinary	745 (23%)	819 (25%)
Breast	545 (17%)	694 (21%)
Gastrointestinal	351 (11%)	255 (8%)
Others	571 (17%)	382 (12%)

*Source: reference 2 and 23.

Table 2. Primary reasons for referral and primary case dispositions of cases seen in RRRP clinic

	1999 – 2003 Cases (%)	2004 – 2008 Cases (%)
Primary reason for referral[c]		
Bone pain	2989 (70%)	1713 (52%)
Brain metastases	583 (14%)	675 (21%)
Others	701 (16%)	879 (27%)
Total	4272	3267
Primary case dispositions[d]		
Prescribed palliative radiation	3571 (84%)	2311 (71%)
Others	701 (16%)	956 (29%)
Total	4272	3267

[a]Case is defined as a patient with one cancer diagnosis.
[c]Secondary reasons for referral may be given along with primary cited list.
[d]Secondary case dispositions may be given along with primary cited list.
*Source: reference 2 and 23.

As the number of new cases increased, it was more difficult to see patients within 1 week of referral. Despite the increase in number of cases, we were able to see 53% within seven days of referral in 2003 (see figure 2). Overall, 38% of new cases were seen in consultation within seven days of referral, and 50% within 7-15 days of referral. For each calendar year from 1999 to 2003, the overall median time from referral to consultation was 8 days, with a range of 5 to 11. Eighty percent who required RT treatment were simulated on the day of their consultation despite the increase in number of cases (Figure 3). Sixty percent of all cases started their RT on the day of their initial consultation.

Table 3. Details of treatment courses for patients seen at RRRP Clinic

	1999 – 2003	2004 – 2008
	Courses[e] (%)	Courses (%)
Treatment regimes for pain due to bone metastases		
800 cGy in one fraction	1336 (45%)	978 (64%)
2000 cGy in five fractions	1256 (42%)	446 (29%)
3000 cGy in ten fractions	113 (4%)	32 (2%)
Others	284 9%)	64 (4%)
Total	2989	1520
Treatment regimes for brain metastases		
2000 cGy in five fractions	512 (88%)	465 (90%)
3000 cGy in ten fractions	26 (4%)	16 (3%)
Others	44 (8%)	36 (7%)
Total	582	517

[e]Course is defined as a series of treatments all related to one total dose/fractionation.

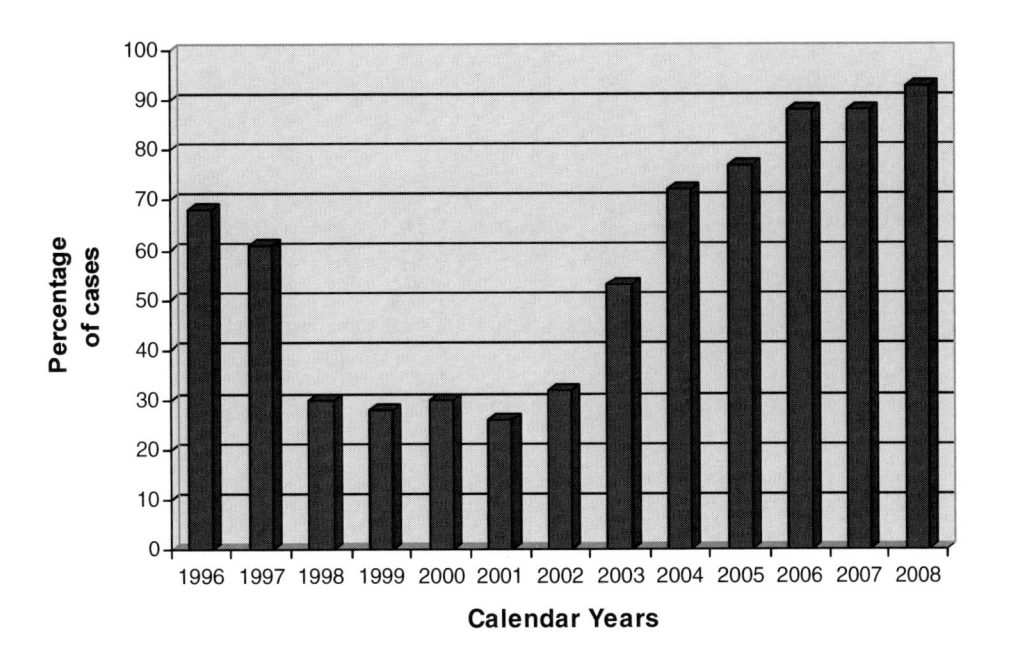

Calendar Years

■days 7>

*Data collected for the calendar year 2008 consists of cases referred to RRRP clinic between January 1 – July 31 inclusive.

*Source: reference 2 and 23.

Figure 2. Interval referral to consult in RRRP by calendar years*.

The second review of the RRRP oversees the period from January 2004 to July of 2008, during which a total of 3,267 cases were referred for palliative RT consultation. Patient descriptive statistics are listed in Table 1. Painful bone metastases accounted for 52.4% of all referrals (Table 2). Of the 3267 cases seen in clinic, 70.7% received palliative RT. The remaining reasons for referral and case dispositions are listed in table 2. A total of 2560 courses of radiation treatment were prescribed with 59.4% of courses for pain relief caused by bone metastases, and 20.2% of courses for brain metastases. The details of treatment courses for patients with bone and/or brain metastases are listed in Table 3. Between January 2004 and July 2008, 49.1% of new cases were seen in consultation within four days of referral, and 1,229 (82.3%) were seen within the first week of referral (Figure 2). The median duration between referral to consultation was 4 days. For patients with metastatic bone pain and/or brain metastases, 81.8% and 69.1%, respectively, were simulated on the same day as consultation (Figure 3).

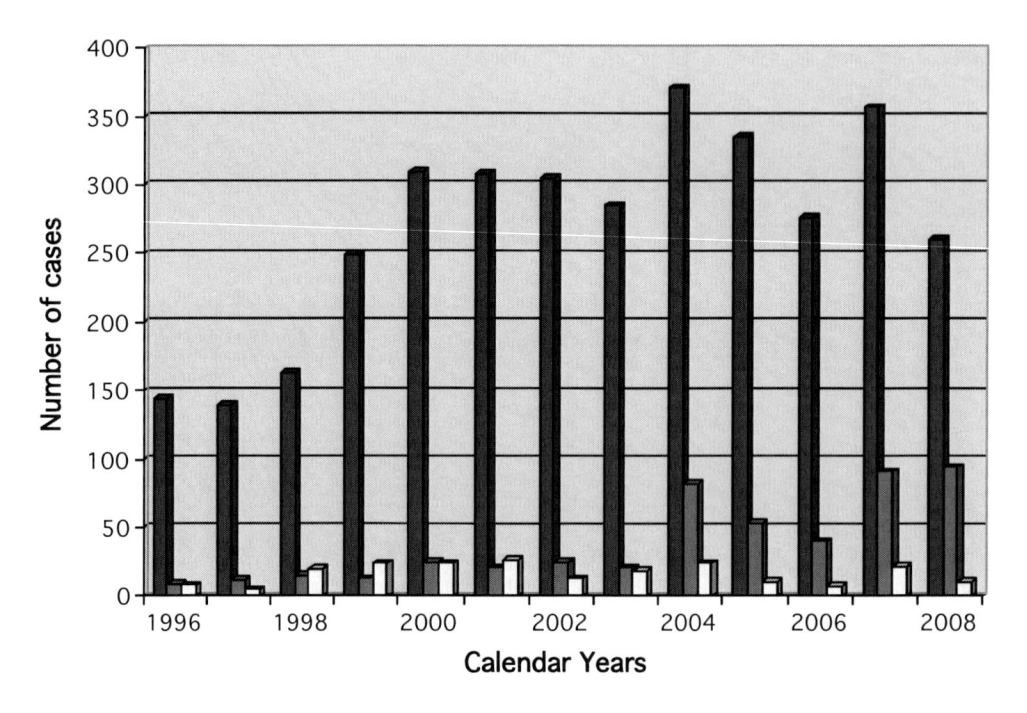

■ 0 days ■ 1-7 days □ >7 days

*Data collected for the calendar year 2008 consists of cases referred to RRRP clinic between January 1 – July 31 inclusive.

Source: reference 2 and 23.

Figure 3. Interval consult to simulation in RRRP by calendar years*.

The goal of palliative radiation is to provide symptomatic relief using a short treatment schedule to minimize treatment related side effects and visits to the cancer centre (16). The longer the treatment duration, the less likely the patient is willing to travel (9). According to the Manpower and Standards of Care formulated by the Radiation Oncology Committee in September 2000, waiting time for initiation of radiotherapy treatment should not exceed 10 working days (7). For the initial eight years of the RRRP, the median interval from referral to consultation was eight days (17). For the time period of January 2004 to July 2008, the overall median interval from referral to consultation decreased to four days. While the clinic is usually able to offer patients the option of starting treatment on the same day as consultation, the patient may request to delay the start of treatment. Reasons may include not wanting to wait at the centre for RT later in the afternoon, needing to arrange drivers to bring them for treatments or having to attend other pre-arranged hospital appointments.

Our experience indicates that changes in the RT referral registration and RT delivery process can shorten waiting times, reduce the number of visits to the cancer centre and provide prompt palliative RT to symptomatic patients in the terminal phase of their illness. Reducing the number of clinic visits before treatment is not only convenient for patients but also reduces the cost to the centre of multiple visits for a single palliative RT treatment.

Referring physician satisfaction

In North America and Europe, approximately 50% of RT administered to cancer patients is palliative in nature. Palliative RT therefore represents a significant portion of cancer care (23). The majority of patients with advanced incurable cancers are cared for by community healthcare providers. We sent out a survey to all referring physicians to explore the strengths and weaknesses of our program in order to improve our services. The results of this survey enabled us to reflect and improve on some of our deficiencies (23).

Out of 126 referring physicians, 64 (51%) returned the completed survey, and 20 practicing physicians were identified who had each referred five or more patients in the study period. Twenty-one (33%) of the 64 reported that they had referred more patients for RT since the inception of our program. The main reasons for physician referral to our program was quick access to services (70%), satisfaction with services provided (59%) and that the referring physician generally refers their oncology patients to the OCC (48%). To assess the referring physicians satisfaction with our program, we asked them to score promptness, communication and overall impression using a scale of 0-10 (0 meaning not at all satisfied and 10 meaning very satisfied). A score of = 7 was reported by 80% of responders. When physicians were asked for their perception of referred patients' and families' satisfaction with our program, 52 of 64 responders (85%) reported a score = 7 (23).

The major strength of the program according to the referring physicians is prompt service. The major weaknesses included poor accessibility for palliative patients in general, difficulty in contacting radiation oncologists, poor communication of information regarding the treatment that patients received at our centre and lengthy time before the dictated consultation notes arrive. Furthermore, there were few patients admitted to our host hospital to receive radiation treatment. Patients treated as outpatients had to travel daily for their fractionated RT. This is a burden for the bed-bound in-patients who have to travel by ambulance.

From the observations of referring physicians, positive feedback from patients/families about our program included the quality of the facilities and caring staff. Some patients/families complained that they were left unattended while they were waiting for the delivery of RT after the consultation with the radiation oncologist. The relative non-provision of any counseling service to these patients by our program was also criticized.

Suggestions from the referring physicians as to how our program might be improved included faster accessibility through the allocation of more resources to palliative RT, and more direct and prompt communications with them. When asked whether they intended to continue referring patients to our program, only one referring physician indicated he would stop referring, and this was because of retirement.

The RRRP was established on the understanding that community care physicians would continue to provide overall palliative care management for referred patients. The recognition that comprehensive palliative services are available to patients in the community, together with the existing heavy workload of our social work and counseling departments, has precluded us from providing routine psychosocial support to patients referred to this program. Although our program has been criticized for the lack of counseling services, we continue to focus on providing rapid access to the radiotherapy service while relying on the referring physicians or facilities to provide complementary palliative care.

Until recently, the Odette Cancer Centre and the Princess Margaret Hospital have been the only two facilities where RT is provided for the population of Greater Toronto. A nurse or nursing assistant escorts patients travelling by ambulance from other hospitals. Therefore, patients are attended by their accompanying nurse while waiting for treatment. However, bed-bound patients travelling from home are treated as other outpatients. While we are aware of the difficulties patients experience when travelling daily by ambulance, gaining access to hospital admission at our host hospital is limited. Needless to say, this situation can only be addressed by restructuring the whole health care system in Ontario.

To improve our communication with referring physicians we re-established our goal of faxing a written report to the referring physician's office on the day of consultation. Previously, we gave this report to patients for delivery. Thus, these notes did not reach the physician until the patient's next office or hospital visit. We have also initiated a quarterly newsletter to all the referring physicians to keep them informed of the activities in our program. To improve the two-way communication, they are invited to submit letters and articles.

The RRRP has been well received by referring physicians. Measures have been taken to correct our deficiencies. We plan to survey our patients' needs and satisfaction to further improve our services, since the patients are the ultimate healthcare consumers.

Model for other centers

The RRRP has served as a template for other rapid radiotherapy clinics. Members from Princess Margaret Hospital's Palliative Radiation Oncology Program (PROP) in Toronto, Juravinski Cancer Centre in Hamilton, Ontario, and the Tom Baker Cancer Centre in Calgary as well as the Cross Cancer Centre in Edmonton, both in Alberta have toured and used the RRRP as a reference centre when establishing their own clinics. Similar programs with the intent of delivering rapid access to palliative radiotherapy have been implemented at other Canadian cancer centres (16), and in Brisbane, Australia.

The Bone Metastases Clinic (BMC)

Skeletal metastases are a frequent complication of cancer, particularly in breast, lung, prostate, thyroid, and renal cancer patients (1,24). Due to advances in systemic treatments, survival in such patients is increasing and, as a result, the prevalence of patients with bone metastases is also expected to increase (1,25). Patients with breast and prostate cancer with bone-only metastases can have a relatively long median survival ranging from 2 to 5 years (24,26), therefore, it is increasingly important to research the appropriate management and prevention of skeletal complications in these patients (27,28). There is a need to reassess the management strategies in patients with bone metastases due to the following reasons (24,27,29-34):

- Pain arising from bone metastases is the most common symptom requiring RT treatment in cancer patients;
- The symptoms of bone metastases are often severe and develop earlier in the clinical course of patients with cancer than symptoms due to either liver or lung metastases;
- Complications of skeletal metastases are common and can seriously impair patient quality of life and function. Pain and impaired mobility occur in 65-75% of patients with bone metastases; fractures of weight-bearing long bones occur in 10-20%; hypercalcemia occurs in 10-15%, and spinal cord or nerve root compression occurs in 5%;
- Increasing incidence of bone metastases and longer survival duration of patients with bone metastases has been observed and;
- The care of this group of patients has been poorly integrated and coordinated.

Pain is the most common symptom resulting from bone metastases, however, bone pain is often under-treated (16,27). Treatment for bone metastases should involve a multidisciplinary approach that includes surgery, radiotherapy, chemotherapy and other treatments (34). Although such therapies are effective in alleviating pain, specialists who deliver the treatments often work independently. Singer commented, "bone pain from mechanical effects often necessitates long term treatment with strong analgesics" (35). In response, Krikler stated that the most effective solution for mechanical pain is surgery (36). Galasko reported that surgical stabilization of such lesions often gives the patient total pain relief and may obviate the need for analgesics (37). Galasko also commented that patients with bone metastases have been inadequately treated, and that oncology education has failed miserably with respect to the optimal management of patients with structurally significant bony metastases (37).

There have been clinical trials and reviews in a variety of disciplines addressing the optimal management of bone metastases, some of which discuss the potential of newer generations of bisphosphonates (26,30,38), the efficacy of RT and the expanding need for effective surgical treatment (34). When bone pain is mechanical in origin, it cannot be adequately treated with RT or systemic therapies and, therefore, surgical stabilization is recommended (24,39). However, due to the risks that come with surgery, particularly in elderly patients, a thorough assessment of all the available treatment options will allow the physicians and the patient to make the best choice (28,31). Surgery and RT are often used in combination with other treatments, therefore, a multidisciplinary approach is especially important in reaching the goals of treatment such as to relieve pain, restore and maintain function and to prevent skeletal related events (SREs). The latter are classified as the need for RT or surgery for palliation of pain, hypercalcemia, pathological fracture, or malignant spinal cord compression (MSCC) (27,29). Effective treatment of SREs in patients with bone metastases is thought to be essential to the preservation of functioning and maintenance of quality of life (QOL).

The Division of Orthopedics at Sunnybrook Health Sciences Centre and the Rapid Response Radiotherapy Program at the OCC initiated a first-of-its-kind clinic, the Bone Metastases Clinic (BMC), at Sunnybrook Odette Cancer Centre in January 1999 (1,25). The clinic aims to provide a coordinated multidisciplinary approach to the management of symptomatic bone metastases patients. This multidisciplinary service is also saving the time and effort that a patient would otherwise spend during separate, sequential, visits to various specialists for consultation.

Review of the Bone Metastases Clinic

The Bone Metastases Clinic (BMC) is managed by a team of various specialties: interventional radiology, nursing, orthopedic surgery, pain and palliative medicine, radiation oncology and radiation therapy. The clinic is held on every second and fourth Friday of every month. Patients are assessed by an orthopedic surgeon, a radiation oncologist and a pain specialist at initial consultation. The team makes a joint recommendation based on their assessments, along with nursing and radiation therapy support. An interventional radiologist is consulted if the patient is considered to be a candidate for percutaneous vertebroplasty or cementoplasty. At initial consultation, patient demographics, reasons for referral and case disposition are recorded. To date, there have been two reviews of the BMC – the first assessing its success from 1999 to 2005, and the second from 2006 to 2008.

Between 1999 and 2005, a total of 272 patients with bone metastases were referred to the BMC (25). Patient demographic data are listed in Table 4. The most common reason for referral was bone pain (42%) (Table 5). Patients identified the spine (41%), pelvis and hips (26%), lower limbs (17%) and upper limbs (13%) as the most painful bony sites. Patients also completed the ESAS at initial consultation, and fatigue and lack of wellbeing were the two most severe symptoms that patients reported. At consultation, the staff orthopaedic surgeons assessment was recorded which involved the functional status of the affected extremity/spine, the presence or risk of fractures and the severity of the risk. The report was completed about 50% of the time. The records show that 35% of patients reported significant limited use of their affected extremity or spine (as evident in the use of prosthesis, walker, cane, crutches and sling) (Table 6). When assessed for the presence or risk of fractures, it was found that 47% of patients were at a high risk of fractures, 34% were at low risk and 12% presented with a fracture at consultation. After thorough examination and evaluation of a patient's symptoms, the BMC team discussed to suggest the best course of action. Of the 272 patients who received consultation, 40% received palliative radiotherapy from 1999 – 2005 (Table 7).

From June 2006 to December 2008, a total of 254 patients with bone metastases were referred to the BMC. Patients identified the spine (43%) to be the most painful bony site (table 4). The major reason for referral was bone pain (69%) (Table 5). The Brief Pain Inventory (BPI) replaced the ESAS scoring system previously used. The median worst, average and current pain score were 7, 4, and 3 respectively (0 = no pain, 10 = worst pain imaginable). Pain interfering with normal work was the most severe problem expressed by patients, with a median score of 8 (0 = no interference, 10 = completely interferes). From May 2008 onward, the bone metastases module (40), the EORTC QLQ-BM22, replaced the BPI to assess patient's quality of life. A number of patients noted that they experience pain in the back, constant pain, pain not relieved by pain medication and pain when walking quite a bit. The orthopedic surgeon's assessment was completed 79% of the time, which has improved since the first six years. The majority of patients reported normal use with pain (37%) (Table 6). At the orthopedic surgeon's assessment for presence or risk of fractures, 17% of patients had a high risk of fractures, 7% had low risk and 25% had a present fracture at initial consultation. After consultation with the BMC physicians, the most common case disposition was palliative radiation (28%) (Table 7).

Table 4. Patient characteristics at the Bone Metastases Clinic from 1999 – 2008

	1999 - 2005	2006 – 2008
Sex	N (%)	N (%)
Male	147 (54%)	132 (52%)
Female	125 (46%)	122 (48%)
Total	272	254
Age (Years)		
Median (Range)	65 (28-95)	64 (29-94)
Locations where cases arrived from		
Home	200 (74%)	216 (85%)
Hospital/Hospice	24 (9%)	12 (5%)
Unknown	39 (14%)	14 (6%)
Primary cancer site		
Breast	84 (31%)	55 (22%)
Lung	56 (21%)	53 (21%)
Renal Cell	20 (7%)	43 (17%)
Prostate	30 (11%)	37 (15%)
Gastrointestinal	16 (6%)	23 (9%)
Unknown	21 (7%)	10 (4%)
Others	45 (17%)	32 (12 %)
Painful bony sites		
Spine	111 (41%)	109 (43%)
Pelvis/Hips	70 (26%)	53 (21%)
Lower limbs	45 (17%)	42 (17%)
Upper limbs	35 (13%)	21 (8%)
Trunk (Ribs, Clavicle, Scapula)	8 (3%)	7 (3%)
Karnofsky performance status		
Median (range)	60 (30 – 90)	70 (10-100)

*Source: reference 36.

From the inception of the BMC in 1999 until 2005, a total of 272 patients were seen (17). The median age and median KPS score at initial consultation were fairly similar to the numbers from 2006 to 2008. Bone pain continues to be the prevalent reason for referral to the

BMC from 2006 – 2008 (69%). Although RT continues to be the most common case disposition seen in 2006-2008, there was an increase seen for patients who required further investigation or imaging (20%) and/or other support services (17%) for this period. During the initial six years at the BMC, the ESAS was used to record patient's symptoms, then the BPI, and finally the EORTC-QLQ-BM22.

Table 5. Reason(s) for referral to the Bone Metastases Clinic

	1999 – 2005[f]	2006 – 2008[g]
	N (%)	**N (%)**
Bone Pain	223 (63%)	175 (58%)
High risk for pathological fracture	41 (12%)	20 (7%)
Pathological fracture	34 (10%)	25 (8%)
Spinal Cord Compression	20 (5%)	2 (0.7%)
Other pain	16 (5%)	8 (3%)
Others	20 (6%)	73 (24%)

[f] 354 reasons in total for n = 272.

[g] 303 reasons in total for n = 254. Eighteen patients' reason(s) for referral were not collected.

*Source: reference 36.

Table 6. Functional status of extremity/spine

	1999 – 2005	2006 – 2008[h]
	N (%)	N (%)
Status		
Normal, pain free use of extremity/spine	19 (14%)	26 (13%)
Normal use with pain	34 (25%)	75 (37%)
Significant limited use	48 (35%)	51 (25%)
Nonfunctional extremity/spine	20 (15%)	14 (7%)
Unknown	16 (12%)	35 (17%)

[h] n = 201 orthopedic assessments filled out.

*Source: reference 36.

Table 7. Case disposition and treatment recommendation(s)

	1999 – 2005[i]	2006 – 2008[j]
	N (%)	**N (%)**
Palliative radiation	108 (40%)	67 (28%)
Further investigation required	18 (7%)	48 (20%)
Referred to other support services	10 (7%)	41 (17%)
Offered surgery	53 (19%)	37 (15%)
No action	69 (25%)	34 (14%)
Others	13 (4%)	13 (5%)

[i] 4 patients received 2 treatment recommendations.

[j] 20 patient's case dispositions are unknown out of 254 patients. 3 patients received 2 treatment recommendations.

*Source: reference 36.

When the total of 272 patients seen from 1999 – 2005 is compared with the 254 patients seen at the BMC from 2006-2008, it is evident that the BMC did approximately the same amount of work in 3 years as it did in its first six years. This is indicative of the increased awareness and need for multidisciplinary care in this group of patients. It is likely that the number of referrals to the BMC will continue to rise, which means there will be also be a need for increased funding as well as human resources. The ultimate goal of the BMC is to improve the overall QOL for patients with bone metastases by maintaining and expanding this one-stop clinic approach for more patients who require this care. This is important given that as the population ages, the burden of cancer and bone metastases may also increase.

The BMC integrated approach to the care of bone metastases patients allows for more streamlined care, in addition to eliminating the inconvenience of separate visits to a variety of specialists for consultation. Patients referred to the BMC receive a multidisciplinary assessment to decide the best course of action in order to maximize the benefits and palliate present symptoms. The fracture risk assessment monitoring of clinical and radiological outcomes allows the treating physicians to learn and modify their treatments, monitor the effect of RT and surgery on painful bony lesions and continually improve our treatment algorithms. In order to further improve patient care at the BMC, it is beneficial to monitor patient's QOL following their clinic visits. Patient satisfaction and cost-effectiveness of the clinic may need to be investigated in order to ensure the BMC continues to give efficient multidisciplinary care to patients with bone metastases.

Prostate Bone Metastases Clinic

Prostate cancer is the fourth most common cancer worldwide and the most common cancer in Canada among men (2,3). In 2009, an estimated 54,500 men will be diagnosed with prostate cancer (PCA) and 4,400 will die of it (2). Most patients with advanced disease will develop metastases.

The most common metastatic site is the bone, with bone metastases being found in approximately 80% of advanced PCA patients (4). Over recent decades, patient survival times have increased due to improved care (41,42). Analgesic therapy and RT to bone have been the cornerstone of palliation in patients with castration-refractory PCA metastatic to bone. The recent addition of taxane-based chemotherapy and bisphosphonates is helpful, but patients may not always be accessing these valuable therapies in a timely manner. The establishment of a prostate bone metastasis clinic in a tertiary care centre provides timely multidisciplinary care to patients with advanced PCA. Cancer metastasis to bone can occur in hormone-sensitive disease, but it may also develop or progress during the castration-refractory stage. In PCA, metastases tend to be rather osteoblastic than osteolytic. In fact, PCA cells produce factors that stimulate osteoblast proliferation, causing increased abnormal bone formation rather than bone breakdown (43). Although androgen deprivation therapy is highly effective in treating hormone-sensitive PCA, almost all patients become resistant after a median of 18–24 months. In the setting of castrate serum testosterone levels, resistance to androgen deprivation is often indicated by a rising level of prostate-specific antigen (PSA) before the appearance of symptoms. With continuing improvement in systemic therapies such as chemotherapy, the overall survival of patients with castration-refractory PCA is increasing

(4). However, recent studies have shown that androgen deprivation therapy might have harmful effects on the skeleton. Treatment-related accelerated bone loss potentially presents men at a higher risk of skeletal complications (4). Management of bone metastases has changed from solely pain relief to improving QOL and survival (44).

Current treatment options for PCA patients with bone metastases include external beam RT, surgery, systemic therapies (bisphosphonates, hormonal therapy, and chemotherapy) and management with pain medications (42,45). The goals of these therapies are to reduce the incidence of SREs, reduce bone pain and morbidity and improve the patient's mobility and overall QOL (3,42). The choice of each of the available treatments depends on the patient's underlying health and performance status, the location of the metastases, the treating physician and the facilities available in the local area (45).

The variety of PCA treatment options has unfortunately translated into a lack of coordination between the specialists responsible for treating the patient. Treating bone pain caused by metastatic disease is a multifaceted task. At the moment, many patients wait for separate appointments to see each specialist, often in sequence, which compounds wait times. Timing is integral to the effective treatment of patients with impending pathologic fracture, spinal cord compression and bone pain. Early diagnosis and treatment are vital for the patient's QOL, and for the prevention of permanent or further neurologic damage (46,47).

The multidisciplinary Prostate Bone Metastases Clinic (PBMC) works with the BMC to help provide patients with the best possible care (5). The PBMC is a one-stop clinic at which patients have the opportunity to see a variety of physicians, based on need. The clinic greatly facilitates direct communication between the health care specialists. Therefore, PBMC addresses the need for a simplified referral to an all-in-one clinic for patients requiring more than one specialist. During the PBMC there is a team of 1 radiation oncologist, 1 medical oncologist, 1 interventional radiologist, 1 orthopedic surgeons, 1 palliative medicine physician, a radiation therapist, a primary nurse coordinator and a research assistant. Each patient has the opportunity to receive specialized care including RT, systemic therapy (chemotherapy, bisphosphonates, and alternative hormonal therapy), pain management, surgical intervention and supportive care where applicable. Hence, the patient benefits from savings in time, money and energy that would otherwise be spent on travel and waits for separate specialist appointments. The PBMC provides optimal service for PCA patients through its multidisciplinary approach. In addition, the venue facilitates clinical research, such as novel bone-targeted therapies, chemotherapies, and improvements in radiation therapy (5).

Need for future research

The Bone Metastases Clinic is expected to address several controversies in the management of patients with impending and complete pathological fractures.

Prophylactic orthopaedic stabilization has reportedly resulted in good pain relief and sustained mobility in up to 90% of patients (48-52). However, this type of prophylactic procedure does not prolong survival (50,53), and relatively high mortality has been reported when multiple fixations are performed during the same operation (51). The need for prophylactic stabilization has, in fact, been questioned by Cheng et al (54) when these patients can be carefully managed with RT. In their retrospective series of 59 patients with metastatic breast cancer, none of the patients with high-risk osteolytic lesions developed pathological fractures after treatment with 30 Gy in 10 daily fractions (54). Few other reports support this experience.

In the literature related to high-risk bony metastases, it is unclear how various RT dose levels and fractionation schedules affect bone healing and prevent fracture. To promote bone healing, radiation oncologists tend to employ single-fraction treatment in patients with very short expected survivals and higher fractionation doses in patients with longer estimated survivals. However, the study by the Radiation Therapy Oncology Group (RTOG) observed an increased risk of pathological fracture after 40.5 Gy as compared with after 25 Gy (55). Unfortunately, there was no analysis on the risk stratification of bone metastases of these two groups of patients receiving different radiation doses. Larger prospective studies are needed to define more precisely the indications for prophylactic RT and to identify an optimal dose.

When a pathological fracture has occurred, the primary goal is to provide pain relief. Secondary intentions are to achieve stability and to restore function. Unless medical contraindications exist, or unless life expectancy is extremely short, surgery is usually recommended. Otherwise, RT alone may be considered.

Postoperative RT is usually recommended; however, the indications for such RT are unclear in the literature. Townsend et al (56) reported normal use of the extremity (with or without pain) in 53% of patients after postoperative RT compared with 11.5% of patients after surgery alone. The actuarial median survival for the surgery-alone group was 3.3 months, compared with 12.4 months for the postoperative RT group. However, this study needs to be interpreted with great caution owing to its retrospective nature and possible unaccountable selection biases.

Postoperative RT has also been challenged on grounds of the risk for poor healing (57). Immediate postoperative RT has been employed to inhibit heterotopic bone formation (58), suggesting an inhibitory effect of RT on bone remodeling and osteoblastic activity. Moreover, immediate postoperative RT can also impair wound healing. Blake (59) suggested that doses above 30 Gy in 10 daily fractions inhibit osteoblastic activity and interfere with bone healing. On the other hand, Ford and Yarnold (60) have successfully employed 40 Gy in 20 daily fractions in patients with longer-than-average prognosis. No good evidence exists regarding the timing of postoperative RT and the best dose fractionation to use. Again, prospective randomized trials are needed to clarify this point.

Patients with lung tumours and adenocarcinomas from other sites have relatively short survival. The role of consolidation with postoperative radiotherapy for this patient population is uncertain. They have to spend part of their limited life span in RT centres. They may also not live long enough for significant tumour progression to occur, resulting in prosthesis or stabilization failure. We should perhaps be selecting a group of patients with longer survival for postoperative RT.

Newer minimally invasive procedures such as vertebroplasty and kyphoplasty have been employed in our clinics. How to optimally integrate such interventions with other treatment options remain to be worked out. To improve our ability to deliver evidence-based, optimal care to this group of cancer patients, these questions need to be answered. The first step is to bring a multidisciplinary approach to the management of patients with bone metastases. Only ongoing research and clinical trials can advance our knowledge and the treatments for patients with bone metastases.

Research as an integral part of the programs

Reviews of the RRRP and the BMC have shown that these clinics are sustainable and successful. However, another important aspect of three clinics is they provide the infrastructure for multidisciplinary collaborative research – a primary focus of the clinics and what distinguishes these programs. The majority of health care providers (HCPs) who work in these clinics produce studies in the field of palliative care. The majority of the patients seen either in the RRRP, BMC, or PBMC are eligible and approached for our ongoing studies. Not only do these clinics offer patients the best evidence-based practice, but also allow patients to contribute to research, which will lead to improving clinical practice. The RRRP has been involved in three cross-Canada randomized National Cancer Institute of Canada (NCIC) clinical trials so far.

One example of original research in palliative radiotherapy that emerged from the RRRP lies in reporting pain flare as a common event following external beam RT for bone metastases. The RRRP has already completed several studies on pain flare after RT (61-65), one of which was a pilot study using dexamethasone to reduce or prevent pain flare (73). Data from this study led to a randomized Phase III Pain Flare Dexamethasone trial sponsored by National Cancer Institute of Canada Clinical Trials Group (NCIC-CTG) due to open in 2009. Another trial currently ongoing at the RRRP in conjunction with the NCIC is a Phase III International Randomised trial of single versus multiple fractions for re-irradiation of painful bone metastases (SC20) (66). The primary objective of this trial is to compare the efficacy of pain relief after re-irradiation with an 8 Gy single fraction or 20 Gy in 5 (or 8) fractions in a simple pragmatic two arm randomised trial. Secondary objectives include determining the overall incidence of pain relief, studying the relationship between pain relief after re-irradiation and response to previous irradiation, as well as determining the characteristics of the group of non-responders (to both the first and second radiation) and the monitoring or acute severe adverse effects.

At the BMC, the orthopedic surgeon and interventional radiologist have an opportunity to interact with the radiation oncologist – which has led to collaborative research (67,68). One example is a study using percutaneous vertebroplasty to improve quality of life in cancer patients with painful spinal metastases or osteoporotic compression (67). Percutaneous vertebroplasty was found to significantly improve pain, mobility and quality of life in 15 cancer patients with bone metastases who failed radiation or with osteoporotic compression fractures. Our group has also developed a bone metastases (EORTC QLQ-BM22) and brain metastases (EORTC QLQ-BN20+2) specific quality of life questionnaire in conjunction with the European Organisation for Research and treatment of Cancer (40).

A bone metastases patient teaching book entitled "Helping you to help yourself" was developed by our group (69). This handbook is a guide for patients with bone metastases, and intends to meet the information needs for patients, caregivers, as well as HCPs. This book lists common medical terminology used, symptoms, diagnostic imaging, treatment options, pain management, as well as resources for coping, and is available to all patients with bone metastases seen at our programs. It has been made available online, and has also been sent out to various cancer centres nation-wide.

Apart from the research and academic activities, teaching plays a big role in the innovative RRRP and BMC. Since 1999, the RRRP team continues to produce a quarterly newsletter named Hot Spot (70), and sends it out to over 2000 HCPs. Hot Spot invites a variety of HCPs to discuss issues of great practical importance and relevance to palliative care, such as cancer pain management, quality improvement in palliative home care programs, as well as Continuing Medical Education (CME). CME can update HCPs on the latest advances for modifications to their clinical practice.

These innovative programs were originally started with the intent to reduce waiting times for palliative patients, and in the case of the BMC/PBMC, to provide multidisciplinary care and meet the needs for lack of resources. The RRRP and the BMC have been reviewed and found to be successful; hence, research and academic activity is becoming the major area of focus for these programs.

Conclusion

This chapter has outlined the innovative programs at the OCC leading to faster and more streamlined care for palliative care patients. Two reviews of the RRRP and the BMC since their inception in 1996 and 1999, respectively, have concluded that there is increased awareness and need for such specialized services for palliative patients. The RRRP has become a model for other centres to provide rapid access to RT for palliative patients. The clinic continues to re-evaluate itself to examine and explore ways to improve our patients' quality of life.

References

[1]   Andersson L, Chow E, Finkelstein J, Connolly R, Danjoux C, Szumacher E, Wong R, Stephen D, Axelrod T. The ultimate on-stop for cancer patients with bone metastases: new combined bone metastases clinic. J Can Nursing Oncol 1999;9(2):103-4.

[2]   (CCS/NCIC) Canadian Cancer Society/National Cancer Institute of Canada. 2008. Canada Cancer Statistics 2008. Toronto, Canada: Canadian Cancer Society/National Institute of Canada.

[3]   Saad F, Karakiewicz P, Perrotte P. The role of bisphosphonates in hormone-refractory prostate cancer. World J Urol 2005;23:14-18.

[4]   Coxon JP, Oades GM, Colston KW, Kirty RS. Advances in the use of bisphosphonates in the prostate cancer setting. Prostate Cancer Prostatic Dis 2004;7:99-104.

[5]   Goh P, Harris K, Napolskikh J, Chow E, Sinclair E, Emmenegger U, Lemon S, Yee A, Wynnychuk L, Myers J, Danjoux C, Ko Y. New multidisciplinary prostate bone metastases clinic: first of its kind in Canada. Curr Oncol 2007;14(1):9-12.

[6]   Schwartz F, Evans W, Sullivan T, Angus H. Cancer quality council of Ontario report – gaining access to appropriate cancer services: a four point strategy to reduce waiting times in Ontario. http://www.cancercare.on.ca/. 2004.

[7]   Canadian Association of Radiation Oncology. Definition of RT waiting. http://www.caro-acro.ca/caro/abt/committees/manp/definition.pdf. September 2000.

[8]   Ash DV. Waiting times for cancer treatment. Clin Oncol 2000;12:140.

[9]   Lehman M, Jacob S, Delaney G, Papadatos G, Jalaludin B, Cail S, McCourt J, Wright S, O'Brien C, Barton M. Waiting times for radiotherapy – a survey of patients' attitudes. Radiother Oncol 2004;70:283-9.

[10]   Mackillop WJ, Fu H, Quirt CF, Dixon P, Brundage M, Yunzheng Z. Waiting for radiotherapy in Ontario. Int J Radiat Oncol Biol Phys 1994;30:221-8.

[11] Mackillop WJ, Zhou Y, Quirt CF. A comparison of delays in treatment of cancer with radiation in Canada and the United States. Int J Radiat Oncol Biol Phys 1995;32:531-9.

[12] Mackillop WJ, Groome PA, Zhang-Solomons J, Zhou Y, Feldman-Stewart D, Paszat L, Dixon P, Holowaty EJ, Cummings BJ. Does a centralized radiotherapy system provide adequate access to care. J Clin Oncol 1997;15(3):1261-71.

[13] Mackillop WJ, O'Brien P, Brundage M, Whitton A, Gallinger D. (2003) Radiotherapy: quality and access issues. In: T Sullivan, W Evans, H Angus, A Hudson (eds) Strengthening the quality of cancer services in Ontario. CHA, Ottawa ON.

[14] Hoelger D. Radiotherapy for palliation of symptoms in incurable cancer (review). Curr Probl Cancer J 1997;21:129-83.

[15] Librach SL. The principles of palliative radiotherapy: palliative care physician's perspective. Can J Oncol 1996;6(Supple 1):2-4.

[16] Danjoux C, Szumacher E, Andersson L, Franssen E, Wong R, Chow E, Connolly R, Pope J, Hayter CR, Finkelstein J, Axelrod T, Stephen D, Sixel K, Thomas G, Schuller T, Stefaniuk K. Palliative radiotherapy at Toronto-Sunnybrook regional cancer centre: the rapid response radiotherapy program. Curr Oncol 2000;7(1):52–6.

[17] Hoegler D. Design and assessment of palliative radiotherapy service structure to patients and referring physician need. Clin Invest Med 1997;A463(Suppl 20):S84.

[18] Mackillop WJ, Zhou S, Groome P, Dixon P, Cummings BJ, Hayter C, Paszat L. Changes in the use of radiotherapy in Ontario 1984-1995. Int J Radiat Oncol Biol Phys 1999;V 22(2):355-362.

[19] Woodward G, Stukel T, Schull M, Gungaj N, Laupacis A. Utilization of Ontario's health system during the 2003 SARS outbreak. Institute for Clinical Evaluative Sciences Report. May 2004.

[20] Chow E, Wong R, Connolly R, Hruby G, Franssen E, Fung K, Vachon M, Andersson L, Pope J, Holden L, Szumacher E, Scheuller T, Stefaniuk K, Finkelstein J, Hayter C, Danjoux C. Prospective assessment of symptom palliation for patients attending a rapid response radiotherapy program: feasibility of telephone follow-up. J Pain Symptom Manage 2001;22(2):649-56.

[21] Danjoux C, Chow E, Drossos A, Holden L, Hayter C, Tsao M, Barnes T, Sinclair E, Farhadian M. An innovative rapid response radiotherapy program to reduce waiting time for palliative radiotherapy. Support Care Cancer 2006;14:38–43.

[22] de Sa E, Sinclair E, Wong J, Danjoux C, Hird A, Hadi S, Barnes E, Tsao M, Chow E. Continued success of the Rapid Response Radiotherapy Program: A review of 2004 – 2008. Support Care Cancer 2009;17(7):757-62.

[23] Chow E, Wong R, Vachon M, Connolly R, Andersson L, Szumacher E, Franssen E, Danjoux C. Referring physicians' satisfaction with the rapid response radiotherapy program. Support Care Cancer 2000;8:405-9.

[24] Coleman RE. Skeletal complications of malignancy. Cancer 1997;80(8 Suppl):1588-94.

[25] Li K, Sinclair E, Pope J, Farhadian M, Harris K, Napolskikh J, Yee A, Librach L, Wynnychuk L, Danjoux C, Chow E. A multidisciplinary bone metastases clinic at Toronto Sunnybrook Regional Cancer Centre – A review of the experience from 1999 to 2005. J Pain Res 2008;1:43-8.

[26] Brown JE, Coleman RE. The present and future role of bisphosphonates in the management of patients with breast cancer. Breast Cancer Res 2002;4(1):24-9.

[27] Janjan NA, Payne R, Gillis T, Podoloff D, Libshitz HI, Lenzi R, Theriault R, Martin C, Yasko A. Presenting symptoms in patients referred to a multidisciplinary clinic for bone metastases. J Pain Sympt Manage 1998;16(3):171-8.

[28] Mystakidou K, Katsouda E, Stathopoulou E, Vlahos L. Approaches to managing bone metastases from breast cancer: The role of bisphosphonates. Cancer Treat Rev 2005;31(4):303-11.

[29] Schachar NS. An update on the nonoperative treatment of patients with metastatic bone disease. Clin Orthop 2001;382:75-81.

[30] Selvaggi G, Scagliotti GV. Management of bone metastases in cancer: A review. Crit Rev Oncol Hematol 2005;56(3):365-78.

[31] Mercadante S, Fulfaro F. Management of painful bone metastases. Curr Opin Oncol 2007;19(4):308-14.

[32] Carlin BI, Andriole GL. The natural history, skeletal complications, and management of bone metastases in patients with prostate carcinoma. Cancer 2000;88(12 Suppl):2989-94.

[33] Lipton A. Future treatment of bone metastases. Clin Cancer Res 2006;12(20 Pt 2):6305s-8s.

[34] Manabe J, Kawaguchi N, Matsumoto S, Tanizawa T. Surgical treatment of bone metastasis: Indications and outcomes. Int J Clin Oncol 2005;10(2):103-11.

[35] Singer CR. ABC of linical haematology. Multiple myeloma and related conditions. BMJ 1997;314(7085):960-3.

[36] Krikler SJ. Multiple myeloma. Surgery is often more effective than analgesia for mechanical pain (letter). BMJ 1997;315(7101):186.

[37] Galasko CS. Multiple myeloma. Surgical stabilization often provides good pain relief (letter). BMJ 1997;315(7101):186.

[38] Kohno N. Treatment of breast cancer with bone metastasis: Bisphosphonate treatment - current and future. Int J Clin Oncol 2008;13(1):18-23.

[39] Coleman RE. Clinical features of metastatic bone disease and risk of skeletal morbidity. Clin Cancer Res 2006;12(20 Pt 2):6243s-9s.

[40] Chow E, Nguyen J, Zhang L, Tseng LM, Hou MF, Fairchild A, Vassiliou V, Jesus-Garcia R, Alm El-Din MA, Kumar A, Forges F, Chie WC, Bottomley A; Euroean Organization for Research and Treatment of Cancer Quality of Life Group. International field testing of the reliability and validity of the EORTC QLQ-BM22 module to assess health-related quality of life in patients with bone metastases. Cancer 2012;118(5):1457-65.

[41] Coleman R, Neville-Webbe H. Prevention of bone metastases. In: Jasmin C, Coleman R, Coia L, Capanna R, Saillant G, eds. Textbook of Bone Metastases. Mississauga, ON: Wiley;2005:387-96.

[42] Brown J, Neville-Webbe H, Coleman R. The role of bisphosphonates in breast and prostate cancer. Endocr Relat Cancer 2004;11:207-24.

[43] Rabbani S, Shukeir N, Mazar A. Prostate cancer: models for developing novel therapeutic approaches. In: Singh G, Orr W, eds. Bone Metastasis and Molecular Mechanisms Pathophysiology. Dordrecht: Kluwer Academic Publishers; 2004:163-86.

[44] McDuffee L, Colterjohn N, Singh G. Bone metastasis and pathological fractures: bone tissue engineering as a novel therapy. In: Singh G, Rubbani S, eds. Bone Metastasis: Experimental and Clinical Therapeutics. Totowa, NJ. Humana Press; 2005:229-41.

[45] Konski A. Radiotherapy is a cost-effective palliative reatment for patients with bone metastasis for prostate cancer. Int J Radiat Oncol Biol Phys 2004;60:1373-8.

[46] Body JJ. Metastatic bone disease: clinical and therapeutic aspects. Bone 1992;13(suppl 1)S57-62.

[47] Tazi H, Manunta A, Rodriguez A, et al. Spinal cord compression in metastatic prostate cancer. Eur Urol 2003;44:527-32.

[48] Fidler M. Prophylactic internal fixation of secondary neoplastic deposites in long bones. Br Med J 1973;1(849):341-3.

[49] Jardines L, Callans LS, TOrosian MH. Recurrent breast cancer: Presentation, diagnosis, and treatment. Semin Oncol 1993;20(5):538-47.

[50] Gristina AG, Adair DM, Spurr CL. Intraosseous metastatic breast cancer treatment with internal fixation and study of survival. Ann Surg 1983;197(2): 128-34.

[51] Tan JL, Lo NN, Tan SK. Surgical treatment of metastatic long bone disease. Singapor Med J 1992;33(4):355-8.

[52] Yazawa Y, Frassica FJ, Chao EY, Pritchard DJ, Sim FH, Shives TC. Metastatic bone disease. A study of the surgical treatment of 166 pathologic humeral and femoral fractures. Clin Orthop 1990;Feb(251):213-9.

[53] Hardman PD, Robb JE, Kerr GR, Rodger A, MacFarlane A. The value of internal fixation and radiotherapy in the management of upper and lower limb bone metastases. Clin Oncol (R Coll Radiol) 1992;4(4):244-8.

[54] Cheng DS, Seitz CB, Eyre HJ. Nonoperatie management of femoral, humeral, and acetabular metastases in patients with breast carcinoma. Cancer 1980;45(7):1533-7.

[55] Tong D, Gillick L, Hendrickson FR. The palliation of symptomatic osseous metastases: Final results of the study by the Radiation Therapy Oncology Group. Cancer 1982;50(5):893-9.

[56] Townsend PW, Rosenthal HG, Smalley SR, Cozad SC, Hassanein RE. Impact of postoperative radiation therapy and other perioperative factors on outcome after orthopedic stabilization of impending or pathologic fractures due to metastatic disease. J Clin Oncol 1994;12(11)2345-50.

[57] Poulsen HS, Nielsen OS, Klee M, Rorth M. Palliative irradiation of bone metastases. Cancer Treat Rev 1989;16(1):41-8.

[58] Sylvester JE, Greenberg P, Selch MT, Thomas BJ, Amstutz H. The use of postoperative irradiation for the prevention of heterotopic bone formation after total hip replacement. Int J Radiat Oncol Biol Phys 1988;14(3):471-6.

[59] Blake DD. Radiation treatment of metastatic bone disease. Clin Orthop 1970;73-89-100.

[60] Ford HT, Yarnold JR. Radiation therapy – Pain relief and recalcification. In: Stoll BA, Parbhoo S, eds. Bone Metastases: Monitoring and treatment. New York: Raven Press; 1983:343-54.

[61] Chow E, Ling A, Davis L, Panzarella T, Danjoux C. Pain flare following external beam radiotherapy and meaningful change in pain scores in the treatment of bone metastases. Radiother Oncol 2005;75:64-9.

[62] Chow E, Loblaw A, Harris K, Doyle M, Goh P, Chiu H, Panzarella T, Tsao M, Barnes E, Sinclair E, Farhadian M, Danjoux C. Dexamethasone for the prophylaxis of radiation-induced pain flare following palliative radiotherapy for bone metastases: a pilot study. Support Care Cancer 2007;15(6): 643-7.

[63] Hird A, Chow E, Zhang L, Wong R, Wu J, Sinclair E, Danjoux C, Tsao M, Barnes E, Loblaw A. Determining the incidence of pain flare following palliative radiotherapy for symptomatic bone metastases: results from three Canadian cancer centres. Int J Radiat Oncol Biol Phys (published online January 22, 2009).

[64] Hird A, Zhang L, Holt T, Fairchild F, DeAngelis C, Loblaw A, Wong R, Barnes E, Tsao M, Danjoux C, Chow E. Dexamethasone for the prophylaxis of radiation-induced pain flare following palliative radiotherapy for symptomatic bone metastases: A phase II study. Clin Oncol (published online February 15, 2009).

[65] Harris K, Chow E. Need for better documentation and definition of pain flare following external beam radiotherapy in the treatment of bone metastases. J Pain Symptom Manag 2007;33(1): 6-8.

[66] Chow E, Hoskin P, Wu J, Roos D, van der Linden Y, Hartsell W, Veith R, Wilson C, Pater J. A phase III international randomized trial comparing single with multiple fractions for re-irradiation of painful bone metastases. National Cancer Institute of Canada Clinical Trials Group (NCIC CTG SC 20). Clin Oncol 2006;18(2):125-8 .

[67] Chow E, Holden L, Danjoux C, Vidmar M, Connolly R, Finkelstein J, Cheung G. Successful salvage using percutaneous vertebroplasty in cancer patients with painful spinal metastases or osteoporotic compression fractures. Radiother Oncol 2004; 70(3):265-7.

[68] Cheung G, Chow E, Holden L, Vidmar M, Danjoux C, Yee A, Connolly R, Finkelstein J. Percutaneous vertebroplasty in patients with intractable pain from osteoporotic or metastatic fractures: a prospective study using quality of life assessment. Can Assoc Radiol J 2006;57(1):13-21.

[69] Fitch, M & Chow, E. Helping you to help yourself. Second edition. Toronto: Odette Cancer Centre; 2008. http://www.sunnybrook.ca/publication/

[70] Sunnybrook Health Sciences Centre. Newsletters and Publications – Hot Spot Newsletter. http://www.sunnybrook.ca/publication/.

In: Advanced Cancer

ISBN: 978-1-62808-239-5

Editors: N. Thavarajah, N. Pulenzas, B. Lechner et al.   © 2013 Nova Science Publishers, Inc.

Chapter 30

Barriers to prescription of sublingual fentanyl tablets for breakthrough cancer pain in an out-patient cancer center

Marissa Slaven, MD[*1], *Frederick A Spencer, MD*[2]
and Edward Chow, MBBS[3]

[1]Division of Palliative Care, Department of Family Medicine,
McMaster University, Hamilton, Canada
[2]Department of Medicine, McMaster University, Hamilton
[3]Department of Radiation Oncology, Sunnybrook Health Sciences Centre,
Toronto, Ontario, Canada

Abstract

Breakthrough cancer pain (BTcP) is a significant source of distress for patients with cancer. Sublingual fentanyl tablets are the first rapid onset opioid targeted to treat BTcP available in Canada. Objectives: In this study we sought to review the use of this product in consecutive patients for efficacy and safety. Methods: A retrospective chart review was conducted of patients attending an out-patient palliative care clinic who received prescriptions for fentanyl tablets over six months. Data extracted included age, gender, palliative performance status (PPS), primary and secondary disease sites, concurrent cancer therapy, concurrent analgesics, and efficacy of sublingual fentanyl. Efficacy was defined as titration of sublingual fentanyl to achieve satisfactory control of pain as per patient report. Results: Twenty charts were reviewed. The mean age of patients was 58 years and the mean PPS score was 77%. The dose range of sublingual fentanyl was 100 micrograms (mcg) up to 800 mcg. The drug was documented to be effective and was

* Correspondence: Marissa Slaven, MD, 699 Concession St, Hamilton, Ontario L9H 1Z8, Canada. E-mail: Marissa.slaven@jcc.hhsc.ca

continued through the follow-up period in nine patients. It was ineffective by ten patients. Only one patient experienced side effects. Conclusion: Successful titration of sublingual fentanyl for BTcP occurred in 50% of patients managed in our clinic. The safety profile in our case review was excellent with only one patient experiencing side effects requiring discontinuation of the medication.Coordinated efforts to improve out-patient titration (e.g. written instructions) as well as research into initiation of drug at higher doses (thereby requiring fewer titration steps) may improve the utility of this agent.

Introduction

Breakthrough cancer pain (BTcP) is a common problem distinct from persistent background pain, which is defined as a constant or continuous pain that is experienced by the patient for more than 12 hours per day. In contrast, breakthrough pain is defined as an exacerbation of pain that occurs on a background of otherwise stable pain in patients receiving chronic opioid therapy (1). Breakthrough cancer pain is characterized by rapid onset, short duration and severe intensity (1).

Breakthrough cancer pain represents a significant burden. A review of the literature demonstrates a prevalence of 51-89% of patients with controlled levels of background pain (1-6). Research shows that cancer patients with chronic pain are less satisfied with their pain control if they have breakthrough pain (9). Cancer patients with breakthrough pain also report higher levels of peak pain, higher levels of depression and anxiety, and greater functional impairment (7-10).

Rapid onset opioids are particularly well suited to address the problem of breakthrough cancer pain. Sublingual fentanyl products are delivered through the oral mucosa rapidly (within a few minutes), avoid first pass metabolism, and are very potent. They are generally well tolerated with side effect profiles similar to other narcotics (11-13).

The fentanyl sublingual tablet was approved for use by Health Canada in 2011 for the treatment of breakthrough pain in opioid-tolerant adult patients who are already receiving around the clock opioid therapy for their underlying persistent cancer pain. Current guidelines suggest patients should be on a minimum of sixty milligrams oral morphine equivalent (MME) in twenty four hours for two weeks before starting on sublingual fentanyl. Regardless of opioid dose prescribed to control chronic pain, sublingual fentanyl must be titrated up from a 100 mcg starting dose whenever it is started, or re-started, by increments (100, 200, 300, 400, 600 and 800mcg). Two clinical trials have shown fentanyl sublingual tablets to be an effective and well-tolerated treatment for the relief of breakthrough pain (11,12).

This paper reviews the use of a fentanyl sublingual tablet in patients in an out-patient palliative care clinic over a six month period. The purpose of this case report is to better understand demographics of patients receiving treatment, efficacy of treatment, potential barriers to use, and side effects of treatment.

Our study

An out-patient pain and symptom management clinic was established in our regional cancer center six years ago. The interdisciplinary team is composed of a physician, an advanced practice nurse, two registered nurses and a social worker. Referrals are for patients eighteen years or above who have a cancer diagnosis and an expected prognosis of one year or less. The clinic operates eight half days each week and sees approximately three hundred and fifty new patients each year. Patients are typically given appointments at one month intervals unless they call the clinic with a request to be seen sooner. All medications are reviewed with patients at each visit for compliance, safety and effectiveness.

Patients with breakthrough pain (BTP) were prescribed a starting dose of 100 mcg of sublingual fentanyl tablet and were instructed that if there was insufficient pain relief after 30 minutes to take rescue medication as allowed. The fentanyl sublingual dosage was then increased by the patient by 100 mcg for subsequent BTP episodes. Patients were instructed to wait two hours before treating subsequent BTP episodes. Patients were asked to call the clinic if they reached a dose of 300 mcg and did not have relief of their breakthrough pain. If there were no adverse effects they were then prescribed tablet strengths of 400, 600 and 800 mcg anddosing continued in this manner until an effective dose was reached or until a maximum dose of 800 mcg is reached. Patients were told they could take up to four doses in a twenty four hour period.

We conducted a retrospective chart review for twenty consecutive patients newly prescribed Abstral, a sublingual rapid onsetfentanyltablet beginning May 1st 2011 through October 31st 2011. Data extracted included age, gender, palliative performance status (PPS), primary and secondary disease sites, concurrent cancer therapy, concurrent analgesics, and use and efficacy of sublingual fentanyl. For the purpose of this study efficacy was defined as patient successful titration of sublingual fentanyl to achieve satisfactory control of breakthrough pain as per patient report. Pain control was deemed inadequate in patients who stopped sublingual fentanyl and/or failed to call for further dose titration despite continued pain. Charts were reviewed through to April 30th 2012. Institutional ethics approval for this retrospective study was obtained.

Findings

Twenty patients were prescribed sublingual fentanyl tablets over a six month period. One chart had insufficient documentation regarding the dosing and efficacy of the fentanyl and was excluded. Of the remaining nineteen patients, ten were male and nine female. The age range was 29-78 years old with a mean age of 58 years. The palliative performance scale (PPS) at the time that sublingual fentanyl was started ranged from 60 to 100% with a mean PPS score of 77%. Primary cancer sites included: sarcoma [3], lung [3], breast [3], renal [2], melanoma, lymphoma, prostate, penile, rectal, mesothelioma, ovarian, and hepatocellular cancer. Eighty percent of patients had metastatic disease with the most common sites being bone [11], lung [4] and liver [4]. Many patients were receiving disease modifying therapy with 11 receiving chemotherapy, 11 received radiation and four received no therapy.

Patients also received co-analgesics including: steroids [6], neurontin [5], NSAIDs [5], pregabalin [1], cannabinoid [1] and tylenol [1]. Patients in this review had a MME range of 60-2250 milligrams with a mean dose of 508 milligrams and a median dose of 200 milligrams prior to starting fentanyl.

The dose range of sublingual fentanyl used ranged from 100 micrograms (mcg) up to the maximum dose of 800 mcg with the median dose being 300 mcg. The drug was documented to be effective and was continued through the follow-up period in nine of the nineteen patients. It was deemed ineffective by ten patients and discontinued by them without consultation with the physician.

The median dose in those for whom it was effective was 300 mcg (range 200to 800 mcg) compared to a medium dose of 100 mcg (range 100 to 800) in those for whom it was deemed ineffective. Six patients for whom the drug was discontinued were not titrated up to maximum dose before discontinuing the drug. The vast majority (90%) of patients for whom it was deemed ineffective were on it for less than one month (median of <1 month, range<1 month to 2 months). For those for whom it was effective half were treated for longer than four months and one was treated for more than one year (median of 18 weeks, range<1 month to 1 year). One of 19 patients had a side effect, delirium, related to the administration of sublingual fentanyl which led to its discontinuation. Three patients for whom it was effective were subsequently transferred to institutions where it was not available and so were forced to discontinue it.

Discussion

Although sublingual fentanyl products have been studied in clinical trial settings it is important to understand what barriers exist to prevent their effective use in real clinical settings.

In our clinic we were successful in managing breakthrough cancer pain in half of the patients for whom the drug was prescribed. The mean effective dose was 300 mcg, well below the maximum recommended dosage of 800 mcg. It is noteworthy that 8 of the 10 patients in whom sublingual fentanyl was deemed "ineffective" in the management of breakthrough pain were not titrated to maximum dose. These patients opted to discontinue the drug without further titration beyond 300 mcg as they lost confidence in sublingual fentanyl products after two to three failures in titration.

It is possible that the overall efficacy would have been higher if more patients had been titrated up to maximum dose before deciding the treatment was ineffective and ceased. Titrating narcotics in an out-patient clinical setting can be challenging. Although patients are given teaching during their clinic visit and are asked to contact the clinic should they have any questions or concerns not all patients remember the teaching on titration or take advantage of the opportunity to receive help. Subsequent to this review we have been providing written instructions to patients for titration in addition to the teaching done in clinic. In clinical trials the mean effective dose of fentanyl sublingual tablet was greater than or equal to 300 mcg (13,14). It would be helpful to identify those patients in whom 100 mcg would not be effective so that a higher initial dose could be used and patients could achieve pain relief with a minimum number of titrations. One study has suggested that it is safe to start titration at higher doses in patients on higher daily MME doses (15). Again; more research is called for in this area.

A limitation of our study is its retrospective design. Other factors that may have impacted successful titration may not have been adequately captured by chart review. Prospective studies evaluating titration strategies and utilizing response to treatment pain scales should be performed. It is noteworthy, that the safety profile in our case review was excellent with only one patient experiencing side effects requiring discontinuation of the medication.

In conclusion, successful titration of sublingual fentanyl tablets for management of breakthrough pain occurred in 50% of patients managed in our out-patient clinic. In the majority of patients for whom it was ineffective it was not titrated to maximal dose before stopping - this was not due to development of side effects. Coordinated efforts to improve out-patient titration (e.g. written instructions) as well as research into initiation of drug at higher doses (thereby requiring fewer titration steps) may improve the utility of this agent.

References

[1] Portnoy RK, Hagen NA. Breakthrough pain: definition, prevalence and characteristics. Pain 1990;41:273-81.

[2] Fine PG, Busch MA. Characterization of breakthrough pain by hospice patients and their caregivers. J Pain Symptom Manage 1998;16(3):179-83.

[3] Mercadante S, Radbruch L, Caraceni A, Cherny N, Kaasa S, Nauck F, et al. Episodic (breakthrough) pain: consensus conference of an expert working group of the European Association for Palliative Care. Cancer 2002;94(3):832-9.

[4] Breivik H, Vherny N, Collett B, Collett B, de Conno F, Filbet M, et al. Cancer-related pain: a pan-European survey of prevalence, treatment and patient attitudes. Ann Oncol 2009;20(8):1420-33.

[5] Zeppetella G, Riberiero M. Pharmacotherapy of cancer-related episodic pain . Expert Opin Pharmacother 2003;4(4):493-502.

[6] Gomez-Batiste X, Madrid F, Moreno F, Gracia A, Trelis J, Fontanals et al. Breakthrough cancer pain: prevalence and characteristics in patients in Catalonia, Spain. J Pain Symptom Manage 2002;24(1):45-52.

[7] Caraceni A, Martini C, Zecca E, Portenoy RK, Ashby MA, Hawson G, et al. Breakthrough pain characteristics and syndromes in patients with cancer. An international survey. Palliat Med 2004;18:177-83.

[8] Portenoy RK, Payne D, Jacobsen P. Breakthrough pain: characteristics and impact in patients with cancer pain. Pain 1999;81:129-34.

[9] Zeppetella G, O'Doherty CA, Collins S. Prevalence and characteristics of breakthrough pain in cancer patients admitted to a hospice. J Pain Symptom Manage 2000;20(2):87-92.

[10] Skinner C, Thompson E, Davies A. Clinical features. In: Davies A. Cancer related breakthrough pain. Oxford: Oxford University Press, 2006:13-22.

[11] Rauck RL, Tark M, Reyes E, Hayes TG, Bartkowiak AJ, Hassman D, et al. Efficacy and long-term tolerability of sublingual fentanyl orally disintegrating tablet in the treatment of breakthrough cancer pain. Curr Med Res Opin 2009;25:2877-85.

[12] Nalamachu S, Hassman D, Wallace M, Dumble S, Derrick R, Howell J. Long-term effectiveness and tolerability of sublingual fentanyl citrate orally disintegrating tablet for the treatment of breakthrough cancer pain. Curr Med Res Opin 2011;27:519-30.

[13] Nalamachu SR, Rauck RL, Wallace MS, Hassman D, Howell J. Successful dose finding with sublingual fentanyl tablet:combined results from 2 open-label titration studies. Pain Pract 2012;12(6):449-56.

[14] Ward J, Laird B, Fallon M; BTcP Registry Group. The UK breakthrough cancer pain registry: Origin, methods and preliminary data. Presented at The Compass Collaboration Annual Scientific Meeting, Edinburgh 2011 Apr 14-15.

[15] Mercadante S, Gatti A, Porizio G, Lo Presti C, Aielli F, Adile C, et al. Dosing fentanyl buccal tablet for breakthrough cancer pain: dose titration versus proportional doses. Curr Med Res Opin 2012;28(6);963-8.

SECTION FOUR:
RADIATION INDUCED NAUSEA
AND VOMITING (RINV)

In: Advanced Cancer   ISBN: 978-1-62808-239-5
Editors: N. Thavarajah, N. Pulenzas, B. Lechner et al.   © 2013 Nova Science Publishers, Inc.

Chapter 31

Review of radiation-induced nausea and vomiting research in the Rapid Response Radiotherapy Program

Natalie Pulenzas, BSc(C), Breanne Lechner, BSc(C),
Nemica Thavarajah, BSc(C) and Edward Chow, MBBS*
Rapid Response Radiotherapy Program, Department of Radiation Oncology,
Odette Cancer Centre, Sunnybrook Health Sciences Centre,
University of Toronto, Toronto, Ontario, Canada

Abstract

Research conducted by the Rapid Response Radiotherapy Program (RRRP) on radiation induced nausea and vomiting (RINV) is examined in this chapter. RINV develops in approximately 50-80% of patients, and severity is dependent on factors such as treatment volume, overall dose, current chemotherapy, and pre-existing nausea and vomiting (N/V). RINV has an acute phase, during and immediately after radiation, and a delayed phase in the days following treatment. The most commonly prescribed anti-emetic in practice was 5-hydroxytryptamine-3 (5-HT3) receptor antagonists (RA), which is also recommended by Multinational Association for Supportive Care in Cancer (MASCC) and the American Society of Clinical Oncology (ASCO). The international patterns of management strategies in RINV, radiation oncologists and trainees were reviewed through an online survey. Awareness of guidelines and standards of practice varied across all groups. Prospective studies that used 5-HT3 RAs for the prophylaxis of RINV resulted in low control rates of N/V, most markedly in the delayed phase. A prospective study used the Functional Living Index of Emesis (FLIE), and developed a daily diary to assess N/V, however had a very low compliance rate due to no follow-up calls and complicated

---

* Correspondence: Professor Edward Chow MBBS, MSc, PhD, FRCPC, Department of Radiation Oncology, Odette Cancer Centre, Sunnybrook Health Sciences Centre, 2075 Bayview Avenue, Toronto, ON Canada. Email: Edward.Chow@Sunnybrook.ca.

instructions. There is no current standardized assessment for RINV that is applicable to palliative cancer patients.

Introduction

Radiation therapy is used to obtain symptom relief for painful bone metastases and improve quality of life (QOL). However, patients may also experience nausea and vomiting as a debilitating side effect of radiation (1). Incidence rate of radiotherapy-induced nausea and vomiting (RINV) is approximately 50-80% of patients receiving radiation treatment (2). Severity of RINV depends on patient and radiation related factors such as treatment volume, overall dose, current chemotherapy, and pre-existing nausea and vomiting (1). RINV may lead to delayed treatment, fear of treatment, and reduced overall QOL (2,3). RINV occurs in two phases; the acute phase immediately after radiotherapy, as well as a delayed phase (1). The Rapid Response Radiotherapy Program (RRRP) provides immediate radiotherapy for palliative cancer patients.

There is extensive research investigating chemotherapy induced nausea and vomiting (CINV), however there is limited data on RINV (3). It is known that the mechanisms underlying CINV are very similar to RINV, as well as the treatment of these symptoms (2). Radiation treatment damages the gastrointestinal mucosa, which subsequently releases serotonin and initiates RINV through binding to 5-hydroxytryptamine-3 (5-HT3) receptors. The most commonly recommended antiemetic for the prophylaxis of RINV are 5-HT_3 receptor antagonists (RA) which prevent the binding of serotonin, and therefore RINV (2,3).

Literature review

A retrospective review of the literature was obtained including all research published from the RRRP involving RINV. There were no exclusion criteria, and RINV data was collected from 2010-present including review articles. A main focus of the RRRP research is the effectiveness and optimal timing of 5-HT_3 RAs in the prophylaxis or rescue of RINV.

Salvo et al (3) conducted a systematic review of the literature in 2012 comparing the efficacy of 5-HT_3 RAs with anti-emetic medications or placebo in randomized controlled trials. Nine trials were identified and included in the review. Majority of the studies reviewed reported superiority of 5-HT_3 RAs when compared with other antiemetic medications or placebo. Two studies reported no significant difference in effectiveness, however these trials had very small sample sizes. Studies reviewed which compared 5-HT_3 RA and other antiemetic medications commonly tested tropisetron versus metroclopramide. Prevention of emesis was statistically more effective for 5-HT3 RAs, however results of prevention of nausea were not statistically significant between treatment options, suggesting nausea is a difficult symptom to control (3).

Dennis et al (2) also conducted a review of the RINV literature in 2011. Major antiemetic guidelines were reviewed from the Multinational Association for Supportive Care in Cancer (MASCC)/European Society of Medical Oncology (ESMO), the American Society of Clinical Oncology (ASCO), and the National Comprehensive Cancer Network (NCCN).

MASC/ESMO and ASCO guidelines recommend pharmaceutical treatment depending on the site of radiation, and consequently the risk of emesis. Moderate and low emetogenic risks from radiation are the most commonly seen groups in a palliative cancer setting. For low emetogenic risk patients (cranium, lower thorax), both guidelines recommend prophylaxis or rescue with a 5-HT$_3$ RA. Treatment for moderate emetic risk (upper abdomen), as recommended by MASC/ESMO is prophylaxis with a 5-HT$_3$ RA with/without concurrent dexamethasone, and ASCO recommends prophylaxis with a 5-HT$_3$ RA alone. NCCN guidelines incorporate all sites of radiation, except whole body, into the same emetic risk category, which therefore lacks validity (2). A study included in the review conducted in Italy determined only 12.4% of patients received prophylactic antiemetic therapy, though there is limited consensus on the implication of this data due to a small amount of literature available. The review by Dennis et al (2) concluded that radiation oncologists frequently underestimate the impact and prevalence of RINV.

Dennis et al (4) conducted a subsequent study investigating the international patterns of practice in RINV of radiation oncologists from twelve countries across the world through a web-based survey. Six clinical radiation therapy scenarios were presented in the survey; one high risk for emesis, two moderate, and two low risk cases. Respondents ranked the case for risks of nausea and vomiting, management strategies, and if applicable chose the anti-emetic medication they would prescribe. Management strategies for RINV varied across the respondents, more prominently in the moderate and low risk cases in deciding between prophylaxis or rescue therapy (4).

Another study conducted by Dennis et al (5) investigated radiation oncology trainee's knowledge in the appropriate management and guidelines of RINV through the same survey used previously. Only 28% of the 176 trainees were aware of the current antiemetic guidelines, and treatment strategies were more variable again in the low and moderate risk cases, as expected (5). These studies show the importance of continuing research in RINV, and developing/establishing appropriate standard antiemetic guidelines.

Presutti et al (1) conducted a prospective study involving 19 patients from the RRRP who received palliative radiation therapy to the upper abdomen and abdominal/pelvic region. The study reported the results of the preliminary analysis. Participants received radiation for painful bone metastases in single or multiple fractions. All patients were prescribed prophylactic Ondansetron (8 mg) (5-HT$_3$ RA) with varying regimens, at the discretion of the physician, and completed daily nausea and vomiting diaries for all days during and ten days post treatment. Exclusion criteria included patients receiving concomitant chemotherapy within the study period, defined as the start of radiation until 10 days post treatment, or other anti-emetic medications. Acute phase RINV was defined as from the commencement of radiation to 24 hours after completion. The delayed phase began from completion of the acute phase (24 hours post-radiation) until 10 days following. Results showed less control of nausea and vomiting in the delayed phase when compared to the acute phase, as the amount of patients with complete prophylaxis decreased (1). Dennis et al conducted the final analysis with 59 enrolled patients, and 32 with complete follow up data from 2007-2010 (6). Twenty-four patients received single fraction radiotherapy, and 8 patients received multiple fractions, of which all received 20Gy in 5 fractions except for one patient who received 30Gy in 10 fractions. Dosing schedules of Ondansetron varied, as patients receiving single fraction radiotherapy were prescribed for a duration of 1 day (n=20), 3 days (n=2), or 5 days (n=2); and multiple fraction radiotherapy prescribed for 5 days (n=6), 10 days (n=1), or 15 days (n=1). Dosage was also variable, as 42% of patients in the single fraction group, and 12% of the multiple fraction group took Ondansetron once daily, as opposed to twice daily dosing. Patients were distinguished as a moderate risk for RINV if radiation included one portion of the upper abdomen (T11-L3 inclusive). Low emetogenic risk was determined to be radiation targeting or involving the pelvis. Similar results to Presutti et al (1) were concluded after final analysis (1,6). Complete prophylaxis of nausea in the moderate risk emetogenic group was achieved by 56% and 31% of patients in the acute and delayed phase respectively for the single fraction group; 71% and 43% for the multiple fraction group. For the low risk emetogenic group, 50% and 43% for single fraction; 100% and 100% for multiple fractions. Complete prophylaxis of vomiting in the moderate risk emetogenic group was achieved by 69% and 44% of patients in the acute and delayed phase respectively for the single fraction group; 57% and 57% for the multiple fraction group. In the low risk emetogenic group, 100% and 57% for single fraction; 100% and 100% for multiple fractions. The authors concluded that despite prophylaxis of RINV with Ondansetron, patients still experienced nausea and vomiting, with higher rates of incidence in the delayed phase (6). Conclusions were lacking in delayed RINV in the systematic review by Salvo et al (3). Of the studies reviewed, a significant limitation of the data collection was the absence of knowledge for the delayed phase (3). A review of the RINV literature in 2011 by Dennis et al (2) concluded that despite $5-HT_3$ RA being recommended for prophylaxis, optimal timing and duration are unknown. Twenty-five trials were reviewed in a subsequent study by Dennis et al (7) to determine optimal timing and duration of $5-HT_3$ RAs. It was determined that $5-HT_3$ RAs were most commonly prescribed for the duration of radiotherapy, but complete control of nausea especially, was low across the majority of trials (7).

Research is lacking in a quality of life questionnaire specific to the RINV setting. One of the most commonly tools used in the RRRP and past studies is the Functional Living Index of Emesis (FLIE). Only two of the nine trials reviewed by Salvo included some measure of QOL, and one study required patients to complete the FLIE preceding and following radiation treatment. The second study used the European Organisation of Cancer Treatment Quality of Life Questionnaire – Core 30 (EORTC QLQ-C30), a general quality of life tool for cancer patients. Results appeared to show a slight increase in QOL of patients who received treatment with 5-HT3 RAs (3). Haid et al (8) created a self reported daily diary to assess for nausea, vomiting, and use of rescue medications based on the MASCC Antiemesis Tool (MAT). Thirty-five patients were accrued and required to complete the daily diary for fifteen days, and the FLIE twice a week during the study period, and a debriefing questionnaire, with no telephone follow up calls. Eligible patients had irradiation to the abdomen, abdomen/pelvis, cranium, or esophagus. However, only four patients completed all follow-ups and the authors concluded this likely occurred due to a lack of follow-up calls throughout the study, and complex instructions and assessments (8).

Discussion

As determined by the literature, there are several guidelines that recommend the use of anti-emetic medications for the prophylaxis of RINV. However, as determined by Dennis et al (4,5) in 2011 and 2012, a low percentage of physicians are aware of the current guidelines.

Further education in these guidelines, especially in radiation oncology trainees, may help in reducing rates of RINV through appropriate prophylactic prescriptions and awareness (4,5). The most commonly used agent for the prophylaxis of RINV has been determined to be 5-HT$_3$ RAs, though despite the use of these medications, nausea and vomiting are still common. Future research should focus on improving the control of nausea and vomiting, particularly in the delayed phase (1,3,6). Determination of optimal timing and duration of 5-HT$_3$ RAs may assist in the control of the delayed phase, but is still unknown (7). The results of these studies show that complete control of nausea is difficult to obtain, therefore complete control of vomiting may be an important endpoint in future studies as this can be viewed as a serious side effect by patients (7). Ondansetron was the most commonly used 5-HT$_3$ RA, and upcoming alternatives may be influential on future research. Specific assessments for measuring QOL and RINV related symptoms have not been standardized. Past prospective studies in the RRRP have used assessments such as the FLIE, and designed new diaries with significant limitations. Such as the diary used by Haid et al (8) resulted in a very low compliance rate. We have been developing a revised daily diary that is applicable for palliative cancer patients, yet optimal in collecting incidences of nausea, vomiting, and use of rescue medication. The use of follow-up calls and reminders may also elevate compliance rate in future prospective studies (8).

Conclusion

RINV still occurs in a significant proportion of palliative cancer patients receiving moderately or low emetogenic radiotherapy. Complete control of nausea has historically been lower than vomiting, suggesting it to be a more difficult symptom to prevent. Further investigation should focus on the use of other 5-HT$_3$ RAs, or use in combination with other medications. Research into the optimal timing and duration of 5-HT$_3$ RA is important to consider so the control of delayed phase RINV can be elevated. A specific QOL questionnaire and daily diary for assessing RINV is important to record symptoms, as well as decrease patient burden and optimize compliance.

Acknowledgments

We thank the generous support of Bratty Family Fund, Michael and Karyn Goldstein Cancer Research Fund, Joseph and Silvana Melara Cancer Research Fund, and Ofelia Cancer Research Fund.

References

[1] Presutti R, Nguyen J, Holden L, DeAngelis C, Culleton S, Mitera G, et al. Radiation-induced nausea and vomiting in a palliative radiotherapy clinic: A preliminary analysis. J Pain Manag 2010;3(3): 301-7.

[2]   Dennis K, Maranzano E, De Angelis C, Holden L, Wong S, Chow E. Radiotherapy-induced nausea and vomiting. Expert Rev Pharmacoecon Outcomes Res 2011;11(6):685-92.

[3]   Salvo N, Doble B, Khan L, Amirthevasar G, Dennis K, Pasetka M, et al. Prophylaxis of radiation-induced nausea and vomiting using 5-hydroxytryptamine-3 serotonin receptor antagonists: a systematic review of randomized trials. Int J Radiat Oncol Biol Phys 2012;82(1):408-17.

[4]   Dennis K, Zhang L, Lutz S, van Baardwijk A, van der Linden Y, Holt T, et al. International patterns of practice in the management of radiation therapy-induced nausea and vomiting. Int J Radiat Oncol Biol Phys 2012;84(1):e49-60.

[5]   Dennis K, Zhang L, Lutz S, van der Linden Y, van Baardwijk A, Holt T, et al. International radiation oncology trainee decision making in the management of radiotherapy-induced nausea and vomiting. Support Care Cancer 2013 Feb 26. [EPub ahead of print]

[6]   Dennis K, Nguyen J, Presutti R, DeAngelis C, Tsao M, Danjoux C, et al. Prophylaxis of radiotherapy-induced nausea and vomiting in the palliative treatment of bone metastases. Support Care Cancer 2012;20(8):1673-78.

[7]   Dennis K, Makhani L, Maranzano E, Feyer P, Zeng L, DeAngelis C, et al. Timing and duration of 5-HT3 receptor antagonist therapy for the prophylaxis of radiotherapy-induced nausea and vomiting: a systematic review of randomized and non-randomized studies. J Radiat Oncol, in press.

[8]   Haid V, Kumar K, Al Duhaiby E, Pang J, DeAngelis C, Pasetka M, et al. Evaluation of a daily diary for assessing the prevalence of radiation-induced emesis (RIE). J Pain Manag 2012;5(3):237-44.

In: Advanced Cancer
Editors: N. Thavarajah, N. Pulenzas, B. Lechner et al.

ISBN: 978-1-62808-239-5
© 2013 Nova Science Publishers, Inc.

Chapter 32

Radiation-induced nausea and vomiting in a palliative radiotherapy clinic

Roseanna Presutti, BSc, Janet Nguyen, BSc,
Lori Holden, MRT(T), Carlo DeAngelis, PhD,
Shaelyn Culleton, BSc, Gunita Mitera, MRT(T), MBA,
May Tsao, MD, Elizabeth A Barnes, MD, Cyril Danjoux, MD,
Arjun Sahgal, MD, Nadia Salvo, MSc (C), Luluel Khan, MD
*and Edward Chow, MBBS**

Rapid Response Radiotherapy Program, Department of Radiation Oncology,
Odette Cancer Centre, Sunnybrook Health Sciences Centre,
University of Toronto, Toronto, Canada

Abstract

In this chapter we report the pattern of radiation induced nausea and vomiting (RINV) after prophylaxis with a 5-hydroxytryptamine-3 (5-HT3) receptor antagonist in patients receiving radiotherapy (RT) to the upper abdomen or abdominal-pelvic region, in the Rapid Response Radiotherapy Program (RRRP). Methods: Patients completed the nausea/vomiting daily diary before, during RT and ten days after RT. Complete prophylaxis (CP) of nausea and CP of vomiting (no nausea/no vomiting and use of no rescue therapy) were determined in both the acute (beginning of RT to 24 hours after completion of RT) and delayed (24 hours after the completion of RT to 240 hours/10 days following RT) phases. RT could be single or multiple treatments. Results: A total of 34 patients were enrolled in this study. Fifteen patients were excluded due to incomplete

* Correspondence: Edward Chow, MBBS, MSc, PhD, FRCPC, Department of Radiation Oncology, Odette Cancer Centre, Sunnybrook Health Sciences Centre, 2075 Bayview Avenue, Toronto, ON M4N 3M5 Canada. Tel: 416-480-4998; Fax: 416-480-6002; E-mail: Edward.Chow@sunnybrook.ca.

diary information and/or non-compliance with prophylactic anti-emetics. The median age was 64 years (range: 48-91) and there were slightly more females (53%) than males (47%). From the acute to delayed phase, CP of nausea declined from 54% to 46% in the single-fraction group and from 67% to 50% in the multiple-fraction group. Similarly, CP of vomiting declined from 92% to 62% in the single-fraction group and from 67% to 50% in the multiple-fraction group. Conclusion: RINV may occur up to ten days post-RT. Due to a small sample size, this is only a preliminary conclusion and further investigation is required.

Introduction

Palliative radiotherapy (RT) is a well-established and effective modality for relieving pain and improving quality of life (QoL) in patients with bone metastases. Patients receiving palliative RT for bone metastases may experience radiation induced nausea and vomiting (RINV), negatively impacting QoL. The experience of RINV is influenced by several treatment-related factors including the irradiated area, dose per fraction, overall dose, treatment volume and the technique of RT used. Patient-related factors including age, sex, history of alcohol use, previous experiences of nausea and vomiting with chemotherapy and/or RT, concurrent or recent chemotherapy, and anxiety also influence the likelihood of patients experiencing RINV (1, 2).

The American Society of Clinical Oncology (ASCO) guidelines for antiemetics in oncology published in 2006 outlined four emetic risk categories (high, moderate, low and minimal) based on radiation treatments. Patients who receive total-body RT are classified as high risk (>90% risk). Moderate risk (60-90% risk) consists of patients receiving RT to the upper abdomen, and low risk (30-60% risk) for RT to the lower thorax and pelvis, cranial radiosurgery or craniospinal RT. The group at minimal risk (<30% risk) of experiencing emesis are those receiving RT to the breast, head and neck, cranium only or the extremities (3,4).

ASCO's guidelines for antiemetic medication regimes are based on which risk category the patient belongs to. The ASCO panel suggests prophylaxis with a 5-hydroxytryptamine-3 (5-HT3) serotonin receptor antagonist (RA), with or without a corticosteroid, with each RT fraction and for at least 24 hours after RT for the high risk group. Prophylaxis with a 5-HT3 RA before each fraction is recommended for the moderate risk group and prophylaxis or rescue with a 5-HT3 RA is recommended for the low risk group. Rescue antiemetics only are recommended for the minimal risk group (4).

The purpose of the present study was to observe the pattern of nausea and vomiting in patients in the moderate risk group receiving prophylaxis with a 5-HT3 RA while undergoing palliative RT for painful bony metastases.

Our study

Patients who received palliative RT to the upper abdomen or abdominal-pelvic region in the Rapid Response Radiotherapy Program (RRRP) were eligible for this study. Radiotherapy could be delivered in single or multiple fractions. All patients were prescribed a 5-HT3 RA (ondansetron 8mg, po) as a prophylactic measure. Prophylaxis regimens varied from patient to patient depending on the prescribing physician's preferences. Basic demographics were collected including age, gender, primary cancer site, and Karnofsky Performance Status (KPS). Ethics approval was obtained from Sunnybrook Health Sciences Centre.

At baseline (day 0), patients completed a diary in which the severity of nausea, vomiting/retching and diarrhea within the past 24-hours was rated on a four-point categorical scale of none, mild, moderate or severe. In the diary, the number of episodes of nausea and vomiting/retching, and the use of prophylactic/regular and rescue anti-emetics within the past 24-hours was also recorded. Following a single treatment, all patients were given the diary to complete daily for a ten-day period (days 1-10). Patients receiving multiple-fraction RT were asked to complete the diary daily for the duration of their treatments, as well as for ten days post-RT (days 1-15). A clinical research assistant contacted the patient on a daily basis either in person at the clinic, or by telephone, to collect the diary information.

For the purpose of this study, the incidence of nausea and vomiting, despite prophylaxis with an antiemetic, in patients receiving single-fraction (8Gy/1) or multiple-fraction RT (20Gy/5) from day 0 (baseline) to day 10 (single-fraction patients) or day 15 (multiple-fraction patients) was investigated. This is expressed as a percentage of patients experiencing at least one episode of nausea and/or vomiting on each specified day.

Complete prophylaxis (CP) of nausea and CP of vomiting, as well as no nausea and no vomiting in both the acute and delayed phase were also investigated. The acute phase was defined as the time period from the beginning of RT to 24 hours after the completion of RT. In patients receiving a single fraction (8Gy/1), this was 0-24hours and in patients receiving multiple-fraction treatment (20Gy/5), this timeframe was 0-144hours. The delayed phase was defined as the time period following the first 24 hours after the completion of RT to 240 hours (10 days) following the completion of RT. Complete prophylaxis of vomiting was defined as no vomiting and use of no rescue therapy, where as no vomiting was defined as no vomiting as a result of the use of rescue therapy [5]. The same definition was applied to nausea, with CP of nausea being defined as no nausea and use of no rescue therapy, and no nausea being defined as no nausea as a result of the use of rescue therapy.

Our findings

A total of 34 patients were enrolled in this study. Since the purpose of the present study was to investigate the pattern of nausea and/or vomiting despite prophylaxis, patients who did not take prophylaxis as prescribed were excluded (n=4). Patients with incomplete nausea and vomiting diary information were also excluded (n=11). As a result, analyses of nausea and vomiting rates were based on 19 patients.

At baseline, the median age was 64 years (range: 48 – 91) and there were slightly more females (53%) than males (47%). The study population consisted primarily of breast and prostate patients, followed by lung, gastrointestinal and renal cell carcinoma as primary cancer sites. All patients were treated for painful bony metastases and received either 8Gy/1 or 20Gy/5 fractions. The vast majority of patients received RT to the spine (mid to lower thoracic spine, lumbar spine, and/or sacrum), followed by the pelvis and ribcage (see table 1).

When investigating the percentage of patients experiencing at least one episode of nausea and/or vomiting from baseline to ten days post-RT, patients were separated by fractionation schedule. In the single-fraction group, approximately 40% of patients had at least one episode of nausea during the study period. The greatest incidence of nausea (46.2%) occurred on days 1, 4, 5, 6 and 7.

Table 1. Patient Demographics (N=19)

Variable	N	Proportion
Age (years)		
Mean ± SD	64.8 ± 12.0	n/a
Median (Range)	64 (48 – 91)	n/a
Gender		
Male	9	(47%)
Female	10	(53%)
Primary Cancer Site		
Breast	8	(42.1%)
Prostate	6	(31.6%)
Lung	3	(15.8%)
GI	1	(5.3%)
Renal Cell	1	(5.3%)
Reason of radiation		
Painful Bone Metastases	19	(100%)
Radiation sites (n=29)		
Spine(excluding cervical spine)	20	(70.0%)
Pelvis	6	(20.7%)
Ribcage	3	(10.3%)
Radiation Dose		
8Gy/1	13	(68.4%)
20Gy/5	6	(31.6%)

n.b. patients may have been treated to more than one site, and all patients receiving RT to multiple sites received the same dose at each site.

Conversely, the mean incidence of vomiting in the single-fraction group was only 6.3%, with the greatest incidence occurring on day 3 with 23.1% of patients having at least one episode of vomiting (see figure 1). In the multiple-fraction group, approximately 29.2% of patients experienced at least one episode of nausea during the study period. The majority of episodes of nausea occurred from days 8 to 14. Fifty percent of patients experienced at least one episode of nausea on days 8, 11, 12, 13 and 14, suggesting that there may be a delayed effect of RT on the experience of nausea. Approximately 23% of patients receiving multiple-fraction RT had at least one episode of vomiting during the study period. Similar to the observed pattern of nausea, the majority of episodes of vomiting also occurred during days 8 to 14. The greatest incidence of vomiting was 50%, occurring on days 11 and 14 (see figure 2).

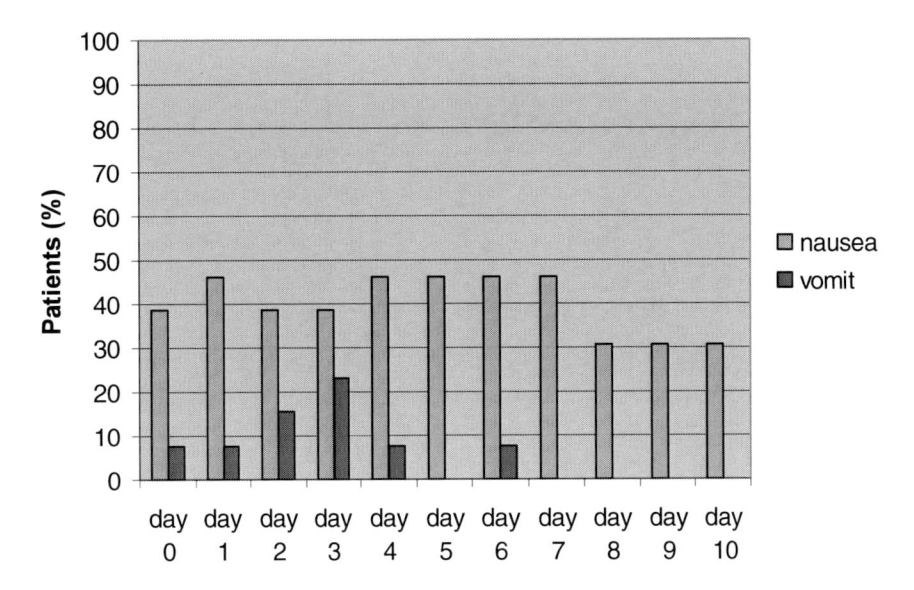

Figure 1. Patients experiencing at least one episode of nausea and/or vomit after receiving single-fraction radiotherapy (8Gy/1) (N=13).

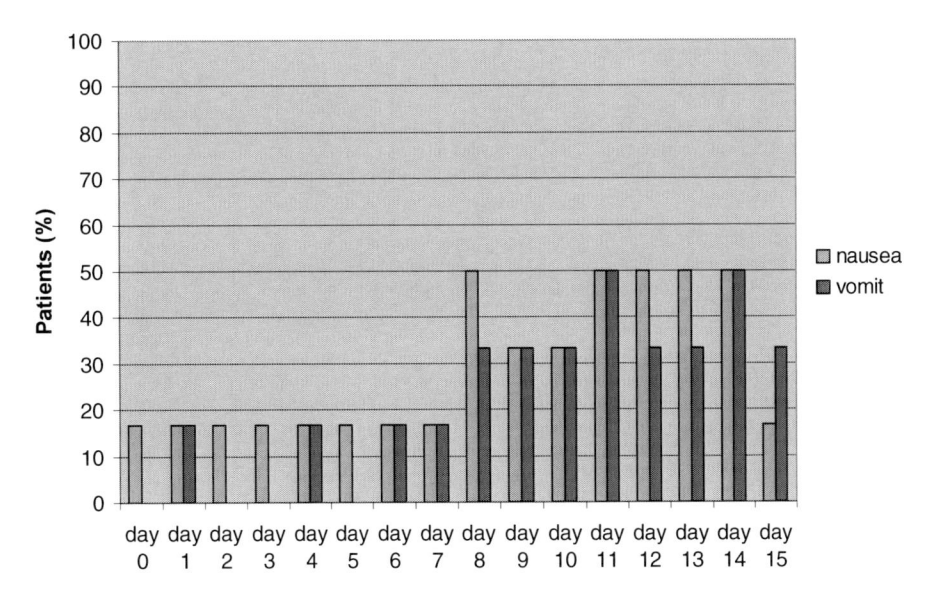

Figure 2. Patients experiencing at least one episode of nausea and/or vomit after receiving multi-fraction radiotherapy (20Gy/5) (N=6).

In the acute phase, the CP rate of nausea was 54% in the single-fraction group versus 67% in the multiple-fraction group. Complete prophylaxis of vomiting was greater in patients receiving single-fraction RT at 92% compared to 67% in patients receiving multiple-fraction RT (see figure 3). During the delayed phase, CP rates for nausea and vomiting in both the single- and multiple-fraction groups declined. Complete prophylaxis of nausea declined from 54% to 46% in the single-fraction group and from 67% to 50% in the multiple-fraction group. Similarly, CP of vomiting declined from 92% to 62% in the single-fraction group and from 67% to 50% in the multiple-fraction group (see figure 4).

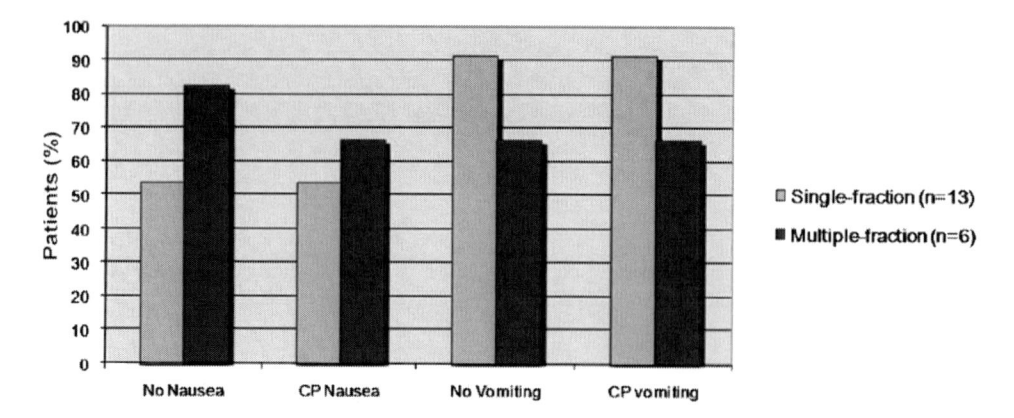

Figure 3. Patients with no nausea and/or vomiting during the acute phase.

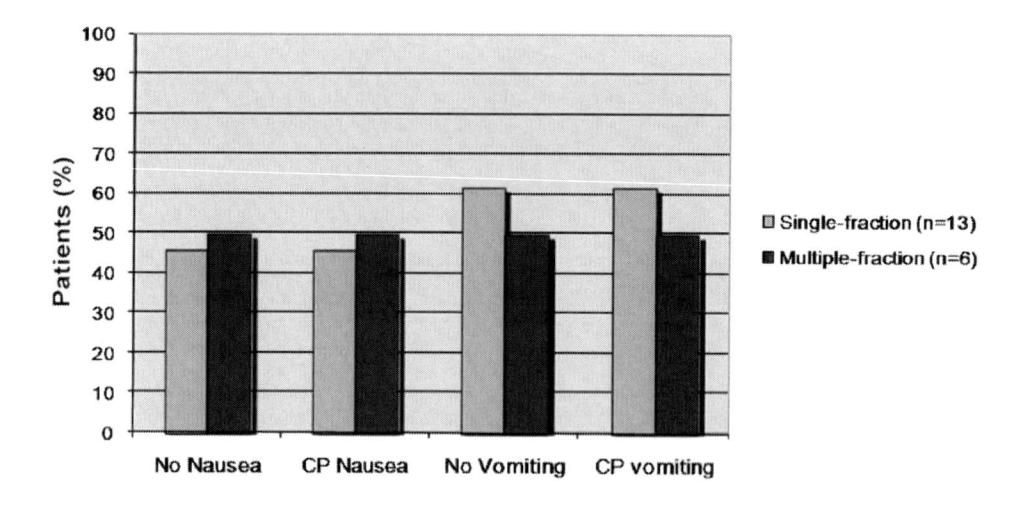

Figure 4. Patients with no nausea and/or vomiting during the delayed phase.

Discussion

The present study investigated the pattern of RINV in patients receiving prophylaxis with the 5-HT3 RA (ondansetron). Several trials have examined the role of ondansetron as a prophylactic agent in the management of RINV (6-11). Two randomized placebo controlled studies (6,7) demonstrated complete protection from emesis in 60-67% of patients in the ondansetron arm versus 10-45% in the control arm. Three further trials (8-11) compared the use of ondansetron to other non-5-HT3 RA anti-emetics (metoclopramide (8,9), prochlorperazine (10) and a combination of chlorpromazine and dexamethasone (11)). The proportion of patients receiving ondansetron experiencing complete protection from emesis ranged from 61-97% compared to 35-46% in patients receiving a non-5-HT3 RA antiemetic. These trials demonstrate that ondansetron is an effective and appropriate agent for use in the prophylaxis of RINV.

Radiation induced nausea and vomiting was first described by Court-Brown in 1953 and was further explained by Danjoux et al (12,13) in 1979 as an acute syndrome. According to Danjoux et al (13) 83% and 39% of patients receiving upper hemi-body and lower hemi-body radiation, respectively, experience radiation induced emesis. Radiation sickness was characterized as having three distinct phases. First, an asymptomatic latent period for 40-90 minutes, followed by an acute bout of nausea and vomiting, and a recovery period (13). Although initially described as an acute syndrome, the results of the present study may suggest otherwise. Our data shows evidence of prolonged RINV, with CP rates of nausea and vomiting declining from the acute to delayed phase in both the single and multiple-fraction groups.

Few trials have previously reported the presence of delayed or prolonged emesis in the radiotherapy setting (11,14). Sykes et al (11) recorded delayed emesis in their study of ondansetron versus a combination of chlorpromazine and dexamethasone for the prevention of nausea and vomiting in patients receiving single-fraction RT (lower hemibody 8Gy/1 or upper lumbar spine 12.5Gy/1). Delayed emesis was described as emesis occurring on days 2-4 of RT, with day 1 being the treatment day. In the ondansetron group (n=33), approximately 96% of patients reported complete or major control of emesis (0-2 emetic episodes) on days 2-4 compared to 42.9%, 39.9% and 37% on days 2, 3 and 4, respectively, in the combination group (n=33). Also, in a pilot study (14) investigating the efficacy of ondansetron plus dexamethasone in patients receiving single-fraction hemi-body RT, a delayed phase was noted. The complete control of emesis was 86% in the first 24 hours post-RT; however, 43% of patients experienced nausea, with or without vomiting, 27-72 hours after RT.

The present study not only confirms the existence of a delayed phase of RINV but also demonstrates that delayed RINV can last up to ten days post-RT. However, this is not without limitations. As a result of non-compliance and attrition, the present study was subject to a small sample size, which is not surprising given the nature of the study population. In order to verify the existence of the delayed phase that our group has described, larger patient numbers would be required. Also, since the present study investigated RINV in patients treated for bone metastases, it is highly likely that the vast majority of patients were on opioids to control bony pain associated with such metastases. Opioids on their own can lead to nausea and/or vomiting, which may contribute to the observed presence of nausea and/or vomiting in the delayed phase. Furthermore, given that this was an observational study, the pattern of prophylaxis was inconsistent both between and within treatment groups. The lack of consistency in anti-emetic prescribing procedures has previously been reported (15), and may have affected the observed incidence and CR rates of nausea and vomiting in the present series.

Despite a small sample size and other limitations, our study does demonstrate that patients receiving palliative RT for bone metastases experience nausea and/or vomiting in the week or so following treatment. If the existence of delayed RINV as defined in the present study can be verified using larger numbers and standard prescribing procedures, a need for improved anti-emetic guidelines may be warranted. The ultimate goal of RT for bone metastases is to relieve pain and improve quality of life, and adequate control of RINV will help to ensure that the latter goal is achieved.

Acknowledgments

This project was funded by Michael and Karyn Goldstein Cancer Research Fund. We thank Stacy Lue for secretarial assistance, Sarah Campos, Jenna VanDraanen, Mark Pasetka, Jocelyn Pang and Erika Stacey for their help. Conflicts of interest notification: None.

References

[1]   Feyer P. The importance of simple, easy-to-follow antiemetic guidelines. Acta Oncologica Suppl 2004;15:5-8.

[2]   The Antiemetic Subcommittee of the Multinational Association of Supportive Care in Cancer (MASCC). Prevention of chemotherapy- and radiotherapy-induced emesis: results of the 2004 Perugia International Antiemetic Consensus Conference. Ann Oncology 2005;17:20-8.

[3]   Gralla R, Osoba D, Kris M, Kirkbride P, Hesketh P, Chinnery L, et al. Recommendations for the use of antiemetics: Evidence-based, clinical practice guidelines. J Clin Oncol 1999;17(9):2971-94.

[4]   American Society of Clinical Oncology, Kris MG, Hesketh PJ, Somerfield MR, Feyer P, Clark-Snow R, et al. American Society of Clinical Oncology guideline for antiemetics in oncology: update 2006. J Clin Oncol 2006;24:2932-47. Erratum J Clin Oncol 2006;24(33):5341-2.

[5]   Rapoport BL, Jordan K, Boice JA, Taylor A, Brown C, Hardwick JS, et al. Aprepitant for the prevention of chemotherapy-induced nausea and vomiting associated with a broad range of moderately emetogenic chemotherapies and tumor types: a randomized, double-blinded study. Support Care Cancer 2010;18(4):423-31.

[6]   Franzen L, Nyman J, Hagberg H, et al. A randomized placebo controlled study with ondansetron in patients undergoing fractionated radiotherapy. Ann Oncol 1996;7:587-92.

[7]   Spitzer T, Bryson JC, Cirenza E, et al. Randomized double-blind, placebo-controlled evaluation of oral ondansetron in the prevention of nausea and vomiting associated with fractionated total-body irradiation. J Clin Oncol 1994;12:2432-8.

[8]   Priestman TJ, Roberts JT, Lucraft H, et al. Results of a randomized, double-blind comparative study of ondansetron and metoclopramide in the prevention of nausea and vomiting following high-dose upper abdominal irradiation. Clin Oncol (R Coll Radiol) 1900;2:71-5.

[9]   Collis CH, Priestman TJ, Priestman S, et al. The final assessment of a randomized double-blind comparative study of ondansetron vs metoclopramide in the prevention of nausea and vomiting following high dose upper abdominal irradiation. Clin Oncol (R Coll Radiol) 1991;3:241-3.

[10]   Priestman TJ, Roberts JT, Upadhyaya BK. A prospective randomized double-blind trial comparing ondansetron versus prochlorperazine for the prevention of nausea and vomiting in patients undergoing fractionated radiotherapy. Clin Oncol (R Coll Radiol) 1993;5:358-63.

[11]   Sykes AJ, Kiltie AE, Stewart AL. Ondansetron versus a chlorpromazine and dexamethasone combination for the prevention of nausea and vomiting: a prospective, ransomised study to assess efficacy, cost effectiveness and quality of life following single-fraction radiotherapy. Support Care Cancer 1997;5:500-3.

[12]   Court-Brown W. Symptomatic disturbance of the single therapeutic dose of X-rays. BMJ 1953;1: 802-4.

[13]   Danjoux CE, Rider WD, Fitzpatrick PJ. The acute radiation syndrome. A memorial to William Michael Court-Brown. Clin Radiol 1979;30:581-4.

[14]   Roberts JT, Priestman TJ. A review of ondansetron in the management of radiotherapy-induced emesis. Oncology 1993;50:173-9.

[15]   Feyer PC, Seegenschmiedt MH. Antiemetic patterns of care for radiotherapy induced nausea and vomiting. ECCO-12 2003;929.

In: Advanced Cancer   ISBN: 978-1-62808-239-5
Editors: N. Thavarajah, N. Pulenzas, B. Lechner et al.   © 2013 Nova Science Publishers, Inc.

Chapter 33

Evaluation of a daily diary for assessing the prevalence of Radiation Induced Emesis (RIE)

*Victoria Haid, BSc(C)[1], Kinshuk Kumar, BSc(C)[1],
Eman Al Duhaiby, MBBS[2], Jocelyn Pang, BSc(C)[1],
Carlo DeAngelis, PharmD[3], Mark Pasetka, PharmD[3],
Yoo-Joung Ko, MD[1], Janet Nguyen, BSc(C)[2],
Kristopher Dennis, MD[2], Edward Chow, MBBS[2]
and Hans T Chung, MD[2]**

[1]Division of Medical Oncology, Odette Cancer Centre, Sunnybrook Health Sciences
Centre, University of Toronto, Toronto, Ontario
[2]Department of Radiation Oncology, Odette Cancer Centre,
Sunnybrook Health Science Centre, University of Toronto, Toronto, Ontario
[3]Department of Pharmacy, Odette Cancer Centre, Sunnybrook Health Science Centre,
University of Toronto, Toronto, Ontario, Canada

Abstract

While radiation-induced emesis (RIE) is relatively common, the use of and designs of patient self-report tools in studies of anti-emetics vary widely. This led us to develop a daily diary to assess RIE. In this chapter we evaluate the feasibility of employing this daily diary amongst patients undergoing radiotherapy. Methods: This was a single-institution prospective study including adult patients receiving radiotherapy to the upper abdomen, whole abdomen, or abdomen and pelvis, or else to the cranium or the

* Correspondence: Hans T Chung MD, FRCPC, Department of Radiation Oncology, Odette Cancer Centre, Sunnybrook Health Sciences Centre, 2075 Bayview Avenue, T-Wing, Toronto, ON Canada M4N 3M5. Email: Hans.Chung@sunnybrook.ca.

esophagus. We developed a 2-page self-assessment daily diary that was composed of a symptom assessment based on the Multinational Association of Supportive Care in Cancer (MASCC) Antiemesis Tool (MAT) and a medication log. Patients completed the daily diary at baseline, during and post-radiotherapy treatment for 15 days. A 7-point Functional Living Index – Emesis (FLIE) self-assessment tool was completed twice a week during and post-treatment. A debriefing questionnaire was completed. Results: Thirty-five patients were accrued; 16 patients did not have any results, 3 had very minimal data, and only 16 patients (46%) had analyzable results. Of these 16 analyzed patients, only 4 completed the entire study. During treatment, 9 patients (56%) experienced nausea, and 2 patients (12.5%) experienced vomiting. Post-treatment 2 (22%) patients experienced nausea and vomiting. Conclusions: Compared to other studies, compliance was poor in our cohort. Possible reasons include the lack of a call-back program, prolonged study period, and lack of simpler formatting.

Introduction

Nausea and vomiting are among the most common and challenging symptoms from cancer therapy which can significantly impact patient quality of life (QOL) (1-4). Due to the relative high incidence of nausea and vomiting in patients who receive radiation therapy, guidelines have been implemented to classify patients into risk groups for nausea and vomiting and to provide evidence-based recommendations for prophylaxis of radiation-induced emesis (RIE) according to risk (5-7).

In 2009, the Multinational Association of Supportive Care in Cancer (MASCC) convened a global expert panel to develop a new international consensus on RIE (7). The MASCC guidelines stratified patients into four risk groups and provided recommendations on the use of prophylactic and rescue anti-emetic treatment.

Results from studies have consistently shown that physicians do not regularly prescribe prophylactic anti-emetics (2,8). In most radiotherapy clinics, patients are seen on an outpatient basis and it is possible that they develop symptoms of nausea and vomiting while at home and do not report it to their physician (2,3). As a result, they may not receive anti-emetic treatment early enough to prevent these symptoms, and the more distressing and perhaps serious side effects that could develop due to untreated nausea and vomiting (2,3). Also, physicians may not be aware of the consequences that arise from not treating RIE and simply regard it as a minor side effect that does not justify anti-emetics (2,4). Results from two studies conducted on radiation-induced emesis demonstrated that only 21% and 17% of all patients on these studies were prescribed antiemetics. Out of these groups 55% and 62% of high risk patients were prescribed antiemetics for RIE, however those in the low risk group were prescribed antiemetics much less frequently (4,8). Furthermore, Enblom et al (4) discovered that 34% of patients who experienced nausea did not feel that what they were prescribed was sufficient (4). In comparison, a study on chemotherapy-induced nausea and vomiting reported that 69.5% and 77.5% of patients were prescribed antiemetics for acute and delayed nausea and vomiting, respectively (3). These studies suggest that physicians may not be using available guidelines, such as those by put in place by MASCC and are often underestimating the effects of RIE (4).

A disconnect exists between what patients experience, what is reported to physicians, and what medication is prescribed by physicians. This disconnect may perhaps be better identified by having self-report tools in practice to assess the occurrence of nausea and vomiting that may not be well-appreciated by physicians (9).

Patient self- report tools, among studies of antiemetics, vary widely; the frequency, format and wording are inconsistent across studies, reflecting the lack of consensus on a self-assessment RIE tool (4,8,10). This led us to develop our own self-assessment RIE tool. The current tool is composed of a daily symptom assessment portion based on the MASCC Antiemesis Tool (MAT) (11), and a daily medication log. We also incorporated the Functional Living Index-Emesis (FLIE) component to measure QOL effects (12). The objectives of this study were to assess the feasibility and compliance of this new tool amongst patients undergoing radiotherapy.

Our study

This prospective observational pilot study was conducted in the outpatient setting at the Odette Cancer Centre (OCC), Sunnybrook Health Sciences Centre. This study was approved by the Institutional Research Ethics Board.

Eligibility criteria

Inclusion criteria included adult patients receiving radiotherapy to the upper abdomen, whole abdomen, or abdomen and pelvis. The area of abdominal radiotherapy was to be at least 80 cm2 in the anterior/posterior direction and located between the upper border of T11 and the lower border of L3, to a total dose of at least 20 Gy in at least 5 fractions. Also eligible were patients receiving radiotherapy to the cranium or to the esophagus. Other inclusion criteria included ability to speak and understand English and provide written consent. Patients who received concurrent chemotherapy with the above described radiotherapy were also eligible for this study.

Study materials

The baseline questionnaire consisted of demographic information, treatment information, and a baseline assessment, which itself consisted of a diary of nausea and vomiting for the 72 hours prior to radiotherapy and a medication log. Basic patient demographic information was collected, including gender and age, previous systemic therapies, and medical conditions.

A seven-day nausea and vomiting/retching self-assessment tool was developed by combining the MASCC Antiemesis Tool (MAT) and the SC19 daily diary (10, 11). It was entitled "Daily Diary of Radiation-Induced Nausea and Vomiting". This assessment tool was based on the MAT because of its ease of use and low compliment of questions (9, 11). It was validated for use once per cycle of chemotherapy (13), but has also been used in other studies. In addition, a daily medication log was developed to record prophylactic or rescue anti-emetics. Together, this formed our daily diary. Appendix 1 contains the sample daily diary and medication log used.

The second questionnaire used in this study is the Functional Living Index-Emesis (FLIE) (12). This questionnaire consisted of 18 questions, 9 each for nausea and vomiting, concerning how these symptoms impacted functional aspects and quality of life. The responses to these questions were to be answered on a 7-point visual analogue scale (Appendix 2).

Study design

Participants in the study were instructed to fill out the daily diary, the FLIE, and the debriefing questionnaire for all of the appropriate days. The daily diary was to be completed every day a participant was on treatment, including weekends, as well as for 15 days after treatment end, to ensure delayed symptoms were recorded. The FLIE was to be completed every Wednesday and Sunday during treatment and every Wednesday and Sunday in the 15 days after treatment, in order to acquire summary information for the preceding three days.

A debriefing form was given at the end of a patient's participation in the study in order to receive their feedback on the questionnaires. Questions consisted of how long it took to complete the dairy, how the patient preferred to complete the dairy, if they felt the study asked too much of them, and also whether any items were difficult, confusing, upsetting, or if they had trouble with the wording or phrasing of the questions. Appendix 3 contains a sample of the debriefing form. Patients were followed up with once a week in clinic. Study personnel reminded patients to complete the questionnaires and answered any questions the patients had. Part-way through the study, prepaid envelopes were given to patients to enable them to send back completed surveys. Telephone numbers of the patients to enable follow-up were given to the study personnel if the patient consented.

Our findings

Between November 2009 and July 2010, 35 patients were enrolled in the study. Sixteen patients (46%) did not send back any data collection forms. Three patients (8%) completed an insufficient amount of diaries that they could not be properly assessed. Sixteen patients (46%) were considered evaluable. The responses were assessed according to completion rates, incidence of nausea and vomiting, and frequency of antiemetic prescriptions. Patient baseline characteristics for the evaluable pateints are given in table 1 and the study profile is given in figure 1.

Daily diary

Sixteen patients were analyzed for their completion of the daily diary; their results are shown in figure 2. Out of these 16 patients, seven patients (44%) completed all of the daily diaries during their study period. This constitutes only a 20% compliance rate amongst all 35 patients. Seven patients (44%) did not complete any post treatment diaries, but completed sufficient on-treatment diaries to be analyzed. An analysis of each question of the diary was also conducted for the 16 patients. The patients complete either of the questions or not of them.

Table 1. Patient Baseline Characteristics

Treatment Site	n	Age	Gender		Treatment Intent		Concurrent Chemotherapy	Prescribed Prophylactic		Baseline Nausea	Baseline Vomiting
			M	F	Palliative	Definitive		Yes	No		
Intracranial	7	24-78	2	5	3	4	0	2	5	1	0
Upper Abdomen	7	47-87	6	1	0	7	4	4	3	0	0
Abdomen/ Pelvis	1	61	1	0	0	1	1	0	1	0	0
Medias-tinum	1	68	1	0	1	0	0	0	1	1	1
Total	16	24-87	10	6	4	12	5	6	10	2	1

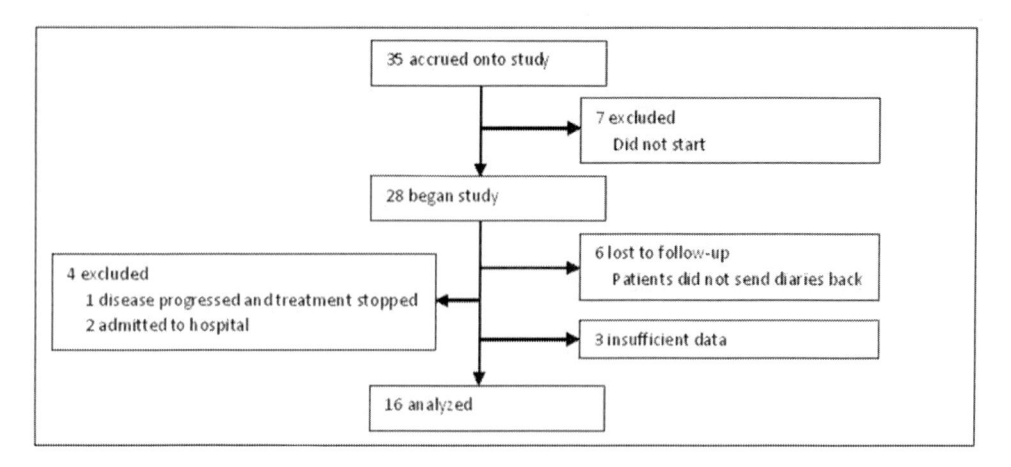

Figure 1. Study profile.

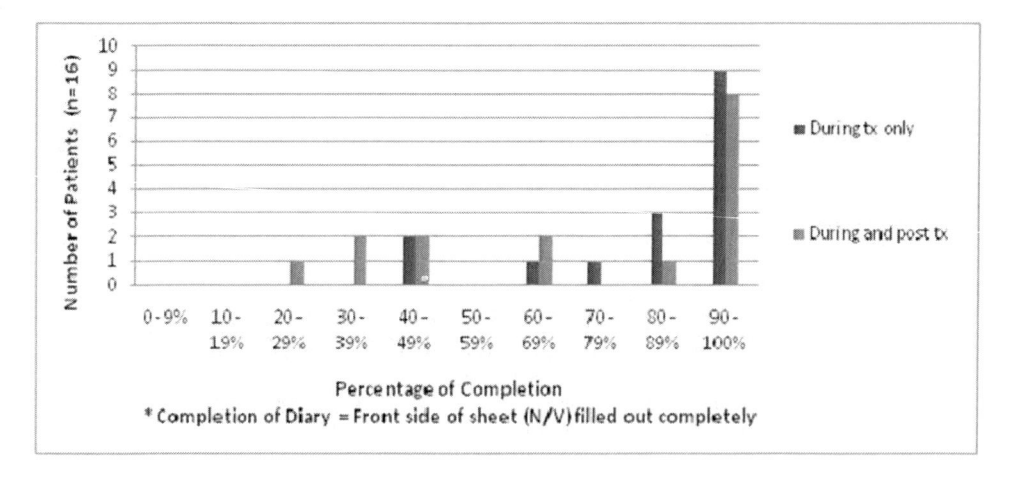

Figure 2. Completion Rates of the Daily Diary.

During treatment, nine patients (56%) reported experiencing nausea at least once and two patients (12.5%) reported experiencing vomiting at least once. Post-treatment, two patients (22%) experienced nausea and vomiting.

Six (67%) patients were prescribed prophylactic anti-emetic medication at baseline. One patient (11%) indicated never taking this medication, and experienced nausea and vomiting. Another patient indicated being prescribed dexamethasone at baseline. However, they did not indicate taking it until partially through treatment along with ranitidine, even though they experienced nausea and vomiting. One of the patients indicated taking dexamethasone, but it was prescribed to reduce intracranial tumor related edema rather than to prevent nausea and vomiting. All other patients are included in table 2.

Of the three patients prescribed prophylactic prochlorperazine only one (11% of all nauseated patients), successfully prevented nausea or vomiting. One patient (11%) who experienced nausea was prescribed Ondansetron part-way through treatment. Two patients (22%) had symptoms of nausea and/or vomiting, but were never prescribed medication. One of these patients only experienced nausea once and took dimenhydrinate for it. The other patient had almost continuous nausea and vomiting.

Table 2. Patients with Nausea and Vomiting and/or Medication

Medication Information	Medication for Nausea / Vomiting	Dose	Site of RT	Planned Dose (cGy / fraction)	Age	# days of nausea	# days of vomiting
Prescribed part-way through treatment	Ondansetron	8 mg	Abdo	4005/15	78	7/10 dtx	0
Prescribed before beginning treatment	Prochlorperazine	10 mg	Abdo	5040/28	47	7/43 dtx	0
	Prochlorperazine	10 mg	Abdo	5400/30	70	2/49 dtx	0
	Dexamethasone	4 mg	Intra-cranial	3000/15	24	2/15 dtx	0
	Prochlorperazine	10 mg	Abdo	5400/30	87	8/36 dtx	0
Prescribed but no N/V	Prochlorperazine	10 mg	Abdo	4500/25	60	0	0
No prescribed medication			Media stinum	2500/5	68	2/7 dtx, 15/16 ptx	4/7 dtx, 16/16 ptx
			Intra-cranial	4005/15	78	1/21 dtx	0

RT = radiation, dtx = during treatment, ptx = post treatment. Abdo = Abdomen/Pelvis

FLIE

16 patients again were analyzed for their completion of the FLIE; their results are shown in figure 3. Two patients (12.5%) did not fill out any FLIEs. Five patients (31%: 14% of total accrued) completed all of the FLIEs. Five patients (31%) did not complete post-treatment FLIEs. Four patients were missing at least one FLIE.

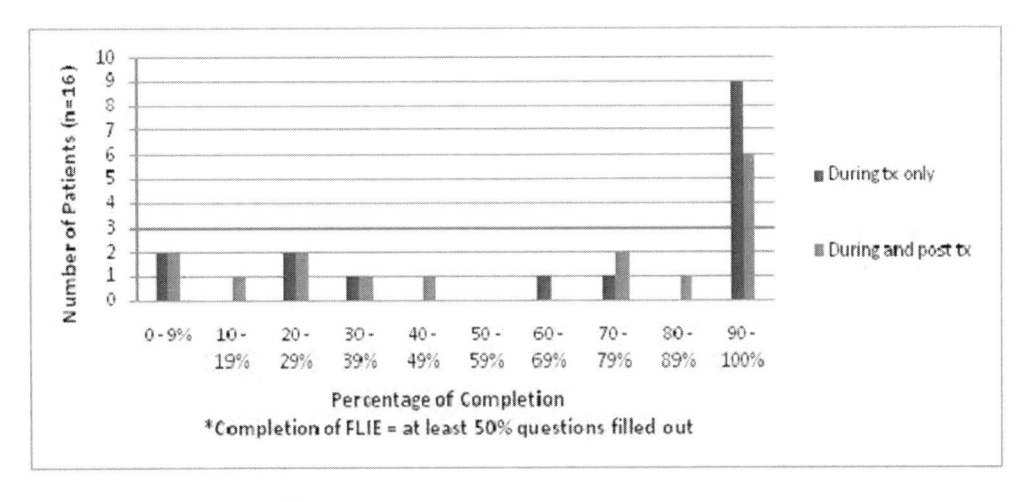

Figure 3. Completion Rates of the FLIE.

The FLIE was also analyzed by question. Fourteen patients completed at least some of the FLIEs. Seven out of the fourteen patients (50%) had all normal results. Three patients (21%) did not fill out the second side of the FLIE at least once. Five patients (36%) left one question blank on only one of the questionnaires. This issue was analyzed more closely to see if there was a consistent question being skipped, but different questions were left blank each time.

Debrief questionnaire

Only ten patients (28.6% of total patients; 62.5% of patients analyzed) completed the debrief questionnaire. The information gathered from the debrief questionnaire gave some useful feedback. The daily diary was found to take between 1 and 10 minutes per day to complete. The majority of the patients completed the questionnaires on their own, except for one patient who completed it by telephone daily. Most patients commented that the questionnaires were not too long, with the exception of two patients, one who commented it went on for too many days, and the other stated the questionnaires were too redundant because they did not experience any nausea or vomiting.

Only one patient said they had difficulty with the questionnaires. This was due to issues with the FLIE. This patient was feeling fine at the time they filled out the FLIE that day, but was sick later on that night. When they went to fill out the next FLIE, the three-day recall did not include the day this patient was sick. No items were found to be confusing, no one had difficulty with the wording or phrasing of any of the items or found any items upsetting. One patient did however comment that their nausea and vomiting was thought to be due to the chemotherapy they were taking, and did not associate any of these symptoms with the radiation.

Overall, taking into consideration all of the results, four patients (25% of analyzed patients, 11% of total patients accrued) completed all of the elements: daily diaries, FLIEs, and debrief questionnaire. Twelve patients were missing some or all of the daily diaries, FLIEs, and/or debrief questionnaires.

Discussion

According to the MASCC guidelines, the risk of radiation-induced nausea and vomiting is 50-80% for the moderate-risk group, including upper abdomen, and 30-60% for the low-risk group, including radiation to the brain. In our study, four out of seven patients (57%) receiving radiation to the upper abdomen experienced nausea. Four out of seven patients (57%) receiving radiation to the brain also experienced nausea. Compared to the MASCC guidelines, the risk percentage found in our study for both groups falls into their appropriate risk range. However, the brain radiation group is on the higher end of the spectrum.

The compliance rate for this study was surprisingly low, compared with other similar studies that have been conducted. Overall, in this study, 35 patients were accrued; only 46% had analyzable results. Out of these, only 4 patients (25%) completed 100% of the study, which compared to the overall total of patients accrued is only 11%.

From those who filled out the debriefing questionnaire, feedback given on the study was very positive, considering many patients did not complete all questionnaires. A few issues were brought to the attention of the study personnel. For patients who did not experience any nausea or vomiting, the questionnaire was felt to be too long and redundant. Another issue was discovered with the FLIE; the three day recall did not cover all episodes of nausea, and as such that issue will be considered when making changes in the next phase of the study. Overall, the majority of those who did give feedback on the questionnaires did not have any issues with them. Due to this feedback, changes to the duration and the length of the daily diary needs to be considered, as well the recall length of the FLIE.

In our study, to increase patient compliance, research assistants visited participants at least once a week while on treatment in order to remind patients to fill out the questionnaires. For the period following treatment, prepaid envelopes were given to participants to make it easier for them to send back completed questionnaires. This was implemented part-way through the study. As well, if participants agreed to give study personnel their phone number, research assistants were able to follow-up via telephone when patients were no longer coming into the OCC. However, a lot of patients did not provide their telephone number, or were not asked. This made it extremely difficult to monitor patients on the study. Despite these attempts to increase patient compliance, completion rates did not dramatically increase.

In contrast, in the National Cancer Institute of Canada Clinical Trials Group SC19 trial on the benefit of adding dexamethasone to the RIE prophylaxis, compliance rates of the EORTC QLQ-C30 questionnaires were 99% at baseline and 97, 93, 95% at fractions 5, 15, and 1 month follow up, respectively. A daily diary was completed by patients every day for the first 15 fractions of treatment. Completion of the EORTC QLQ-C30 was mandatory for this study, and although it is not stated if the daily diary they used was mandatory as well, there seemed to be more pressure from the study team to complete the forms (10).

The Italian Group for Antiemetic Research in Radiotherapy (IGARR) study on emesis in radiotherapy also reported very high compliance rates, with only 16 patients out of 1020 (98%) not evaluable for the study (14 of which did not fill out the diary card). Daily diary cards were filled out every day during treatment and for a week after stopping radiotherapy treatment, rather than 15 days, as was the case in our study. On these diary cards patients recorded the occurrence and intensity of nausea, and any episodes of vomiting or retching. Antiemetic drugs were also recorded. A simple three-grade scale was used for nausea, rather than the seven-point scale used in this study, other than the shortened scale both diaries asked a similar amount of questions (8).

In a third study by Enblom et al demonstrated that 93% of 396 patients completed the questionnaire (28 patients did not). These patients received the questionnaire at their regular radiotherapy treatment session and sent it in to the study coordinator using prepaid envelopes. Participants were also given a phone call reminder if they had not sent their questionnaires back within two weeks of the end of treatment, which increased answering rates. According to the study, this high response rate was thought to be due to patients finding the study valuable, the questionnaire relevant, having reminders by phone, and inclusion of a variety of cancer types (4).

Cohen et al (3) assessed patients receiving chemotherapy rather than radiotherapy. Patients were asked to complete a daily diary for the first 8 days after treatment during each cycle; the FLIE was also administered before chemotherapy, at the end of day 1 and at the end of day 6 after chemotherapy. This study included 151 patients; 97% had complete diaries for the first cycle, 89% had complete diaries for the second cycle, and 70% had complete dairies for the third cycle (3) .

These few studies on RIE, as well as one study on chemotherapy-induced nausea and vomiting, all have shown significantly high compliance rates. Many of these previously completed studies were shorter than this study by at least seven days. When patients consider their involvement more mandatory and valuable, they may feel more inclined to participate fully (10). One study involved a call-back program which was used to remind patients to fill in forms at home. This is an important step in obtaining high accrual rates (4,8).

Many amendments need to be made for this study to improve upon its completion rates. A call-back program should be implemented. Thorough explanation of the relevance of the study and the importance of patient completion needs to be emphasized. The questionnaire itself needs to be shortened and the duration of the study should also be shortened for the next phase of this study.

References

[1]   Coates A, Abraham S, Kaye S, et al. On the receiving end -- patient perception of the side-effects of cancer chemotherapy. Eur J Cancer Clin Oncol 1983;19(2):203-8.

[2]   Horiot J. Prophylaxis versus treatment: Is there a better way to manage radiotherapy-induced nausea and vomiting? Int J Radiat Oncol 2004;60(4):1018-25.

[3]   Cohen L, de Moor CA, Eisenberg P, et al. Chemotherapy-induced nausea and vomiting: Incidence and impact on patient quality of life at community oncology settings. Support Care Cancer 2007;15(5):497-503.

[4]   Enblom A, Axelsson B, Steineck G, et al. One third of patients with radiotherapy-induced nausea consider their antiemetic treatment insufficient. Support Care Cancer 2009;17(1):23-32.

[5]   Urba S. Radiation-induced nausea and vomiting. J Natl Compr Canc Netw 2007;5(1):60-5.

[6]   Feyer P, Stewart A, Titlbach O. Aetiology and prevention of emesis induced by radiotherapy. Support Care Cancer 1998;6(3):253-60.

[7]   Feyer PC, Maranzano E, Molassiotis A, et al. Radiotherapy-induced nausea and vomiting (RINV): MASCC/ESMO guideline for antiemetics in radiotherapy: Update 2009. Support Care Cancer 2011;19(Suppl 1):S5-14.

[8]   Maranzano E, De Angelis V, Pergolizzi S, et al. A prospective observational trial on emesis in radiotherapy: Analysis of 1020 patients recruited in 45 italian radiation oncology centres. Radiother Oncol 2010;94(1):36-41.

[9]   Brearley SG, Clements CV, Molassiotis A. A review of patient self-report tools for chemotherapy-induced nausea and vomiting. Support Care Cancer 2008;16(11):1213-29.

[10]   Wong RKS, Paul N, Ding K, et al. 5-hydroxytryptamine-3 receptor antagonist with or without short-course dexamethasone in the prophylaxis of radiation induced emesis: A placebo-controlled randomized trial of the national cancer institute of Canada clinical trials group (SC19). J Clin Oncol 2006;24(21):3458-64.

[11]   MASCC Assessment Tool. 2004. Retrieved: August 2009 from Multinational Association of Supportive Care in Cancer Website: http://www.mascc.org/mc/page.do?sitePageId=88036

[12]   Lindley CM, Hirsch JD, O'Neill CV, et al. Quality of life consequences of chemotherapy-induced emesis. Qual Life Res 1992;1(5):331-40.

[13]   Molassiotis A, Coventry PA, Stricker CT, et al. Validation and psychometric assessment of a short clinical scale to measure chemotherapy-induced nausea and vomiting: The MASCC antiemesis tool. J Pain Symptom Manag 2007;34(2):148-59.

SECTION FIVE:
BONE METASTASES

In: Advanced Cancer
Editors: N. Thavarajah, N. Pulenzas, B. Lechner et al.

ISBN: 978-1-62808-239-5
© 2013 Nova Science Publishers, Inc.

Chapter 34

Review of bone metastases research in the Rapid Response Radiotherapy Program (RRRP)

*Breanne Lechner, BSc(C), Natalie Pulenzas, BSc(C),
Nemica Thavarajah, BSc(C) and Edward Chow, MBBS**
Rapid Response Radiotherapy Program, Department of Radiation Oncology,
Odette Cancer Centre, Sunnybrook Health Sciences Centre,
University of Toronto, Toronto, Ontario, Canada

Abstract

Bone metastases are a common occurrence in patients with advanced cancer. Complications of bone metastases can include pain, hypercalcemia, pathological fractures, spinal instability, spinal cord compression and immobility. Palliative radiotherapy (RT) is a well-established and effective treatment option for symptomatic bone metastases. The Rapid Response Radiotherapy Program (RRRP) provides timely RT for palliative cancer patients, focusing on quality of life (QOL) as an important endpoint. This paper reviewed the past research conducted in the RRRP on bone metastases. Studies in the RRRP have focused on topics including QOL in patients with bone metastases, the incidence and methods to prevent pain flare following RT, optimal treatment regimens for bone metastases and various patient population subgroups.

* Correspondence: Professor Edward Chow MBBS, MSc, PhD, FRCPC, Department of Radiation Oncology, Odette Cancer Centre, Sunnybrook Health Sciences Centre, 2075 Bayview Avenue, Toronto, ON Canada. Email: Edward.Chow@Sunnybrook.ca.

Introduction

Bone metastases are a common occurrence in patients with advanced cancer, and are found in 70%-85% of patients at autopsy (1). Metastases to the bone are particularly common in patients with primary breast, lung and prostate carcinomas (1). The morbidity associated with metastatic bone disease includes pain, hypercalcemia, pathological fractures, spinal instability, spinal cord compression, and immobility (2). Pain is the most prevalent symptom of bone metastases and is experienced by 60-70% of patients (3). Symptoms of bone metastases can have a significant negative impact on patients' quality of life (QOL). Palliative radiotherapy (RT) is a well-established and effective treatment option for symptomatic bone metastases (3). The overall pain response rate is approximately 80% (4-7). Controversy over the optimal treatment schedules and fractionation of RT still exists, with patterns of practice in radiation oncologists consistently showing reluctance to adopt single fraction as a preferred practice despite research demonstrating the equivalence of single and multiple fractions for pain relief in uncomplicated bone metastases (7). A significant side effect associated with RT is pain flare. Pain flare is a temporary worsening of pain in the treated bony metastatic site following RT (3). Treatment for the prophylaxis of pain flare is an important topic of research in the field of radiation oncology. Promising research has been conducted on the use of the corticosteroid dexamethasone for the prophylaxis of pain flare following RT to bone metastases (8, 9).

There have been many studies that have focused on patients with bone metastases in the Rapid Response Radiotherapy Clinic (RRRP) at the Sunnybrook Odette Cancer Centre. The RRRP is a specialized clinic developed in 1996 to provide timely palliative RT with the purpose of improving or maintaining QOL in patients with advanced cancer (6). Extensive research regarding all aspects of palliative RT has been conducted in the RRRP since its establishment. This paper reviews the past research in the RRRP examining various aspects of bone metastases research.

Literature search

A literature search was conducted to identify studies investigating bone metastases in cancer patients conducted in the RRRP from 2000 to present. All publications pertaining to patients with metastatic bone disease were included. The methods and results of the studies were summarized, and important areas of bone metastases research were discussed in detail.

Studies examining the impact of bone metastases on QOL, the incidence of pain flare, the use of dexamethasone for pain flare prevention, bone metastases treatment regimens, and various patient population subgroups were examined.

Quality of life

Patients with bones metastases are often very symptomatic, and thus the improvement of QOL is a very important treatment outcome. One central area of research in the RRRP is the development of tools to assess QOL. A literature review by Tharmalingam et al (2), published in 2008, focused specifically on QOL measurement in bone metastases patients. This review included any studies measuring QOL in patients with bone metastases from 1966 to June 2006, which resulted in 47 relevant trials identified (2). A total of 24 different instruments were used to evaluate QOL including pain assessment scales, validated QOL instruments, and study-designed questionnaires (2). Most studies employed study designed questionnaires (ten of the studies) or the European Organization for Research and Treatment of Cancer (EORTC) Core Questionnaire (EORTC-C30) (ten of the studies). The Functional Assessment of Cancer Therapy-General questionnaire (FACT-G) was used to evaluate QOL in five of the studies, the Edmonton Symptom Assessment System (ESAS) was used in four of the studies, and the Brief Pain Inventory (BPI) was used in four of the articles. The use of a variety of study-designed assessments did not allow for outcome comparison between studies. The authors of this review concluded that these results demonstrate the need for a standard instrument specific to bone metastases incorporating pain, skeletal complications, and psychosocial domains to assess QOL (2).

In 2009, a study published by Chow et al (10) supported the development of a bone metastases module to supplement the EORTC QLQ-C30 or the EORTC Palliative Quality of Life Questionnaire (QLQ C15-PAL) for patients with bone metastases. Phases one and two of module development were conducted in Canada, Australia, and Germany in accordance with EORTC QOL group guidelines. Phase one involved identifying relevant health-related quality of life (HRQOL) issues for patients with bone metastases by reviewing the Medline and Psych info databases, existing HRQOL questionnaires for bone metastases, and interviews of patients and health care professionals. This study found 61 health-related quality of life (HRQOL) issues generated from 152 health care professionals and 413 patients. In Phase two, a list of these issues was presented to health care professionals and patients to determine which items were most relevant. This resulted in the construction of a 22 item provisional module. Phase three involved further testing in 170 patients from nine countries, which resulted in the twenty-two item bone metastases module (QLQ-BM22). This BM22 module contained symptom scales, with five painful site items and three pain characteristic items, and also functional scales, with eight functional interference items and six psychosocial aspects. The study successfully developed the EORTC QLQ-BM22 module to measure HRQOL in cancer patients with bone metastases. This single module was developed to facilitate reliable comparisons in bone metastases clinical trials.

Further research was conducted to test the reliability and validity of the EORTC QLQ-BM22 internationally by Chow et al (11). A total of 400 patients undergoing a variety of treatments for bone metastases were accrued from March 2010 to January 2011 in seven countries including Brazil, Canada, Cyprus, Egypt, France, India, and Taiwan. The QLQ-BM22 was administered with the QLQ-C30 at baseline and a one month follow-up. A debriefing questionnaire was administered to determine patient acceptability and understanding. Multi-trait scaling analyses confirmed 4 scales in the 22-item module. The scales were able to discriminate between clinically distinct patient groups, such as patients with varying performance status. The QLQ-BM22 was well received in all seven countries and the majority of patients did not recommend any significant changes from the module in its current form. The results of this study confirmed the validity, reliability, cross cultural applicability, and sensitivity of the EORTC QLQ-BM22 (11).

Further study by Zeng et al (12) aimed to establish the minimal clinically important difference (MCID) for the EORTC QLQ-BM22 to aid in determining the relevance of QOL changes after treatment and in sample size determination in clinical trials. A total of 93 out of the 400 patients enrolled with bone metastases across seven countries completed the QLQ-BM22 and the QLQ-C30 at baseline and at a one month follow up and had performance status assessed at both time points. The MCID was calculated for each QOL scale for determining improvement and deterioration using both an anchor-based, which used performance status, and a distribution-based approach. Improvements of 30.5, 20.1, 30.5, and 19.6 in the pain, painful site, painful characteristic, and functional interference scales, respectively, demonstrated clinical relevance. Decreases of 12.4, 22.4, and 13.5 in emotional functioning, global health status, and financial issues, respectively, were required to represent clinically relevant deterioration. MCIDs for improvement were closest to 0.5 standard deviations, while for deterioration, closer to 0.3 standard deviations on the QLQ-BM22. These results suggest that a clinically meaningful improvement requires a greater change in QOL than a meaningful deterioration for the QLQ-BM22. For the QLQ-C30, the MCIDs were similar for improvement and deterioration. Ultimately, this study presented a set of MCIDs for the QLQ-BM22, though the study is limited by a small sample size and the use of only one anchor (12).

An additional study in the RRRP conducted by Campos et al (13) tested the reliability of patient perceptions in important bone metastases QOL items. In 2005, 130 patients completed the EORTC QLQ-BM61, the 61 item QOL questionnaire precursor to the QLQ-BM22, and 27 of the patients were re-approached when they returned to clinic between 2007 and 2008. For each item of the QLQ-BM61, patients indicated if it was relevant to be included in the final version of the bone metastases questionnaire. Additionally, any treatment the patient received between baseline and re-approach was collected. There was no significant change in the items that patients selected for the final questionnaire between baseline and re-approach, indicating that patient perceptions of relevant QOL items did not change over time, which showed good reliability of patients' perceptions of important QOL issues. It was found that 10 of the 61 items had a significant value when assessing the relationship of the change in items patients selected and complications and treatment. This indicated that increased complications of disease and changes in treatment can affect patients' perceptions of important QOL items. This research is important to keep in mind as many QOL measurement tools are based on patient perceptions of generated QOL issues (13).

In 2009, a study by Chow et al (14) was completed to validate what constitutes a meaningful change in pain scores following palliative RT for bone metastases. A total of 178 patients treated with external beam RT scored their worst pain on a scale of zero to ten before treatment, daily during treatment, and for ten days after RT as well as indicating if their pain was "worse", "the same", or "better" compared to pre-treatment. A total of 1431 pain scores were obtained. The results demonstrated that patients perceived an improvement in pain when their self-reported pain score decreased by at least two points. The authors concluded that this study validated the previous finding that a meaningful change in pain score is represented by a decrease in patient self-reported pain score by at least two points. This was an important confirmation for the use of pain scores in clinical trial endpoints for partial treatment responses (14).

A literature review by Presutti et al (15) focused on examining bone metastases and QOL, addressing previous clinical trials assessing QOL in bone metastases patients receiving palliative RT. This review included aforementioned studies by the RRRP in the development of the EORTC QLQ-BM22 and further analyzed the development process. This review also examined the relevant international research on randomized trials examining single versus multiple fractions of RT for patients with bone metastases assessing QOL. Additionally, the review included external research on the development of the of the 16-item Functional Assessment of Cancer Therapy-Bone Pain (FACT-BP) scale to assess cancer related bone pain. The FACT-BP showed high internal consistency and was closely correlated with the pain intensity scales of the BPI, thus the FACT-BP was found to be a robust tool for assessing cancer related bone pain. Ultimately this review by Presutti et al (15) concluded that QOL is a valuable endpoint in clinical trials for determining the success of an intervention for bone metastases.

An additional study in the RRRP published in 2011 examined the reported rates and predictive factors for sleep disturbance in patients with bone metastases (16). A total of 400 patients with symptomatic bone metastases treated with palliative RT were enrolled between May 2003 and June 2007, of which 235 completed all follow up points. The BPI questionnaire and analgesic consumption were recorded at baseline, and follow up BPI was completed post RT at week four, eight, and twelve.

Ordinal logistic regression analysis was used to search for the relationship between sleep disturbance and other covariates. At baseline, 99 (25%) of patients had moderate sleep disturbance and 144 (36%) of patents had severe sleep disturbance. There was improvement in sleep scores for both responders and non-responders at week four and week eight, but scores worsened for non-responders at week twelve. Age, Karnofsky Performance Scale (KPS), pain score, and lung primary were the significant variables associated with sleep disturbance (16).

Research by Zeng et al (17) assessed the levels of functional interference caused by pain after treatment with conventional RT using the BPI. After RT, a total of 159, 129, and 106 patients completed the BPI over the phone at week four, eight, and twelve respectively. To assess the validity of the BPI, Cronbach's alpha, confirmatory factor analysis, and discriminant validity tests were performed. One-way analysis of variance was used to compare BPI scores.

The combination of different analyses confirmed the validity of the BPI over the telephone since reasonably high levels of internal consistency, composite reliability, and convergent validity were present at weeks four, eight, and twelve. Functional interference scores were worse in patients with lower skeletal pain, thus functional interference may be inherently higher in patients with pain in the lower body. After treatment with RT, there was no longer a statistically significant difference between patients with upper and lower body pain, thus RT reduces functional interference due to pain regardless of location on the body (17).

A study by Dennis et al (18) aimed to determine the efficacy of RT for the palliation of pain from bone metastases among patients in their last three months of life. This study reviewed past ESAS and BPI databases compiled from patients with bone metastases receiving palliative RT, identifying patients who died within three months of receiving RT. From a total of 918 patients, 232 dying within three months of beginning treatment were identified. A pain response was evaluable for the 109 (47%) patients with available follow-up information.

The overall response rates were 70% at one month and 63% at two months, which included complete and partial responses in accordance with the International Bone Metastases Consensus definitions. Patients responding to treatment at one month reported significantly less interference due to pain in their general activity, walking ability, normal work, and enjoyment of life than patients not responding to treatment. Thus, it was concluded that despite being near the end of life, patients responding to palliative RT for painful bone metastases may benefit from improvement of functional abilities prior to passing away in addition to pain relief alone.

Pain flare

Pain flare is defined as a temporary worsening of pain in radiated bony metastatic sites immediately after RT (19). The incidence of pain flare following palliative RT for bone metastases is an area of interest for research in the RRRP.

An initial study conducted by Chow et al (20) in 2005 examined the incidence in pain flare following RT by recording patients' daily pain scores and oral morphine equivalent dose. Pain flare was defined as a two point increase in pain score compared to baseline with no decrease in analgesic intake, or a 25 % increase in analgesic intake with no decrease in pain score. This study resulted in an overall incidence of pain flare ranging from 2% to 16%. This finding added to the results of previous studies, with a wide range of reported incidence of pain flare in the literature spanning from 2% to 44%. A joint study was thus initiated to further investigate the incidence of pain flare.

Hird et al (1) conducted a multicenter study to more definitively determine the incidence of pain flare in patients with bone metastases being treated with RT. A total of 111 patients with painful bone metastases, the majority of which received either 8Gy in one fraction (64%) or 20Gy in five fractions (25%), were enrolled. Overall, pain flare occurred in 44 of the 111 patients (40%) during RT and within ten days following RT. Patients treated with a single 8Gy fraction reported pain flare incidence of 39% (27/70) and for those treated with multiple fractions the incidence was 41% (17/21). Pain flare occurred within the first five days following RT in 80% of all evaluable patients. Thus, this study was able to document the incidence of pain flare in patients with bone metastases receiving RT.

Additional investigations regarding pain flare in the RRRP examined the incidence of pain flare, its impact on patients, and prophylaxis of pain flare. Results of previous investigations, including those previously mentioned, were reviewed by Presutti et al (19). The review also included a study by Hird et al (3) published in 2009 that involved administering a five item Pain Flare Qualitative Questionnaire to 35 patients, 13 of which completed the questionnaire. Overall, 10/13 (77%) of patients indicated some level of functional interference due to the pain flare experienced. More than three quarters of the patients had to increase their pain medications in order to cope with pain flare. Despite this, still 9/13 (69%) of the patients failed to achieve adequate pain control. It was stated by 11/13 (85%) of patients that they would prefer the prevention of the pain flare as opposed to management with pain medication. One significant limitation of this study was the small sample size.

Dexamethasone

One treatment option for the prophylaxis of pain flare is the prescription of dexamethasone, a corticosteroid, prior to treatment. Essential research has been done in the RRRP regarding dexamethasone and its ability to reduce the instance of pain flare in patients receiving RT for bone metastases. Initially, a pilot study was published in 2007 examining dexamethasone for the prophylaxis of radiation-induced pain flare, which included 33 patients. Dexamethasone was found to be well tolerated, though further investigation was indicated to confirm the efficacy of dexamethasone in preventing pain flare (8). Subsequently, a phase two study was completed in the RRRP and published in 2009 by Hird et al (21). Patients with bone metastases treated with a single 8Gy were prescribed 8mg of dexamethasone just before palliative RT and for three consecutive days after treatment. Worst pain score and analgesic consumption converted into total daily oral morphine equivalents were collected at baseline and daily for ten days after treatment. A total of 41 patients were evaluable. The overall incidence of pain flare was 9/41 (22%) within ten days of completing RT. Most (55%) of these pain flares occurred on day five. It was concluded that dexamethasone is effective in the prophylaxis of RT-induced pain flare after palliative RT for bone metastases, though further randomized studies are necessary to confirm this finding.

Treatment regimens

The optimal regimen for palliative RT of bone metastases has been the subject of much debate throughout the literature. A significant amount of research has been conducted in RRRP regarding single versus multiple fractionation schedules for RT. A review by Culleton et al (22) examined conventional RT to bone metastases in the literature, specifically focusing on studies comparing a single fraction (SF) versus multiple fractions (MF). The most common treatment schedules delivered for palliation of bone metastases include single 8Gy treatment and multi-fractioned low dose regimes consisting most commonly of 20Gy in five fractions and 30Gy in ten fractions. Upon review of past meta-analyses and studies with a variety of endpoint definitions used, it was evident that an international consensus on endpoint definitions was needed. In response to the need for endpoint definition for future trials, the International Bone Metastases Consensus working party was established in 2000 to reach a consensus. Conclusions that the party agreed upon were published in 2002 by Chow et al (23). One of the most important findings was the definition of complete response as a pain score of zero at the treated site with no concomitant increase in analgesic intake, and partial response as pain reduction of two or more points on a scale of ten without increase in analgesic intake or analgesic reduction of 25% or more without an increase in pain score (23). This international consensus was updated again in research published by Chow et al in 2011 (24). Changes from the original consensus included the suggestion that only worst pain at the index site should be measured, not average pain in addition to worst pain. Also, the more recent consensus suggested the use of an additional response category, indeterminate response, to represent cases that could not be classified as complete response, partial response, or pain progression. In 2004, a study in the RRRP was conducted comparing response rates from palliative RT of bone metastases employing the international consensus endpoints and traditional endpoints for 518 patients. It was found that the international consensus endpoints lowered the complete and partial response rates compared to the traditional endpoints and more accurately reflected the true efficacy of radiation (25). In 2007, a systematic review was conducted of randomized palliative RT trials updating previous meta-analyses (7). The purpose of this study was to compare response rates for trials evaluating SF versus MF regimens. A total of 16 randomized trials were identified, and the overall SF response rate was 58% which was similar to the MF response rate, at 59 %. The complete response rates were found to be 23% for a SF and 24% for MF with no significant differences between the two groups. This review was updated in 2011 by Chow et al (26). In total, 25 randomized controlled trials were identified. The overall response rate was similar in patients receiving SF (1696 of 2818; 60%) and MF (1711 of 2799; 61%). Complete response rates were 620 of 2641 (23%) in the SF arm and 634 of 2622 (24%) in the MF arm. No significant difference was seen in overall or complete response rates. Retreatment rates favored patients in the MF arm, where the likelihood of requiring re-irradiation was 2.6-fold greater in the SF arm. Thus, it was concluded that SF and MF regimens provided equal pain relief; however, significantly higher retreatment rates occurred in those that received a SF.

In 2006, our group conducted a study to examine how patients categorize their pain with both the verbal descriptor scale and eleven-point visual analogue scale (27). It was found that patients scored pain as 'mild' if pain was equal to four or less, 'moderate' if pain was between five and seven, and 'severe' if pain was equal to eight or more (27). Similarly in 2007, Li et al (28) also conducted a study to establish cut off points for 'mild', 'moderate', and 'severe' pain by grading pain intensity with functional interference using the BPI. The optimal cut points were 1-4 for mild pain, 5-6 for moderate and 7-10 for severe pain. Li et al (29) also conducted a study, published in 2008, to determine the most appropriate time to evaluate the response to palliative RT for bone metastases. It was concluded that two months was the most appropriate time to measure response rates because maximum pain relief may take more than one month for some patients to achieve, and attrition is a major problem after two months.

Another important topic addressed in the review by Culleton et al (22) was the examination of patterns of practice. In 2000, the results of a survey of 172 Canadian radiation oncologists made up of case scenarios were published by Chow et al (30). The most common dose prescribed was 20Gy in five fractions (72%) followed by 8Gy in one fraction (16%). It was found that 70% of practitioners used standard dose fractions to palliate painful bone metastases irrespective of site and tumor type. When evaluating the pattern of practice in the RRRP from 1999 to 2005, there was a significant increase in the prescription of SF for bone metastases. The noted increase in SF went from 51% in 1999 to 66% in 2005 (31). In 2008, a survey was distributed internationally to 962 practicing radiation oncologists (32). It was found that a SF was used most often by the Canadian Association of Radiation Oncology (CARO) members but overall, the most common palliative dose prescribed in all cases was 30Gy in ten fractions. SF regimens were prescribed most often frequently by Canadian Association of Radiation Oncology (CARO) members and they were two to three times more likely to recommended it when compared with American Society for Radiation Oncology (ASTRO) members who overall, were the least likely to use a SF. This international survey concluded that despite evidentiary support, SF has not been widely accepted as a treatment for uncomplicated painful bone metastases (32).

Recently, a review by Dennis et al (33) was conducted to determine the optimal dose of SF conventional palliative RT for the relief of pain caused by bone metastases. Relevant randomized controlled trials were included. A total of 26 articles were found for review, and 24 trials cumulatively randomized 3233 patients to 28 SF arms: two arms received 4Gy, one 5Gy, one 6Gy, twenty-two 8Gy, one 10Gy and one 8–15Gy. Efficacy endpoints and pain assessment times varied. In general, higher doses produced better pain response rates. In trials that directly compared different SF doses, 8Gy was statistically superior to 4Gy. Also, 8Gy was by far the most commonly administered SF dose within 24 randomized trials of conventional RT for the palliation of bone metastases. Thus, the authors concluded that 8Gy should be the standard dose against which future treatments are compared due to its reproducible pain response rate and its established safety profile (33).

In addition to studies regarding palliative RT for bone metastases, research completed in the RRRP has analyzed various methods for the detection and treatment of bone metastases. A review by Bedard et al (34) examined the literature to evaluate the accuracy, specificity, and sensitivity of Positron Emission Tomography (PET) used in the diagnosis of bone metastases. Out of the 44 publications identified, all studies except for one demonstrated that PET scan with the use of fluorodexyglucose (FDG) is superior to a bone scan. While FDG detects osteolytic lesions with great accuracy, it is unsuccessful in detecting osteoblastic lesions suggesting use for other modalities.

A review by Culleton et al (35) examined the clinical benefits of combining bisphosphonates with RT for the treatment of bone metastases. A search of publications from 1950 to 2008 identified thirteen relevant studies. Three studies were in-vitro cell studies, which found a significant synergistic effect when the treatments were combined, by means of a reduction in cell viability via inducted apoptosis. Two of the studies involved animal tumor models which found that combined treatment may lead to improved mineralization compared to RT alone. The remaining eight were human studies. Two of the human studies were randomized trials comparing combination therapy versus a placebo and RT, which both showed greater long term benefits in the arm that received both RT and bisphosphonates in terms of recalcification and the development of new bony lesions. Thus, the authors concluded that this preliminary evidence demonstrates that patients with bone metastases may significantly benefit from treatment with bisphosphonates and RT concurrently.

Patient populations

Research in the RRRP has also focused on various patient populations affected by bone metastases and RT for these patient populations. A study by Hird et al (36) was completed to examine if bone metastases from gastrointestinal (GI) cancers show response rates similar to those of bone metastases from other primary cancers after RT in the RRRP. A total of 69 patients with bone metastases from GI primaries who received palliative RT in the RRRP clinic during 1999 to 2006 were identified, patients between 1999-2003 were assessed with ESAS and patients from 2003-2006 were assessed with the BPI. Response rates for this cohort of metastatic GI cancer patients were then compared to rates for 479 patients receiving palliative RT for bone metastases from other primary cancer sites. No statistically significant differences were observed in RT response rates for bone metastases from GI cancers than from other primary cancer sites.

A study by Campos et al (37) was published in 2010 that examined the efficacy of palliative RT in relieving metastatic bone pain in elderly patients. The response to RT for palliation of metastatic bone pain was evaluated in 558 patients between 1999 and 2008. No significant difference was found in the response rate in patients aged ≥ 65, ≥ 70, and ≥ 75 years compared with younger patients at one, two, and three months after RT. The response was found to be significantly related to the performance status of the patient. Elderly patients should be referred for palliative RT for their painful bone metastases, regardless of age, because they receive equal benefit from treatment.

A study conducted by Culleton et al (38) evaluated the effect of gender on symptoms among patients with bone metastases controlling for gender specific-malignancies. This retrospective review included 900 patients who received palliative RT and completed the ESAS (n=508) or the BPI (n=392) from 1999 to 2004 at baseline and follow up. In all patients who completed the ESAS, females had significantly greater severity of tiredness, nausea, depression, anxiety, and breathlessness. In sub-analysis when gender-specific primary cancers were removed, no significant differences in ESAS symptoms were found between genders. The BPI walking ability item was significantly worse for females in both the overall and sub-analysis. Females had worse symptoms at follow up prior to the removal of gender specific primaries in both the ESAS and BPI. Conclusions of this study resolved that that gender specific cancers may significantly bias gender studies of cancer-related symptoms when primary tumor type is not taken into account.

Zeng et al (39) published a study to compare functional interference and pain response outcomes using the BPI for patients treated with palliative RT to spine versus non-spine bones. A total of 386 patients were analyzed, 62% were treated with a SF, 38% with MF. Pain and functional interference scores significantly improved over time in both spine and non-spine sites. At three months, 42% of all patients had a partial response, and 25% had a complete response. Location of bone metastases and RT dose were not predictive factors for pain response or functional interference following radiation treatment.

Discussion

An extensive amount of research has been conducted in the RRRP regarding all aspects of treatment for bone metastases. Studies in the RRRP have focused on QOL in bone metastases patients, optimal treatment regimens, pain flare in its prophylaxis with dexamethasone, and the comparison of different populations. Many significant findings have been established based on research in the RRRP.

In terms of QOL research in patients with bone metastases, studies in the RRRP have been successful in defining standards for future clinical trials. In coordination with the EORTC, a bone metastases specific module, the QLQ-BM22, was developed and validated to assess QOL in patients with bone metastases using questions specifically relevant for patients with bone metastases (10). Additionally, research in the RRRP has helped to establish standardized methods of assessing partial and complete response to RT, definitions of meaningful changes in pain scores, and associating verbal descriptors with analogue scales (12, 14, 23). These findings have great significance for future research by allowing large scale reviews and analyses to yield comparable studies and significant results.

Research in the RRRP has also analyzed patterns of practice for RT by radiation oncologists and has compared different fractionation schedules for RT. Research in the RRRP has demonstrated that despite evidence demonstrating SF as equivalent to MF in pain response rate, many practicing radiation oncologists still prescribe MF (7, 26, 32). Research in this area is of great clinical importance, as it would be ideal to balance fewer appointments for patients with efficacy of treatment. Current research in the RRRP is examining the results of patients randomized to either a SF or MF to determine equivalence between the two fractionation schedules on pain relief in re-irradiation.

Another important area of research in the RRRP has investigated pain flare following RT and the prevention of pain flare with the use of steroids. Previous pilot and phase two studies in the RRRP have demonstrated promising results for the use of dexamethasone in pain flare prevention (8, 21). Currently, a randomized trial in the RRRP is underway to assess the efficacy of dexamethasone in the prophylaxis of radiation-induced pain flare when compared with a placebo.

Conclusion

There has been an ample amount of research on bone metastases conducted in the RRRP. Substantial work has been accomplished over the years in the RRRP to aid in the development of a bone metastases specific QOL module, establish standard definitions for RT response and pain assessment, determine ideal RT treatment schedules, and prevent or treat pain flare in patients with bone metastases receiving RT. Further research concerning bone metastases is underway in the RRRP, and should continue to investigate optimal treatment regimens and methods to diminish pain flare in patients with bone metastases treated with RT.

Acknowledgments

We thank the generous support of Bratty Family Fund, Michael and Karyn Goldstein Cancer Research Fund, Joseph and Silvana Melara Cancer Research Fund, and Ofelia Cancer Research Fund.

References

[1]   Hird A, Chow E, Zhang L, Wong R, Wu J, Sinclair E, et al. Determining the incidence of pain flare following palliative radiotherapy for symptomatic bone metastases: Results from three canadian cancer centers. Int J Radiat Onc Biol Phys 2009;75(1):193-7.

[2]   Tharmalingam S, Chow E, Harris K, Hird A, Sinclair E. Quality of life measurement in bone metastases: A literature review. J Pain Res 2008;1:49-58.

[3]   Hird A, Wong R, Flynn C, Hadi S, De Sa E, Zhang L, et al. Impact of pain flare on patients treated with palliative radiotherapy for symptomatic bone metastases. J Pain Manage 2009;2(4):401-6.

[4]   Chow E, Wong R, Hruby G, Connolly R, Franssen E, Fung KW, et al. Prospective patient-based assessment of effectiveness of palliative radiotherapy for bone metastases. Radiother Oncol 2001;61(1):77-82.

[5]   Berk L. Prospective trials for the radiotherapeutic treatment of bone metastases. Am J Hospice Palliat Med 1995;12(4):24-8.

[6]   Arcangeli G, Giovinazzo G, Saracino B, D'Angelo L, Giannarelli D, Arcangeli G, et al. Radiation therapy in the management of symptomatic bone metastases: The effect of total dose and histology on pain relief and response duration. Int J Radiat Oncol Biol Phys 1998;42(5):1119-26.

[7]   Chow E, Harris K, Fan G, Tsao M, Sze WM. Palliative radiotherapy trials for bone metastases: A systematic review. J Clin Oncol 2007;25(11):1423-36.

[8]   Chow E, Loblaw A, Harris K, Doyle M, Goh P, Chiu H, et al. Dexamethasone for the prophylaxis of radiation-induced pain flare after palliative radiotherapy for bone metastases: A pilot study. Support Care Cancer 2007;15(6):643-7.

[9]   Hird A, Zhang L, Holt T, Fairchild A, DeAngelis C, Loblaw A, et al. Dexamethasone for the prophylaxis of radiation-induced pain flare after palliative radiotherapy for symptomatic bone metastases: A phase II study. Clin Oncol (R Coll Radiol) 2009;21(4):329-35.

[10]   Chow E, Hird A, Velikova G, Johnson C, Dewolf L, Bezjak A, et al. The European Organisation for Research and Treatment of Cancer quality of life questionnaire for patients with bone metastases: The EORTC QLQ-BM22. Eur J Cancer 2009;45(7):1146-52.

[11]   Chow E, Nguyen J, Zhang L, Tseng LM, Hou MF, Fairchild A, et al. International field testing of the reliability and validity of the EORTC QLQ-BM22 module to assess health-related quality of life in patients with bone metastases. Cancer 2012;118(5):1457-65.

[12]   Zeng L, Chow E, Zhang L, Tseng LM, Hou MF, Fairchild A, et al. An international prospective study establishing minimal clinically important differences in the EORTC QLQ-BM22 and QLQ-C30 in cancer patients with bone metastases. Support Care Cancer 2012;20(12):3307-13.

[13]   Campos S, Zhang L, Chow E. Determining reliability of patient perceptions of important bone metastases quality of life issues. J Pain Manage 2009;2(4):453-64.

[14]   Chow E, Hird A, Wong R, Zhang L, Wu J, Barbera L, et al. Validation of meaningful change in pain scores in the treatment of bone metastases. J Pain Manage 2009;2(4):407-11.

[15]   Presutti R, Nguyen J, Hird A, Fairchild A, Clemons M, Kerba M, et al. Bone metastases and quality of life. J Pain Manage 2011;4(1):117-31.

[16]   Khan L, Uy C, Nguyen J, Chow E, Zhang L, Zeng L, et al. Self-reported rates of sleep disturbance in patients with symptomatic bone metastases attending an outpatient radiotherapy clinic. J Palliat Med 2011;14(6):708-14.

[17]   Zeng L, Sahgal A, Zhang L, Koo K, Holden L, Jon F, et al. Patterns of pain and functional improvement in patients with bone metastases after conventional external beam radiotherapy and a telephone validation study. Pain Res Treat 2011; 601720.

[18]   Dennis K, Wong K, Zhang L, Culleton S, Nguyen J, Holden L, et al. Palliative radiotherapy for bone metastases in the last 3 months of life: Worthwhile or futile? Clin Oncol (R Coll Radiol) 2011;23(10):709-15.

[19]   Presutti R, Hird A, DeAngelis C, Fairchild A, Holt T, Loblaw A, et al. Palliative radiotherapy of bone metastases and pain flare. J Pain Manage 2011;4(1):105-1.

[20]   Chow E, Ling A, Davis L, Panzarella T, Danjoux C. Pain flare following external beam radiotherapy and meaningful change in pain scores in the treatment of bone metastases. Radiother Oncol 2005;75(1):64-9.

[21]   Hird A, Zhang L, Holt T, Fairchild A, DeAngelis C, Loblaw A, et al. Dexamethasone for the prophylaxis of radiation-induced pain flare after palliative radiotherapy for symptomatic bone metastases: A phase II study. Clin Oncol (R Coll Radiol) 2009;21(4):329-35.

[22]   Chow E, Culleton S, Kwok S. Conventional radiation treatment and bone metastases. J Pain Manage 2010;4(1):23-32.

[23]   Chow E, Wu JS, Hoskin P, Coia LR, Bentzen SM, Blitzer PH. International consensus on palliative radiotherapy endpoints for future clinical trials in bone metastases. Radiother Oncol. 2002 Sep;64(3):275-80.

[24]   Chow E, Hoskin P, Mitera G, Zeng L, Lutz S, Roos D, et al. Update of the international consensus on palliative radiotherapy endpoints for future clinical trials in bone metastases. Int J Radiat Oncol Biol Phys 2012 ;82(5):1730-7.

[25]   Chow E, Davis L, Holden L, Schueller T, Wong R, Hayter C, et al. A comparison of radiation therapy outcomes of bone metastases employing international consensus endpoints and traditional endpoints. Support Cancer Ther 2004;1(3):173-8.

[26]   Chow E, Zeng L, Salvo N, Dennis K, Tsao M, Lutz S. Update on the systematic review of palliative radiotherapy trials for bone metastases. Clin Oncol (R Coll Radiol) 2012;24(2):112-24.

[27] Chow E, Doyle M, Li K, Bradley N, Harris K, Hruby G, et al. Mild, moderate, or severe pain categorized by patients with cancer with bone metastases. J Palliat Med 2006;9(4):850-4.

[28] Li KK. Harris K. Hadi S. Chow,E. What should be the optimal cut points for mild, moderate, and severe pain? J Palliat Med 2007;10(6):1338-46.

[29] Li KK, Hadi S, Kirou-Mauro A, Chow E. When should we define the response rates in the treatment of bone metastases by palliative radiotherapy? Clin Oncol (R Coll Radiol) 2008;20(1):83-9.

[30] Chow E, Danjoux C, Wong R, Szumacher E, Franssen E, Fung K, et al. Palliation of bone metastases: A survey of patterns of practice among Canadian radiation oncologists. Radiother Oncol 2000;56(3):305-14.

[31] Bradley NM, Husted J, Sey MS, Sinclair E, Li KK, Husain AF, et al. Did the pattern of practice in the prescription of palliative radiotherapy for the treatment of uncomplicated bone metastases change between 1999 and 2005 at the rapid response radiotherapy program?. Clin Oncol (R Coll Radiol) 2008;20(5):327-36.

[32] Fairchild A, Barnes E, Ghosh S, Ben-Josef E, Roos D, Hartsell W, et al. International patterns of practice in palliative radiotherapy for painful bone metastases: Evidence-based practice?. Int J Radiat Oncol Biol Phys 2009;75(5):1501-10.

[33] Dennis K, Makhani L, Zeng L, Lam H, Chow E. Single fraction conventional external beam radiation therapy for bone metastases: A systematic review of randomised controlled trials. Radiother Oncol 2013;106(1):5-14.

[34] Bedard G, Zeng L, Lam H, Lauzon N, Hicks K, Chow E. Positron emission tomography and bone metastases – A review of the literature. J Pain Manage 2012;5(4):331-345.

[35] Culleton S, Hird A, Nguyen J, Emmenegger U, Verma S, Simmons C, et al. Bisphosphonates in combination with radiotherapy for the treatment of bone metastases: A literature review. J Pain Manage 2009;2(4):375-8.

[36] Hird A, Chow E, Yip D, Ross M, Hadi S, Flynn C, et al. After radiotherapy, do bone metastases from gastrointestinal cancers show response rates similar to those of bone metastases from other primary cancers? Curr Oncol 2008;15(5):219-25.

[37] Campos S, Presutti R, Zhang L, Salvo N, Hird A, Tsao M, et al. Elderly patients with painful bone metastases should be offered palliative radiotherapy. Int J Radiat Oncol Biol Phys 2010;76(5):1500-6.

[38] Culleton S, Dennis K, Koo K, Zhang L, Zeng L, Nguyen J, et al. Gender difference in symptom presentations among patients with bone metastases in gender-specific and gender-neutral primary cancers. World J Oncol 2011;2(3):102-112.

[39] Zeng L, Chow E, Zhang L, Culleton S, Holden L, Jon F, et al. Comparison of pain response and functional interference outcomes between spinal and non-spinal bone metastases treated with palliative radiotherapy. Support Care Cancer 2012;20(3):633-9.

In: Advanced Cancer
Editors: N. Thavarajah, N. Pulenzas, B. Lechner et al.
ISBN: 978-1-62808-239-5
© 2013 Nova Science Publishers, Inc.

Chapter 35

Conventional radiation treatment and bone metastases

Shaelyn Culleton, BSc (C), Sheldon Kwok, BA (C)
and Edward Chow, MBBS*
Rapid Response Radiotherapy Program, Department of Radiation Oncology,
Odette Cancer Centre, Sunnybrook Health Sciences Centre,
University of Toronto, Toronto, Canada

Abstract

With approximately half of all advanced cancer patients developing bone metastases during the course of their disease, palliative radiation has become an important first line treatment in managing painful bony lesions. The most common palliative regimens used in treating painful bone metastases consist of 8Gy in a single fraction (frx), 20Gy in 5 frx and 30Gy in 10 frx. The optimal regimen (single versus multiple frxs) has been subject to much debate over the years. Earlier studies and meta-analyses published in the 80s and 90s provided mixed results without a clear consensus to support either fractionation scheme. One confounding factor in these analyses lay in inconsistent endpoint definitions for pain, and it became apparent that a consensus on endpoint definitions was a necessity. This resulted in a series of studies evaluating international patterns of practice, correlation of various pain scales, determining what meaningful change in pain response is for patients and the response shift phenomenon. It appears that despite evidence supporting equal efficacy of fractionation schemes using standardized endpoints, that the use of multiple fractionation schemes is still the most common dose-fractionation prescription for uncomplicated bone metastases.

* Correspondence: Edward Chow, MBBS, PhD, FRCPC, Department of Radiation Oncology, Odette Cancer Centre, Sunnybrook Health Sciences Centre, 2075 Bayview Avenue, Toronto, ON M4N 3M5, Canada. E-mail: Edward.Chow@sunnybrook.ca.

Introduction

Approximately 50-75% of patients with advanced cancer will develop bone metastases during the course of their disease (1). The most common primary cancer sites that develop secondary spread to bone are prostate (54-85%), breast (47-85%), lung (32-40%), thyroid (28-60%) and renal cell (33-40%) carcinomas (2). With recent advances in systemic therapies and supportive care, a certain proportion of patients (particularly those with breast and prostate primaries) are living longer with a diagnosis of bone metastases, and this has important implication on initial management. For example, a greater risk of experiencing skeletal related events (including hypercalcemia, cauda equina compression, pathological fractures and bony pain) has been observed and an increased need for radiation and re-irradiation with prolonged survival (3).

The most common treatment schedules delivered for palliation of bone metastases includes a single 8Gy treatment and multi-fractionated low dose regimes consisting of most commonly 20Gy in 5 fractions (frx) and 30Gy in 10 frx (4). There has been a long standing debate regarding the most appropriate treatment schedule to palliate painful bone metastases. This has triggered several randomized trials and meta-analyses evaluating the effectiveness of a single frx (SF) versus multiple frxs (MF), which altogether (especially when considering earlier analyses) have produced mixed results (5). The lack of concensus could be explained by the variety in endpoints used for local control and pain control, and the need for better endpoint definitions and validation of assessment tools was clearly needed for palliative radiotherapy trials to move forward.

This paper will include an overview of the studies surrounding SF versus MF treatment for bone metastases and highlight the transition from traditional endpoints to a more concise endpoint definition for palliative radiation treatment of bone metastases. In addition, correlation of pain scales with 'mild', 'moderate' and 'severe' pain as well as establishing the most clinically significant timing to determine response rate will also be discussed. From a patient perspective, the 'response shift phenomenon' and what a patient perceives as meaningful change following radiation treatment for bone metastases will also be highlighted. Lastly, the trend in the pattern of practice of radiation oncology in both Canada and internationally will be discussed along with future projects regarding research in palliative radiotherapy for bone metastases.

Single fraction versus multiple fraction treatment schedules

Past meta-analyses and studies

Since the 1980s, randomized studies have been published evaluating the effectiveness of SF versus MF schedules for the palliation of symptomatic bone metastases. The results of these earlier studies varied based on their response definitions as well as their study endpoints. For example, in one of the first randomized studies by the Radiation Therapy and Oncology group (RTOG) published in 1982, they reported no difference between long and short MF schedules. However upon reanalysis using a different response criteria (which took analgesics into consideration), a separate group reported an advantage using longer MF schedules for bone metastases (6). Adding to the controversy of SF versus MF schemes, in 1998 two systematic reviews of the literature were published independently by Ratanatharathorn et al (7) and McQuay et al (8), which yielded two separate conclusions. Ratanatharathorns et al. analysis found that MF schedules were better at palliating painful bone metastases than SF whereas McQuay et al's analysis showed that there was no difference between the efficacy of SF and MF courses (7,8). However, both studies cited the poor reporting and highly variable endpoint definitions as problems with their overall analyses. In 2002-2003, two separate meta-analyses by Wu at al (9) and Sze et al (10) both showed that there was no advantage of MF versus SF schedules with respect to pain relief but retreatment rates were significantly lower in the MF group. Even with the concordant results of these meta-analyses, it was clear that consensus was needed to define more meaningful endpoints for future radiotherapy trials in order to come to a more meaningful and accurate conclusion regarding SF versus MF schedules.

Development of international consensus endpoints

Because of the variety of endpoint definition used in many of the previous studies assessing SF versus MF treatment, it became clear that an international consensus on endpoints definitions needed to be established and promoted for consistency in future trials for palliative radiation of bone metastases. As part of defining an appropriate endpoint, in 2002 Wu et al (11) compared the primary endpoints definitions from a total of twelve randomized studies conducted between 1980 though 2001. All of the studies used pain reduction as a primary endpoint, with only 2 studies incorporating analgesics into the primary definition. Five of the twelve studies defined a one-point reduction or more in pain score as the primary response and the majority of studies defined a complete response as a pain score of 0. Nine studies used patient self-assessed pain scores whereas three of the studies opted to use physician assessed pain scales. Only three studies defined a set time at which a patient's response was assessed whereas the other nine trials simply evaluated pain response at any time when pain score improved during follow-up. None of the twelve trials accounted for any concurrent systemic therapies or subsequent changes in therapies at or following radiation treatment.

Table 1 shows the primary endpoint definition, complete response definition as well as the pain scales used to evaluate patients in all twelve trials. From this table, one can appreciate the vast number of primary endpoint definitions and types of pain scales employed for all twelve studies. Clearly in order to appropriately evaluate the difference in efficacy between SF and MF, a consensus in primary endpoint definitions was needed. Wu et al (11) concluded that although the data suggests similarities in pain relief among various dose-fractionation schedules, direct comparison of all twelve studies would lack validity and internal consistency. It would not be appropriate for systematic reviews to compare the response rates across different studies primarily because of the high variability between response definitions (11).

Table 1. Endpoint definitions and pain scales used in trials (11)

Author	Primary Response	Complete Response	Pain Scale
Bone Pain Working Party	Any decrease in pain category	0 pain	0-3
Steenland et al.	Pain score decrease by 2 or more	0-1 pain score	0-10
Nielsen et al.	50% decrease on VAS or decrease by 1 of 5	0 pain	0-10 (VAS) and 0-4
Jeremic et al.	Any decrease in pain category	0 pain	0-3
Gaze et al.	Any decrease in pain category	0 pain, 0 analgesic	0-4
Niewald et al.	'At least partial'	Not used	0-3
Rasmussen et al.	Decrease in size of lesion on XR or osteosclerosis	Normal bone architecture on XR	(Relief scale 0-4)
Hoskin et al.	Any decrease in pain category	0 pain	0-3
Price et al.	Any decrease in pain category	0 pain	0-3
Tong et al.	Pain score reduced to 4 or less	0 pain	0-9
RTOG 9714	Combined pain and narcotic score = 0	Combined pain and narcotic score = 0	0-10 (BPI)
Kirkbride et al.	0 pain score without increase in analgesic score or decrease in pain and analgesic scores	Not used	0-5 (Mcgill-Melzack)

In response to the need for a single endpoint definition for future trials, in April 2000 the International Bone Metastases Consensus Working Party was established. Investigators were invited to meet and reach a consensus on a set of optimal endpoint measurements for future external beam radiotherapy trials in bone metastases.

In addition to defining response, the party explored the inherent difficulty of measuring a response to localized radiotherapy when cancer pain can come from multiple sites and can palliated by other systemic agents, including analgesics, chemotherapy, hormonal therapy and bisphosphonates. Other issues included the role of analgesic consumption, the definition of 'partial' response and the interpretation of re-treatments (6).

Endpoints employed in previous bone metastases trials evaluating fractionation schedules were first identified. Participants were then invited to rank their preference of choice and then they discussed results in depth. A second survey, consisting of two parts (items of general agreement and items with no majority agreement), were sent to all participants for further opinions. The results of the second survey were analyzed critically and endorsed by all participants. These results led to an acceptable set of endpoints that could be used for future clinical trials to promote consistency in reporting. Conclusions that the party agreed upon were published in June 2002 and were categorized into: 1) Eligibility criteria for future trials, 2) Pain and analgesic assessments, 3) Radiation techniques, 4) Follow-up and timing of assessments, 5) Parameters at follow-up, 6) Endpoints and 7) Re-irradiation (6).

The resulting consensus regarding patient eligibility for future trials included several parameters. It was decided that patients should have measurable pain, with a minimal pain score of 2/10 at the time of enrollment. Also, systemic chemotherapy, hormonal therapy, and the use of biphosphonates should not be changed four weeks before and after the delivery of radiotherapy for an appropriate evaluation of response to radiation. In addition, all narcotic analgesic doses are to be scored and converted to daily oral morphine equivalents. Minimal follow-up assessment was agreed to be at two weeks then at one month with monthly follow-ups thereafter until six months post radiation treatment. Pain score, analgesic use and any changes in systemic treatment (including biphosphonates, surgical intervention, skeletal related events, and radiation-related acute toxicities) should be recorded for each follow-up. Lastly, re-irradiation should be recorded but should not be included as part of the outcome from the first radiation treatment. The response to re-irradiation should also be separately analyzed.

One of the most important contributions to future radiotherapy trials involving bone metastases was the International Bone Metastases Consensus Working Party's definition of response rates which were to be determined at 1, 2 and 3 months following radiation treatment. They defined a complete response as a pain score of zero at the treated site with no concomitant increase in analgesic intake (measured in daily oral morphine equivalents). Subsequently, partial response is defined as either:

- Pain reduction of 2 or more at the treated site on a 0-10 scale without analgesic increase
- Analgesic reduction of 25% or more from baseline without an increase in pain score

Pain progression was defined as an increase in pain score of 2 or more points above baseline with stable analgesic use or an increase of 25% or more with baseline in analgesic use (measured in daily oral morphine equivalents) with the pain score stable or 1 point above baseline. Overall the developed consensus was created to determine the minimum features of trial design and endpoint criteria that should be incorporated and/or reported in future clinical trials for palliative radiotherapy in bone metastases (6).

Results of first analysis using international consensus endpoints

Once an international consensus on endpoint definitions had been established, in 2004 our group conducted a study comparing response rates from palliative radiation therapy of bone metastases employing international consensus endpoints and traditional endpoints (3). From January 1999 to January 2002, a total of 518 patients that were English speaking and able to complete the symptom assessment scale were enrolled into the study. Patients were asked to rate their pain intensity on a categorical score of 0-10 and analgesic intake was recorded and converted into daily oral morphine equivalents. Follow-up interviews after radiation treatment were conducted by telephone at weeks 1, 2, 4, 8 and 12 (12).

Response rates were assessed three different ways for a direct comparison. First, response rates were assessed by pain score only with a complete response (CR) defined as a pain score of 0 and a partial response (PR) defined as a reduction in pain score of 2 or more, or a decrease of at least 50% from the baseline score. The second method integrated pain and analgesic scores where a response was simply defined as either a reduction of pain score of 2 or greater with no increase in analgesics or a stable pain score with at least a 50% reduction in analgesic intake. Lastly, the response rates were analyzed employing international consensus endpoints. Table 2 shows the response rates using more traditional endpoints. When radiation therapy outcomes were evaluated by pain score only, PR rates at 1, 2, 4, 8 weeks were 41%, 41%, 39%, 35%, and 41% respectively and CR rates were 21%, 30%, 32%, 35% and 32% respectively. When determined by integrated pain and analgesic scores, response rates were 51%, 50%, 52%, 45% and 48% respectively.

Table 2. Response evaluation using traditional endpoints (12)

Number of weeks after Radiation Therapy	Evaluated Patients	Pain Score Only Number of Patients (I/E)*			Integrated Pain and Analgesic Scores Number of Patients (I/E)*	
		CR	PR	CR + PR	Response	CCR
1	272 (53%)	58 (12%/21%)	112 (23%/41%)	(35%/62%)	140 (28%/51%)	23 (5%/8%)
2	297 (57%)	88 (18%/30%)	121 (25%/41%)	(43%/71%)	147 (29%/50%)	38 (8%/13%)
4	266 (51%)	86 (18%/32%)	105 (22%/39%)	(40%/71%)	137 (27%/52%)	42 (8%/16%)
8	231 (45%)	80 (17%/35%)	80 (17%/35%)	(34%/70%)	104 (21%/45%)	35 (7%/15%)
12	193 (37%)	61 (13%/32%)	80 (17%/41%)	(30%/73%)	92 (18%/48%)	28 (6%/15%)

*The denominators for "I" represent the evaluable study population (n=481 for pain score only and n = 500 for integrated pain and analgesic scores) for "E", those patients were evaluable by telephone interview at assigned intervals.

Abbreviation CCR = combined complete response (zero pain score and zero morphine equivalent).

Table 3 shows response rates using international consensus endpoints. Partial response rates were 32%, 28%, 26%, 22% and 28%, respectively while CR rates were 17%, 23%, 24%, 25% and 23%, respectively. This study showed when traditional endpoint definitions were employed, they were congruent with previously reported rates. As anticipated, this study also showed that the international consensus endpoints lowered the CR and PR rates when compared with the traditional endpoints.

Table 3. Response evaluation using international endpoints (12)

Number of weeks after Radiation Therapy	Evaluated Patients	Number of Patients (I/E)*			
		CR	PR	CR + PR	Progression
1	272 (53%)	45 (9%/17%)	87 (17%/32%)	(26%/49%)	22 (4%/8%)
2	297 (57%)	67 (13%/23%)	82 (16%/28%)	(29%/51%)	20 (4%/7%)
4	266 (51%)	64 (13%/24%)	70 (14%/26%)	(27%/50%)	20 (4%/8%)
8	231 (45%)	58 (12%/25%)	51 (10%/22%)	(22%/47%)	18 (4%/8%)
12	193 (37%)	44 (9%/23%)	54 (11%/28%)	(20%/51%)	11 (2%/6%)

*The denominators for "I" represent the evaluable study population (n = 500) for "E", those patients were evaluable by telephone interview at assigned intervals.

As shown, response rates obtained regarding radiation therapy outcomes are a direct result of the endpoint definition used. One of the benefits of using the international consensus endpoints is that it takes into account both pain score and analgesic consumption and thus more accurately reflects the true efficacy of radiation. For example, a patient with an initial pain score of 7/10 who is taking 15mg of morphine per day receives palliative radiation treatment and at 1 month his pain score decrease to 0. However, the patient's analgesic consumption increased significantly during this same time to 90mg. When assessed by pain score only, the patient would be categorized as a CR. However, when using international consensus endpoints, the patient would not be classified as either PR, CR or progression because of the difficulty regarding the relative contribution of analgesics and radiation therapy. Based on the findings of this study, we encouraged all other study investigators to re-evaluate their study findings by employing international consensus endpoint definitions (12).

Most updated systematic review of the literature on SF versus MF

In addition to comparing radiotherapy outcomes based on different endpoint definitions, in 2007 our group conducted a systematic review of randomized palliative radiotherapy trials updating previous meta-analyses. The purpose of this study was to compare response rates for trials evaluating SF versus MF regimens. Sixteen randomized trials were identified that compared SF to MF, with the oldest dating back to 1986 (5).

The sixteen studies that were used in the review were found to differ greatly in endpoint definitions. When assessing all studies using the random-effects model, the overall SF response rate was 58% (1468/2513 patients), which was similar the MF response rate at 59% (1466/2487 patients). The overall odds ratio of 0.99 indicated that there is no difference between SF and MF for relief of symptomatic bone metastases. The CR rates were found to be 23% for a SF and 24% for MF treatment with no significant differences between the two groups (5).

The re-treatment rates for both intention-to-treat and assessable patients treated with a SF were significantly higher than those with MF treatment (odds ratios were both 2.50). However, it is important to note that physicians may be more willing to re-treat patients after a SF treatment. Despite the increased risk of re-treatment with SF, the burden of multiple hospital appointments for the patient and amount of machine time required to treat is minimized with SF. Additionally, SF treatment is advantageous for patients with a short life expectancy as they are not expected to live long enough to require re-treatment. Despite increasing evidence from this meta-analysis and others that a SF and MF treatment are equally effective in relieving pain from symptomatic bone metastases, surveys on patterns of practice worldwide still demonstrate reluctance among radiation oncologists to adopt single frx as a standard practice (13). A future challenge would be to identify which subset of patients would most benefit from MF so that the allocation of resources can be distributed most effectively amongst patients requiring treatment for symptomatic bone metastases(5).

Analysis of mild, moderate and severe pain endpoints

In addition to using the 0-10 analogue scale to record pain score, other scales can be used to evaluate pain intensity, including verbal descriptor scales (VDS). The VDS allows patients to describe their pain verbally, i.e. 'no pain', 'mild', 'moderate' or 'severe' pain. This method may be preferable for patients and valuable for clinical evaluation, research and public policy. However, there is a lack of consensus on how VDS correlates with a 11-point visual analogue scale resulting in problems in following treatment guidelines, interpreting study outcomes and aiding policy or clinical practice guidelines. In 2006, our group conducted a study to examine how patients categorize their pain with both the VDS and 11-point visual analogue scale. Each patient was asked to rate their current pain on a numerical scale [0-10] and categorize their pain as 'none', 'mild', 'moderate' or 'severe' according to the VDS. When analyzed, it was found that patients scored pain as 'mild' if pain = 4, 'moderate' if pain was 5-7 and 'severe' if pain was = 8. Similarly in 2007, our group also conducted a study to establish cut off points for 'mild', 'moderate', and 'severe' pain by grading pain intensity with functional interference using the Brief Pain Inventory (BPI). Our results indicated a non-linear relationship between cancer pain severity and functional interference. Following multivariate analysis of variance (MANOVA), the optimal cut points were 1-4 for mild pain, 5-6 for moderate and 7-10 for severe pain. More research is still needed to see if these three pain categories are adequate for clinical and randomized trials; what the meaningful reduction in VDS score is; and how it would correlate with the more traditional 11-point visual analogue scale (14,15).

Most useful follow-up for end-point analysis

Besides finding an appropriate endpoint to measure response rates, when response is determined is also equally important in defining criteria. The International Consensus Working Party agreed that response should be evaluated at 1 to 3 months following radiation treatment. However, little is known about the differences in response rates when measured at 1, 2 and 3 months. In 2007, our group conducted a study to determine the most appropriate time to evaluate the response to palliative radiotherapy for bone metastases. Patients were assessed with BPI at baseline, 1, 2 and 3 months after radiation therapy. Analgesic consumption was recorded and converted to oral morphine equivalents. Response rates were then calculated using the International Consensus endpoints at 1, 2 and 3 months of follow-up. Overall response rates for evaluable patients were found to be 58% at one month, 66% at two months and 67% at three months. However, when intention-to-treat patients were included in the analysis, overall response rates were found to be 35% at one month, 32% at two months and 24% at three months. These results compared favorably with response rates reported in other palliative radiotherapy trials for bone metastases. Our group concluded that two months was the most appropriate time to measure response rates because a) maximum pain relief may take more than one month for some patients to achieve; and b) attrition is a major problem when response rates are measured after two months (16).

Meaningful change for patients

Pain intensity levels are mainly assessed and measured by pain scores and patients are often not informed of their previous pain score at baseline. As a result a patient may provide a pain score at follow-up interview which has increased from baseline despite reporting to the investigator that their pain has gotten better. One way to better assess the consistency of a reported pain score to ask whether the pain is 'worse', 'the same' or 'better' when compared to the pre-treatment level. This would indicate whether a 'meaningful' improvement has occurred from a patient perspective following radiation treatment. In 2009, our group conducted a study to validate the meaningful change in pain scores for patients receiving palliative radiotherapy for bone metastases by asking patients to score their pain on the 0-10 scale, and if their pain was getting 'better', 'worse' or 'the same'. The results of the study evaluating 178 patients concluded that patients perceived an improvement in pain when their pain score decreased by at least two points. This study supports the partial response definition in clinical trials and the international consensus endpoints (17).

Patient expectations and response shift phenomenon

Another issue that should be taken into account when defining and assessing pain intensity levels of patients receiving palliative radiotherapy for bone metastases are patient expectation and 'response shift' phenomenon. Partial response definitions are arbitrarily defined and do not take into account the individual differences in what each patient may consider as a meaningful pain response. Patients can perceive and assess pain differently depending on their own health status, and this can change with time and experience. Medical psychologists have recently defined what a 'response shift' is in quality of life research. The response shift phenomenon refers to the change in internal standards that accompany changes in health state. The response shift could significantly affect estimates of treatment efficacy and side effects as patients adapt to treatment toxicities and changes in their disease status over time. The effects of the response shift can be measured using the 'then test'. Patients are asked to not only score their current pain, but also rate their level of pain prior to radiation therapy, thus providing an estimate of treatment effectiveness.

This study conducted once again by our group in 2006 included 217 patients with bone metastases who receive palliative radiotherapy for symptomatic boney lesions. Patients reported that they expected a 50-70% reduction in pain score from baseline in order to consider radiation to be worth-while for them. Response shifts were observed in both directions creating a bell-shaped curve, with only 11% of patients (31/114) demonstrating no response shift. When taking response shift into account, CR and PR response rates were not affected. Since only 114 evaluable patients were able to be assessed, the effects of response shift should be analyzed further to determine its effects on assessing pain intensity levels and perhaps it could be considered as a factor in future partial response definitions (18).

Pattern of practice

Canadian survey regarding pattern of practice in 2000

In 2000, 172 Canadian radiation oncologist (156 in academic practice) responded to a survey presenting a series of five case scenarios, two of which were taken from two previous US surveys. Each of the five cases scenarios included a patient with a diagnosis of breast, lung or prostate cancer presenting with symptomatic bone metastases. The most common dose prescribed for all five cases was 20Gy in 5 frx (72%) followed by 8Gy in 1 frx (16%). The shorter 20Gy in 5 frx and 8Gy in 1 frx schedules were far more often employed in all five cases (81%) when compared with a longer course of 30Gy in 10 frx (10%). It was also found that 70% of practitioners used a standard dose frx to palliate painful bone metastases irrespective of site and tumor type. In comparison, the two previous US surveys showed that practicing American radiation oncologists tended to use longer fractionated schemes, with the most common prescribed dose being 30Gy/10. Reimbursement was postulated to be one of the contributing factors for this discrepancy in practice between American and Canadian radiation oncologists. All three of these surveys were conducted before the publication of two major bone metastases trials comparing SF and MF schemes. These two trials, conducted by the Dutch Bone Metastasis Study Groups and the UK Bone Pain Trial Working Party, consisted of a combined study population of 1,936 patients. They both independently concluded that there was no advantage in terms of response rate with using MF over SF schedules (1).

Review of the pattern of practice in the RRRP

Following the publication of various meta-analyses and trials from our group as well as various others, a growing consensus has shown that MF and SF schemes are equally effective in the palliation of painful bone metastases. When evaluating the pattern of practice in the RRRP from 1999 to 2005, there was a significant increase in the prescription of SF for bone metastases.

The noted increase in SF went from 51% in 1999 to 66% in 2005 (P = 0.0001), with the odds of prescribing a SF in 2005 being 1.5 times greater than in 1999. Our analysis found that patients who were older, had a lower KPS or lived very distant from the cancer centre were more likely to receive a SF. It was also more likely to be utilized if the treatment site was in the limb, hips, pelvis or ribs. The increase in the use of a SF at the RRRP corresponded nicely with the mounting of published evidence demonstrating the equal efficacy of MF when compared to SF (19).

International pattern of practice survey conducted in 2008

Shortly after the pattern of practice was evaluated in the RRRP, a survey similar to the Canadian pattern of practice survey issued in 2000 was distributed internationally in 2008. This survey consisted of a 19-item demographic questionnaire and five hypothetical case studies and was pilot tested for validity, ease and timing of completion as well as relevance. A total of 962 practicing radiation oncologists who were members of either the American Society for Radiation Oncology (ASTRO), the Canadian Association of Radiation Oncology (CARO) or fellows of the Royal Australian and New Zealand College of Radiology (RANZCR) responded to the survey. It was found that a SF was used most often by CARO members but overall, the most common palliative dose prescribed in all cases was 30Gy in 10 frx. The frequency of radiation oncologists prescribing 30Gy in 10 frx remained relatively stable over time when the results of this survey was compared to previous pattern of practice surveys conducted in Europe, UK, Canada, United States, Australia/NZ and Asia. Single frx regimens were prescribed most often by CARO members and they were 2-3 times more likely to recommended it when compared with ASTRO members who overall, were the least likely to use a SF. When looking a predictive factors that influenced the decision to treat with a SF, radiation oncologist who were trained outside the U.S. or were university affiliated (as opposed to being in private practice) were significantly more likely to prescribe a SF. Despite convincing evidence that a SF of radiation is just as effective as MF, the international community still relies on MF treatment schedules, which may put selected patients at a disadvantage (13).

The advantages of using a SF for patients with painful bone metastases over MF are considerably favourable. Not only do they have an equal chance of achieving a CR or PR with one treatment verses several treatments, but they also invest considerably less time in their medical appointments (5). The duration of response and progression rates following SF treatment are also very similar to MF treatment, with no significant difference between the two regimens. Single frx treatments also benefit practitioners as it decreases machine wait times, which in turn benefits all patients in need of radical or palliative radiation treatment. One of the augments refuting the use of SF treatment is when a high performance status patients with a life expectancy measured in years requires palliative radiation for bone metastases (13).

Some radiation oncologists will argue that with retreatment rates being approximately 2.5-fold higher for a SF, in a high performance status and high-longevity population it is better to use a MF course of treatment (5). However, even when re-treatment is taken into account, a SF is still more cost-effective than MF and re-treatment with another SF would still amount to less machine time and less medical appointments for patients (23). The reasons cited by radiation oncologists for using MF were presence of a solitary bone lesion, tumor histology, department policy, reduction of side effects, disease progression, and addressing neurologic compromise. Overall, this international survey concluded that despite evidentiary support, a SF has not been widely accepted as a treatment for uncomplicated painful bone metastases (13).

Future projects

Regarding future projects, an emerging preference for more trials to include patient centred endpoints as opposed to clinically significant trial endpoints is starting to arise. Particularly in the palliative patient population, assessing quality of life has become a more pertinent issue as newer palliative treatments are being developed and require assessment.

The current International Consensus end-point definitions for radiotherapy only takes into account pain and analgesic scores and does not address a patients functional status or overall feeling of well-being. Incorporating the use of the BPI into future trial endpoint definitions may provide a more meaningful patient centred endpoint for future radiotherapy trials. The BPI has the advantage of assessing not only pain and analgesics, but functional impact on daily activities, sleep, mobility and psych-social well being. With the development of better and more patient centred endpoint definitions, not only would we be able to assess clinical significance but patient impact as well; which has become a very important part of palliative trials (21,22).

Other future projects also include the weighting of co-analgesics with no morphine equivalency in future radiotherapy trials as well as the validation of bone metastases-specific quality of life instruments like the bone metastases module (BM22) (6).

Conclusion

With the establishment of international consensus endpoints for palliative radiotherapy trials for bone metastases the evidence quite clearly shows equal efficacy of SF and MF treatment (3,5). Despite this well founded evidence, the international community of radiation oncologists still relies on MF schedules to palliate uncomplicated bone metastases (13). We encourage practicing radiation oncologists to incorporate the use of a SF when warranted to reduce patient burden and decrease machine wait times. With increasing awareness of the importance for incorporating functional and quality of life in endpoint assessments, future endpoint definitions may include tools like the BPI or BM22 and are in development.

References

[1]   Chow E, Danjoux C, Wong R, Szumacher E, Franssen E, Fung K, et al. Palliation of bone metastases: A survey of patterns of practice among Canadian radiation oncologist. Radiol Oncol 2000;56:305-14.

[2]   Hird A, Chow E, Yip D, Ross M, Hadi S, Flynn C, et al. After radiotherapy, do bone metastases from gastrointestinal cancer show response rates similar to those of bone metastases from other primary cancers? Curr Oncol 2008;15(5):18-24.

[3]   Chow E, Hoskin P, Roos D, van der Linden Y, Hartsell W, Vieth R, et al. A phase III international randomized trial comparing single with multiple frxs for re-irradiation of painful bone metastases: National cancer institute of canada clinical trials group (NCIC CTG) SC 20. Clin Oncol 2006;18: 125-8.

[4]   Chow E, Finkelstein J, Coleman R. Metastatic cancer to the bone. In: Devita V, Lawrence T, Rosenberg S, eds. Cancer: Principle and practice of oncology. Philadelphia, PA: Lippincott Williams Wilkins, 2008:2510-22.

[5]   Chow E, Harris K, Fan G, Tsao M, Sze W. Palliative radiotherapy trials for bone metastases: A systematic review. J Clin Oncol 2007;25(11):1423-36.

[6]   Chow E, Wu J, Hoskin P, Coia L, Bentzen S, Blitzer P. International consensus on palliative radiotherapy endpoints for future clinical trials in bone metastases. Radiother Oncol 2002;64:275-80.

[7]   Ratabatharathorn V, Powers W, Moss W. Bone metastases: Review and critical analysis of random allocation trials of local field treatment. Int J Radiat Oncol Biol Phys 1999;44:1-18.

[8]   McQuay H, Collins S, Carroll Dea. Radiotherapy for the palliation of painful bone metastases. Cochrine Database Syst Rev 1999;3.

[9]   Wu J, Wong R, Johnston Mea. Meta-analysis of dose-fractionation radiotherapy trials for the palliation of painful bone metastases. Int J Radiat Oncol Biol Phys 2003;55:594-605.

[10]   Sze W, Shelley H, Held Iea. Palliation of bone metastastatic bone pain: Single fraction versus multifraction radiotherapy: A systematic review of randomized trials. Clin Oncol 2003;15:345-52.

[11]   Wu J, Bezjak A, Chow E, Kirkbride P. Primary treatment endpoint following palliative radiotherapy for painful bone metastases: Need for a consensus definition? Clin Oncol 2002;14:70-7.

[12]   Chow E, Davis L, Holden L, Schueller T, Wong R, Hayter C, et al. A comparison of radiation therapy outcomes of bone metastases employing international consensus endpoints and traditional endpoints. Support Cancer Ther 2004;1(3):173-8.

[13]   Fairchild A, Barnes E, Ghosh S, Ben-Josef E, Roos D, Hartsell W, et al. International patterns of practice in palliative radiotherapy for painful bone metastases: Evidence based practice? Int J Radiat Oncolo Biol Phys 2009, in press.

[14]   Li K, Harris K, Hadi S, Chow E. What should be the optimal cut points for mild, moderate and severe pain? J Palliat Med 2007;10(6):1338-46.

[15]   Chow E, Doyle M, Li K, Bradley N, Harris K, Hruby G, et al. Mild, moderate, or severe pain categorized by patients with cancer with bone metastases. J Palliat Med 2006;9(4):850-4.

[16]   Li K, Hadi S, Kirou-Mauro A, Chow E. When should we define the response rates in the treatment of bone metastases by palliative radiotherapy. Clin Oncol 2008;20:83-9.

[17]   Chow E, Hird A, Wong R, Zhang L, Wu J, Barbera L, et al. Validation of meaningful pain scores in the treatment of bone metastases. Submitted.

[18]   Chow E, Chiu H, Doyle M, Hruby G, Holden L, Barnes E, et al. Patient expectation of the partial response and response shift in pain score. Support Cancer Ther 2007;4(2):110-8.

[19]   Bradley N, Husted J, Sey M, Sinclair E, Li K, Husain A, et al. Did the pattern of practice in the prescription of palliative radiotherapy for the treatment of uncomplicated bone metastases change between 1999 and 2005 at the rapid response radiotherapy program? Clin Oncol 2008;20:327-36.

[20]   Szumacher E, Llewellyn-Thomas H, Franssen E, Chow E, Deboer G, Danjoux C, et al. Treatment of bone metastases with palliative radiotherapy: Patients' treatment preferences. Int J Radiat Oncol Biol Phys 2005;61(5):1473-81.

[21]   Harris K, Liying Z, Chow E. Reliability of brief pain inventory (BPI) in patients with bone metastases. J Pain Sympt Palliat 2007;2(2):3-15.

[22]   Li K, Chow E, Chui H, Bradley N, Doyle M, Barnes E, et al. Effectiveness of palliative radiotherapy in the treatment of bone metastases employing the brief pain inventory. J Cancer Pain Sympt Manage 2008;2(3):19-29.

[23]   van der Hout W, van der Linden Y, Steeland E, et al. Single versus multiple-fraction radiotherapy in patients with painful bone metastases: Cost-utility analysis based on a randomized trial. J Natl Cancer Inst 2003;95:222-9.

In: Advanced Cancer
Editors: N. Thavarajah, N. Pulenzas, B. Lechner et al.   ISBN: 978-1-62808-239-5
© 2013 Nova Science Publishers, Inc.

Chapter 36

Palliative radiotherapy of bone metastases and pain flare

Roseanna Presutti, BSc[1], Amanda Hird, BSc[1],
Carlo DeAngelis, PharmD[2], Alysa Fairchild, MD[3],
Tanya Holt, MBBS[4], Andrew Loblaw, MD[5]
*and Edward Chow, MBBS[*1]*

[1]Rapid Response Radiotherapy Program, Department of Radiation Oncology,
Odette Cancer Centre, Sunnybrook Health Sciences Centre, University of Toronto,
Toronto, Ontario, Canada
[2]Department of Pharmacy, Odette Cancer Centre, Sunnybrook Health Sciences Centre,
University of Toronto, Toronto, Ontario, Canada
[3]Rapid Access Palliative Radiotherapy Program, Department of Radiation Oncology,
Cross Cancer Centre Institute, Edmonton, Alberta, Canada
[4]Palliative Radiotherapy Outpatient Clinic, Southern Area Radiation Oncology
Services—Mater Centre, University of Queensland, Brisbane, Australia
[5]Department of Radiation Oncology, Odette Cancer Centre, Sunnybrook Health Sciences
Centre, University of Toronto, Toronto, Ontario, Canada

Radiotherapy is an effective modality for the palliation of symptomatic bone metastases with pain relief experienced by up to 80% of patients. Immediately following irradiation treatment, some patients experience an increase in pain, which is identified as a pain "flare". Approximately forty-percent of patients experience pain flare and can be greatly impacted by this phenomenon. Pain flare may have a debilitating effect on general functioning and quality of life, and the majority of patients prefer prevention of pain flare. Recent research has shown dexamethasone, a corticosteroid, to be an effective prophylactic agent reducing the incidence of pain flare to approximately 20% within a

* Correspondence: Edward Chow, MBBS, PhD, FRCPC, Department of Radiation Oncology, Odette Cancer Centre, Sunnybrook Health Sciences Centre, 2075 Bayview Avenue, Toronto, ON M4N 3M5, Canada. E-mail: Edward.Chow@sunnybrook.ca.

ten-day period following radiation treatment. Despite advances in reducing the incidence of pain flare, the mechanism behind this phenomenon is still largely unknown but may be related to inflammatory cytokines. Research is ongoing on pain flare urinary markers and dexamethasone metabolism to better understand the mechanism and experience of pain flare despite prophylaxis. This paper explores the incidence of pain flare, its impact on patients and the role of dexamethasone prophylaxis. Future investigations are also discussed.

Introduction

Bone metastases are highly prevalent in patients with cancer, found at autopsy in 70%–85% of patients (1). Pain is the most common symptom associated with bone metastases, and it is estimated that severe pain is experienced by 50-75% of all patients (1). Defined by Stern et al (2) in 1995, severe pain refers to a pain score of $\geq 7/10$, employing an 11-point numerical rating scale.

The mechanism of cancer-induced bone pain is complex. When tumor metastasizes to bone, primary nerve afferents are directly activated resulting in pain. At the cellular level, the balance of osteoblasts and osteoclasts is altered and inflammatory infiltrates are produced. Indirectly, macrophages, osteoblasts, osteoclasts and tumour cells can all release growth factors, cytokines, chemokines, prostaglandins, and endothelins which in turn stimulate local sensory afferent and sympathetic nerve fibers resulting in pain (3-5). More specifically, growth factors released by cancer cells invading bone can promote osteoclast growth and activity, which is directly related to bone pain (6).

Palliative radiotherapy (RT) is a well-established and effective modality for relieving pain and improving quality of life in patients with bone metastases. The overall pain response rate is approximately 80% (7-11). Several randomized clinical trials have been conducted to determine the optimal total dose and fractionation to maximize pain relief. Three recent meta-analyses summarizing the randomized trials have concluded that there is no significant difference in terms of pain relief from single fraction compared with multiple fractions of RT (11-13).

In addition, palliative RT is associated with few treatment-related side effects, most of which are dependant on the site exposed to radiation (14). However, in some cases, a transient increase in bone pain at the irradiated metastatic site immediately following RT may be experienced, termed a "flare reaction." Pain flare has been a well-recognized side effect from treatment of painful bone metastases with either external beam RT or radiopharmaceutical therapy (15-23) and even with chemotherapy.

The incidence of pain flare has been well-documented following radiopharmaceutical and hormonal treatment in patients with bone metastases (23-30). The reported incidence ranges from 7 to 39% in radiopharmaceutical trials (22, 31-33), and occurs in 10–20% of patients at approximately 48 hours post-treatment. Interestingly, pain flare from radiopharmaceuticals is usually predictive of a clinical response (34). Although some RT trials have mentioned pain flare as a potential side effect of treatment for patients with bone metastases, the incidence of this phenomenon has, until recently, been poorly documented.

This chapter discusses the advances that have been made into understanding the phenomenon of pain flare. Research on the incidence, impact, prevention and mechanism of pain flare are presented.

Studies

The following section outlines the results of previous investigations conducted on the incidence of external beam RT-induced pain flare in patients with symptomatic bone metastases.

In 1996, Kirkbride and Aslanidis were among the first to document the pain flare phenomena. They monitored short-term toxicity and pain relief at two weeks, and at one month, following treatment with 12 Gy in a single fraction to a bone metastases site (35). Thirty-one percent of patients (5/16) experienced an increase in pain immediately following treatment. Loblaw et al (36) continued work in this area at the University of Toronto. He reported the incidence of pain flare following palliative RT in patients participating in the Canadian Bone Metastases Study. Response rates were compared prospectively for patients receiving 8 Gy in one fraction versus 20 Gy in five fractions. Forty-four patients recorded their average pain using the Present Pain Intensity (PPI) scale of the McGill-Melzack pain questionnaire, and daily analgesic medications, for seven days immediately following RT. Pain flare was defined as "a two-point increase in the PPI with no decrease in analgesic score, or a 50% increase in analgesic score with no decrease of PPI, on at least two consecutive days". Pain flare was reported by thirty-four percent (15/44) of patients with a median duration of three days. Reportedly, 10/23 (44%) patients receiving a single 8 Gy, and 5/21 (24%) patients treated with 20 Gy in five fractions experienced a pain flare (p=0.085). Investigators concluded that pain flare is common following palliative RT for bone metastases, and patients receiving a single fraction may be at higher risk (36).

Pain flare is a common side effect of external beam RT, with an incidence rate ranging from 31-44%. This range can be attributed to differing pain flare definitions, different measures of pain intensity and variable methods of capturing the occurrence of pain flare. For this reason, it was recognized that better documentation and a clearer definition of a pain flare was needed.

Results of recent investigations

Two studies investigating the incidence of pain flare following palliative RT have been recently conducted. In 2005, the incidence of pain flare following single fraction or a fractionated course of RT was investigated (37). Patients were asked to rate their pain on a scale of zero (the absence of pain) to ten (worst possible pain) prior to treatment, daily during treatment and for ten days immediately following the completion of RT.

At each daily follow-up, patients rated their current pain as worse, same or better in comparison to their baseline pain. Analgesic intake was recorded and converted into an oral morphine equivalent dose (OMED). Pain flare was defined a priori as a two-point increase in pain score compared to baseline, with no decrease in analgesic intake, or a 25% or more increase in analgesic intake with no decrease in pain score. If baseline pain was nine, pain flare was defined as a follow up pain score of ten accompanied by the perception of current pain as worse than baseline. If baseline pain was ten, pain flare was a follow up pain score of ten, with current pain described as worse than the baseline. In order to distinguish pain flare from pain progression, both pain score and analgesic intake had to return to baseline following the increase in pain/pain flare.

In this study, the overall incidence of pain flare ranged from 2% to 16% (see table 1). Pain flares were reported by 12/88 patients (14%) on day 1 and 14/88 (16%) on day two. High occurrences of pain flares were experienced on days 1 and 2 for those patients receiving single doses of 8-10 Gy (14% each day). From day 3 and onwards, the incidence of pain flare declined to <7%. In patients receiving 20 Gy in five fractions, the pain flare incidence ranged from 3% to 23% during and immediately following RT, with the highest rates of pain flare experienced on days 2 and 7 (21% and 23%, respectively). Pain flare in the five-fraction group was described most often between days 6 and 8, which were experienced within the first three days following the completion of radiation. A total of five patients received 30 Gy in 10 daily treatments, with only one patient noticing a pain flare on day three.

Table 1. Incidence of pain flare

Incidence of pain flare

| Day | Radiation dose fractionation regimes | | | |
	Single treatment ($n=43$)	Five daily treatments ($n=40$)	Ten daily treatments ($n=5$)	Overall ($n=88$)
1	6 (14%)	6 (15%)	0	12 (14%)
2	6 (14%)	8 (21%)	0	14 (16%)
3	2 (5%)	6 (15%)	1 (20%)	9 (10%)
4	3 (7%)	5 (13%)	0	8 (9%)
5	2 (5%)	5 (13%)	0	7 (8%)
6	3 (7%)	6 (15%)	0	9 (10%)
7	2 (5%)	9 (23%)	0	11 (13%)
8	3 (7%)	7 (18%)	0	10 (11%)
9	1 (2%)	6 (15%)	0	7 (8%)
10	2 (5%)	7 (18%)	0	9 (10%)
11	0 (0%)	6 (15%)	0	6 (7%)
12	-	4 (10%)	0	4 (9%)
13	-	5 (13%)	0	5 (11%)
14	-	4 (10%)	0	4 (9%)
15	-	2 (5%)	0	2 (5%)
16	-	1 (3%)	0	1 (2%)
17	-	-	0	0
18	-	-	0	0
19	-	-	0	0
20	-	-	0	0
21	-	-	0	0
22	-	-	0	0
23	-	-	0	0
24	-	-	0	0
25	-	-	0	0

From day 12 onwards, the denominator for overall pain flare became 44 (patients on five and 10 daily treatments).

* reference (37)*.

This study confirmed the occurrence of pain flare in patients receiving palliative RT for symptomatic bone metastases. When the initial results (overall incidence of 2% to 16%) are amalgamated with the results of previous investigations (overall incidence ranging from 10% to 44%), the spectrum of reported pain flare widens, ranging from 2% to 44%. As a result of this large discrepancy, three Canadian outpatient palliative RT clinics —the Odette Cancer Centre (OCC) in Toronto, the Princess Margaret Hospital (PMH) in Toronto and the Tom Baker Cancer Centre (TBCC) in Calgary—initiated a joint study in February 2006 to confirm the incidence of pain flare (38). This study employed the same methodology as the previous study (37). The Brief Pain Inventory (BPI) was the pain measurement tool also employed prior to treatment and for the ten days following RT.

Across all three centres, the incidence of pain flare was 44/111 (40%). There was no significant difference in pain flare incidence for patients treated with a single or multiple fractions. In patients receiving a single 8 Gy, the incidence of pain flare was 27/70 (39%) compared to incidence of 16/41 (41%) in patients treated with multiple fractions. The median duration of the pain flare was 1.5 days. Eleven of forty-four (25%) patients experienced more than one pain flare, with the total number of flares totaling 60. Most pain flares were reported on days 1-5 (80%) following RT, as opposed to days 6–10 (20%) (Figure 1). Patients with breast cancer were more likely to experience pain flare (52%) compared to 25% in prostate cancer and 23% in lung cancer (p=0.0227).

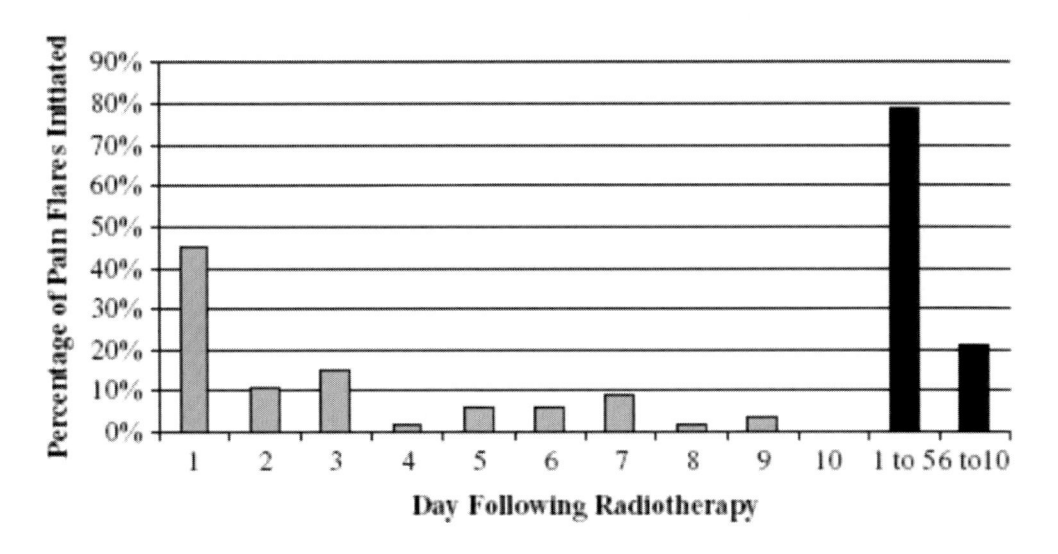

Figure 1. Percentage of pain flares appearing on Days 1-10 immediately following the completion of radiotherapy. Reference (38).

Our multi-centre investigation is the largest pain flare incidence study to date. With an overall incidence of 40%, it is important for health care professionals to be aware of this phenomenon and to treat patients accordingly at times of pain flare.

Impact of pain flare

Pain flare occurs in a significant proportion of patients treated with external beam RT for symptomatic bone metastases. Although examining the incidence of pain flare is crucial, understanding the impact of pain flare on a patient's life is equally as important. In light of this, a qualitative questionnaire was developed and administered to patients who were identified to have experienced a pain flare in the previous multi-centre pain flare incidence trial (38). The aim was to investigate the impact of pain flare on bone metastases patients treated with external beam RT. A five-item Pain Flare Qualitative Questionnaire was produced by brainstorming with palliative radiation oncologists. All patients identified as having a pain flare from an October 2007 interim analysis (35/93) were approached to participate, and were interviewed (via telephone) by a trained research assistant (39).

Patient perspective

The Pain Flare Qualitative Questionnaire was completed by 13/35 (37%) patients. Ten out of 35 (29%) were deceased/hospitalized, 8/35 (23%) were unreachable and 4/35 (11%) were from TBCC and not included in the analysis. Patient responses to each item are summarized in the following sections (39).

> "What did the pain increase mean to you at the time of the flare? (For example, what went through your mind when you were experiencing the flare?)"

Many patients indicated a fear that the "cancer was getting worse", and that their "cancer pain was never going to end". Some believed that it meant the RT was ineffective, with one patient experiencing confusion since RT was meant to improve pain. In general, patients well informed of the possibility of an increase in pain were not concerned by the experience. In fact, one mentioned a sense of optimism, believing that pain flare indicated that RT was "working". Nevertheless, some patients informed of the possibility of experiencing pain flare reported feeling that the experience was unexpected, leading to significant worry and stress.

> "Did the increase in pain interfere with your daily functioning? (For example, general activity, mood, walking ability, normal work, relations with others, sleep, enjoyment of life?)"

Overall, 10/13 (77%) patients indicated some level of functional interference due to the pain flare. The majority indicated that the pain flare completely interfered with their daily activities. Daily activities had to be modified considerably during the flare to avoid aggravation of the pain they were experiencing.

> "What did you do to manage the increase in pain? (For example: extra pain medications, sitting, lying down, etc)"

More than three quarters of patients indicated that they had to increase their pain medications in order to cope with the pain flare. Despite this, 9/13 (69%) patients failed to achieve adequate pain control. Additionally, some patients were reluctant to take additional breakthrough pain medications due to unfavourable side effects (i.e. constipation, dry mouth, and fatigue). Some patients simply rested, limited their movement and/or used a hot water bottle or other maneuvers to manage their increased pain.

"In retrospect, what does the pain flare mean to you now?"

The majority of patients had not thought about their pain flare experience retrospectively. One patient indicated that pain relief from RT comes with discomfort, while another described an awareness of the feeling and duration of pain flare. Patients able to adequately manage the pain flare experience with breakthrough pain medications did not respond to this item. One patient was unable to recall the pain flare experience and stated, "I don't know what the pain flare means at all".

"Overall, do you feel the radiation treatment was worthwhile?"

Despite experiencing pain flare, the majority of patients indicated that RT was useful. Although pain flare was problematic for one patient, RT was ultimately able to improve the patient's daily functioning. Another patient expressed that in order to improve functioning there was no choice but to experience the pain flare. Another patient felt that hormone therapy provided adequate pain relief, and therefore, would have delayed RT. For one patient, RT did not result in any subsequent pain relief and the pain flare caused a significant amount of stress. The remaining patients were unable to attribute pain relief to RT alone, as it may have been due to the use of analgesics.

Implications of the patient perspective

At the end of the interview, patients were also asked if they would have preferred the prevention of the pain flare altogether as opposed to management with pain medications. It was explicitly stated by 11/13 (85%) patients that they would prefer the prevention of the pain flare (39).

Pain flare has a debilitating effect on patients by interfering with daily activities and general functioning. In addition, thinking about treatment success leads to patients experiencing a great deal of anxiety and stress. Furthermore, increasing analgesic intake is not always adequate when trying to control a radiation-induced pain flare. From the patient perspective, prevention of pain flare rather than management with the use of breakthrough pain medications is overwhelmingly preferred.

Preventing radiation-induced pain flare

As discussed, pain flare is a common occurrence, and has a debilitating effect on patients. There is evidence that this patient group has a preference for prevention rather than treatment of radiation induced pain flare. Prevention of pain flare would eliminate additional and unnecessary suffering in patients receiving palliative RT for bone metastases and would prevent the increased use of breakthrough analgesics and the associated side-effects, including constipation, dry mouth and drowsiness (39).

Dexamethasone

Dexamethasone, a synthetic glucocorticoid used as an anti-inflammatory or immune-suppressive agent, has also been employed as an adjuvant analgesic in pain management. At the molecular level, unbound glucocorticoids readily cross cell membranes and bind with high affinity to specific cytoplasmic receptors. This binding induces a response by modifying transcription and ultimately protein synthesis to achieve the steroid's intended action.

In the treatment of brain metastases with whole brain RT, dexamethasone has been used as a prophylactic medication to reduce tumour-associated edema (40, 41). It is an effective prophylactic antiemetic for patients receiving RT to the upper abdomen (40, 42) and in the prevention of pain flare dexamethasone is a good choice as a prophylactic agent because of its long half-life (36-54 hours).

Pilot study

As a pilot study, our group investigated the efficacy of dexamethasone prophylaxis against pain flare for patients receiving a single 8 Gy for their bone metastases. The definition of pain flare and methodology from our previously mentioned pain flare incidence study was employed (37). Patients were given a single dose of dexamethasone (two 4mg tablets orally) at least one hour prior to RT. In total, 45 patients were enrolled and complete follow-up data were available for 33 patients (23 men, 10 women). Eight patients (24%) experienced pain flare during the 10 day follow-up period. They were all male, with a median age of 68.5 years. Two patients experienced a one-day pain flare on day 3. Three patients had a one day pain flare on day 7. Three other patients had a prolonged pain flare: one had a three-day pain flare on days 2-4, one had a three-day pain flare on days 4-6 and the other a six-day pain flare on days 3-8 (43).

Optimal regimen of dexamethasone

Given the half-life of dexamethasone, in the pilot study one would expect the dexamethasone to exert its maximum effect in the first two days after administration. Indeed, only one patient (3%) experienced a pain flare in the first two days (43). Three other patients had pain flare starting on day 3, beyond the expected half-life of a single dose of dexamethasone. These three patients may have benefited from an additional dose of dexamethasone on day 2 or 3 (43). Building on our initial findings, a phase II trial was initiated in a joint effort involving the Odette Cancer Centre in Toronto, the Cross Cancer Centre in Edmonton and the Mater Hospital in Brisbane, Australia to investigate the benefit of increasing the duration of dexamethasone from one dose prior to RT (as in the pilot study) to four doses—baseline (day 0) and days 1-3 immediately following external beam RT (14). In a phase III trial of dexamethasone vs placebo for the prophylaxis of radiation-induced emesis, significantly more insomnia was reported in patients who received dexamethasone (42). Therefore, in this trial patients were instructed to take dexamethasone in the morning with breakfast to minimize insomnia.

Overall, 61 patients were enrolled, with 41 evaluable. Nine out of forty-one patients (22%) experienced eleven episodes of pain flare (6 men, 3 women). The median duration of pain flare was one day. Pain flares lasting for one day occurred on days 1, 2, and 4, while two separate three-day pain flares were experienced on days 6 to 8. Six of eleven (55%) observed pain flares occurred on day 5 (Figure 2). In total, 7/41 patients (17%) experienced pain flare in the first 5 days after RT and 2/41 (5%) experienced pain flare sometime during days 6-10 after the completion of RT. The complete absence of pain flare during treatment and in the 5 days following treatment was 34/41(83%) and 39/41 (95%) for days 6-10 following RT (14). Given that patients received their last dose of dexamethasone on the morning of day 3, and given the half-life of dexamethasone, the protective effect of the last dexamethasone dose likely lasted to the morning of day 5 and possibly accounted for the surge in pain flares experienced on day 5.

Both our pilot study and phase II trial suggest that dexamethasone is an effective agent in the prevention of pain flare following RT for bone metastases (14,43). Nonetheless, some patients still experience pain flare despite dexamethasone prophylaxis.

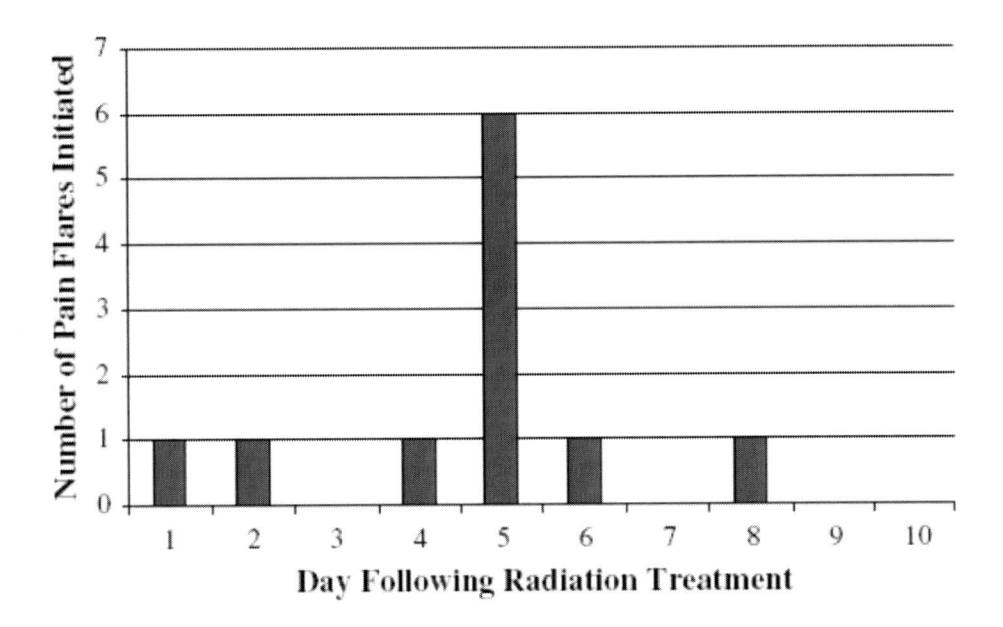

Figure 2. Distribution of pain flare 10 days immediately after the completion of radiotherapy. Total number of patients experiencing a pain flare= 9/41. Total number of pain flares= 11. Reference (14).

Discussion related to international literature

A randomized trial by Foro et al. evaluated response rates in patients receiving a single 8 Gy, 15 Gy in three fractions, or 30 Gy in ten fractions. A visual analog scale was used to evaluate pain relief every three months for a total of one year. Fifteen percent of patients receiving a single dose reported a temporary increase in pain following treatment (44).

Advances in research and treatment published and presented from other institutions

In their randomized trial of treatment with a single 8 Gy versus 20 Gy in five fractions for neuropathic pain due to bone metastases, Roos et al. added "flare effect" to the record form 15 months after initiating the trial. Flare effect was defined as "a temporary increase in pain at the index site within a week of commencing radiation treatment", and was evaluated using a 3-point numerical scale (1=mild, 2=moderate, 3=severe increase in pain). The overall incidence of flare effect was 10% (20/194). There were 2, 5, and 7 patients in the single dose arm and 2, 2, and 2 in the multifraction arm who experienced mild, moderate, and severe flare effect, respectively (P=0.029 comparing trends vs. grades) with the flare rate worse in the single versus multifraction arm (45).

Unanswered questions/controversies

Research on the incidence, impact and prevention of pain flare has been conducted. Although breakthrough analgesics can be prescribed for patients to take in the event that they experience a pain flare, and the use of dexamethasone as prophylactic agent has been shown to be effective in some cases, understanding how and why this phenomenon occurs is vital.

Future research and directions

The precise mechanism of pain flare is unknown; however, it may be related to an imbalance between pro-inflammatory and anti-inflammatory cytokines (46). Taking this into account, research investigating the correlation between pain flare and inflammatory mediators in the urine of patients undergoing RT for painful bone metastases is ongoing. Although the inflammatory markers of interest are often measured in serum, several studies have used urine samples and enzyme-linked immunosorbent assays (ELISA) for analysis of these cytokines (47,48). To achieve this, urine and saliva samples are collected at baseline (day 0) and two urine samples are collected during the first five days following RT. Pain scores, analgesic intake and functional interference are recorded in a diary for ten days upon the completion of RT. Upon completion, our group hopes to come to a better understanding of the mechanism behind pain flare, in turn allowing us to develop the optimal management and prevention strategy for potential sufferers of pain flare.

Urinary markers of dexamethasone metabolism

In addition to investigating the correlation of pain flare with urinary inflammatory markers in patients receiving a single 8Gy of RT, research on the correlation of pain flare with the urinary levels of dexamethasone metabolites in patients receiving dexamethasone prophylaxis is also being conducted. The effectiveness of dexamethasone as an adjuvant analgesic is evident; however, its precise mechanism of action is still largely unknown. From our Phase II trial, 9/41 (22%) patients still experienced pain flare despite the use of dexamethasone, while others were protected from the increase in pain (14). These patients still experiencing a pain flare despite dexamethasone prophylaxis may be rapid metabolizers of dexamethasone.

When oxidized, dexamethasone yields two 6-hydroxylation by-products: 6β-Hydroxy-dexa-methasone and 6α-Hydroxydexamethasone, which can be obtained in an 85:15 ratio (49, 50). Using the major metabolite of dexamethasone, 6β-Hydroxydexamethasone, to measure dexamethasone metabolism has been proven to be highly appropriate (49, 51, 52). The urinary ratio of 6β-hydroxydexamethasone/dexamethasone has been reported at 5.2 (50). A one-compartment, first-order elimination model can be applied to explain urinary dexamethasone concentration (50). 6β-Hydroxydexamethasone is commonly measured in urine by using high performance liquid chromatography (HPLC) (46, 49, 50, 53, 54).

Significant inter-individual variability in the pharmacokinetic response to dexamethasone exists (49, 50). Investigating this variability will allow for balance between therapeutic effects of the drug and side effect management, since specific individual dosing requirements for dexamethasone have not been well established. As dexamethasone has an extensive side effect profile (including hyperglycemia, peripheral edema, infections, proximal myopath, and gastritis), determining optimal dosing based on individual characteristics would potentially increase quality of life for individuals taking this medication (40, 41).There is, therefore, a need to explore the possibility of individual variation in dexamethasone metabolism, which will be applicable to other clinical uses of this drug. Dexamethasone metabolism can be affected by different single nucleotide polymorphisms (SNPs) of the enzymes responsible for its degradation, specifically CYP 3A4 or SNPs of glucorticoid receptors (46, 49, 55). We will measure the relevant SNPs to look for correlations between specific polymorphisms and pain flare.

It is hypothesized that the patients on dexamethasone who experience pain flare will have higher levels of inflammatory cytokines, lower levels of parent drug in urine and a SNP that predisposes them to metabolize dexamethasone more quickly. Conversely, it is expected that the patients on dexamethasone who do not experience pain flare will have lower levels of inflammatory cytokines, higher levels of parent drug in urine, and an SNP that predisposes them to metabolize dexamethasone more slowly, offering greater protection from pain flare.

Understanding the mechanism of pain flare and preventing this phenomenon is of great importance for the palliative patient receiving RT. Our previous investigations have demonstrated the incidence of pain flare and the effectiveness of dexamethasone as a prophylactic agent. Due to the surge of pain flares observed on day 5 of our Phase II trial (55%), extending the duration of oral dexamethasone from 4 days (as in the phase II trial) to 5 days may be an effective way to prevent this (14).

Randomized control trial

A Phase III trial comparing the effectiveness of protection from radiation-induced pain flare with dexamethasone (8mg in five daily doses) versus placebo is in development. The tablets will be administered orally in both arms at least one hour prior to palliative RT (day 0) and in the morning on days 1-4 following RT. This investigation hopes to provide solid evidence for the efficacy of dexamethasone prophylaxis and further information on the optimal duration of dexamethasone. It is hypothesized that the incidence of pain flare experienced on day 5 post-RT will be significantly reduced with this dosing schedule.

Conclusion

Pain flare is a common occurrence in patients receiving RT for symptomatic bone metastases. Our investigations have suggested an overall pain flare incidence rate of 40%. From the patient's perspective, pain flare has a pronounced effect both physically and psychosocially. Evidence shows that patients overwhelmingly prefer the prophylaxis of pain flare to managing pain flare with increased breakthrough pain medications.

Advances have been made in the prevention of pain flare with the use of dexamethasone as a prophylactic adjuvant agent in RT trials. In phase II studies prophylactic dexamethasone has been shown to reduce the incidence of pain flare; results of a phase III study are awaited. However, despite prophylaxis, pain flare is still experienced by some, with the majority occurring within the first 5 days after RT. Ongoing research is being conducted on urinary inflammatory markers and pain flare. In order to better manage and prevent pain flare, the mechanism of action needs to be better understood. Our ongoing studies may help to shed light on this.

References

[1]   InSightec Image Guided Treatment. Pain palliation of bone metastases—overview. 2005; April 1. Available at: http://www.insightec. com/135-en-r10/BoneMetastases.aspx. Retrieved May 2, 2009.

[2]   Serlin RC, Mendoza TR, Nakamura Y, et al. When is cancer pain mild, moderate, or severe? Grading pain severity by its interference with function. Pain 1995;61:227-84.

[3]   Goblirsch MJ, Zwolak PP and Clohisy DR. Biology of bone cancer pain. Clin Cancer Res 2006;12(20 Suppl):6231s-35.

[4]   Luger NM, Mach DB, Sevcik MA, et al. Bone cancer pain: From model to mechanism to therapy. J Pain Sympt Manage 2005; 29:S32-46.

[5]   Urch C. The pathophysiology of cancer-induced bone pain: Current understanding. Pall Med 2004;18:267-74.

[6]   Goblirsch M, Mathews W, Lynch C, et al. Radiation treatment decreases bone cancer pain, osteolysis and tumor size. Rad Res 2004;161:228-34.

[7]   Chow E, Wong R, Hruby G, et al. Prospective patient-based assessment of effectiveness of palliative radiotherapy for bone metastases in an outpatient radiotherapy clinic. Radiother Oncol 2001;61:77-82.

[8]   Nielsen OS. Palliative radiotherapy of bone metastases: there is now evidence for the use of single fractions. Radiother Oncol 1999;52:95-6.

[9]   Berk L. Prospective trials for the radiotherapeutic treatment of bone metastases. Am J Hosp Palliat Care 1995;12:24-8.

[10]   Arcangeli G, Giovinazzo G, Saracino B, et al. Radiation therapy in the management of symptomatic bone metastases: the effect of total dose and histology on pain relief and response duration. Int J Radiat Oncol Biol Phys 1998;42:1119-26.

[11]   Chow E, Harris K, Fan G, et al. Palliative radiotherapy trials for bone metastases: a systematic review. J Clin Oncol 2007;25:1423-36.

[12]   Sze WM, Shelley M, Held I, Mason M. Palliation of metastatic bone pain: Single fraction versus multifraction radiotherapy. A systemic review of randomized trials. Clin Oncol 2003;15:345-52.

[13]   Wu JSY, Wong R, Johnston M, et al. Meta-analysis of dosefractionation radiotherapy trials for the palliation of painful bone metastases. Int J Radiat Oncol Biol Phys 2006;55:594-605.

[14]   Hird A, Zhang L, Holt T, et al. Dexamethasone for the prophylaxis of radiation-induced pain flare after palliative radiotherapy for symptomatic bone metastases: a phase II study. Clin Oncol 2009;21: 329-35.

[15]   Silberstein EB. Teletherapy and radiopharmaceutical therapy of painful bone metastases. Semin Nucl Med 2005;35(2):152-8.

[16]   Kraeber-Bodere F, Campion L, Rousseau C, et al. Treatment of bone metastases of prostate cancer with strontium-89 chloride: efficacy in relation to the degree of bone involvement. Eur J Nucl Med 2000;27(10):1487-93.

[17]   Roka R, Sera T, Pajor L, et al. Clinical experience with rhenium-188 HEDP therapy for metastatic bone pain. Orv Hetil 2000;141(19):1019-23.

[18]   Slovin SF, Scher HI, Divgi CR, et al. Interferon--gamma and monoclonal antibody 131I-labeled CC49: outcomes in patients with androgenindependent prostate cancer. Clin Cancer Res 1998;4(3):643-51.

[19]   Schoeneich G, Palmedo H, Dierke-Dzierzon C, et al. Rhenium-186 HEDP: palliative radionuclide therapy of painful bone metastases. Preliminary results. Scand J Urol Nephrol 1997;31(5):445-8.

[20]   Limouris GS, Shukla SK, Condi-Paphiti A, et al. Palliative therapy using rhenium-186-HEDP in painful breast osseous metastases. Anticancer Res 1997;17(3B):1767-72.

[21]   de Klerk JM, van het Schip AD, Zonnenberg BA, et al. Phase 1 study of rhenium-186-HEDP in patients with bone metastases originating from breast cancer. J Nucl Med 1996;37(2):244-9.

[22]   Dafermou A, Colamussi P, Giganti M, et al. A multicentre observational study of radionuclide therapy in patients with painful bone metastases of prostate cancer. Eur J Nucl Med 2001;28(7):788-98.

[23]   Bubley GJ. Is the flare phenomenon clinically significant? Urology 2001;58:5-9.

[24]   Ackery D, Yardley J. Radionuclide-targeted therapy for the management of metastatic bone pain. Semin Oncol 1993;20:27-31.

[25]   Brunelli C, Constantini M, Di Giulio P, et al. Quality-of-life evaluation: when do terminal cancer patients and health-careproviders agree? J Pain Symptom Manage 1998;15:151-8.

[26]   Cella D, Hahn EA, Dineen K. Meaningful change in cancer specific quality of life scores: differences between improvement and worsening. Qual Life Res 2002;11:207-21.

[27]   Chow E, Wu J, Hoskin P, Coia L, Bentzen S, Blitzer P on behalf of the International Bone Metastases Consensus Working Party. International consensus on palliative radiotherapy endpoints for future clinical trials in bone metastases. Radiother Oncol 2002;64:275-80.

[28]   Coleman RE, Mashiter G, Whitaker KB, Moss DW, Rubens RD, Fogelman I. Bone scan flare predicts successful systemic therapy for bone metastases. J Nucl Med 1988;29:1354-9.

[29]   De Haes J, Stiggelbout A. Assessment of values, utilities, and preferences in cancer patients. Cancer Treat Rev 1996;22:13-26.

[30]   Grossman SA, Sheidler VR, Swedeen K, Mucenski J, Piantadosi S. Correlation of patient and caregiver ratings of cancer pain. J Pain Symptom Manage 1991;6:53–7.

[31]   Tian JH, Zhang JM, Hou QT, et al. Multicentre trial on the efficacy and toxicity of single-dose samarium-153-ethylene diamine tetramethylene phosphonate as a palliative treatment for painful skeletal metastases in China. Eur J Nucl Med 1999;26:2–7.

[32] Turner JH, Claringbold PG, Hetherington EL, Sorby P, Martindale AA. A phase I study of samarium-153 ethylenediaminetetramethylene phosphonate therapy for disseminated skeletal metastases. J Clin Oncol 1989;7:1926-31.

[33] Turner SL, Gruenewald S, Spry N, Gebski V, Metastron Users Group. Less pain does equal better quality of life following strontium-89 therapy for metastatic prostate cancer. Br J Cancer 2001;84:297-302.

[34] Robinson RG, Preston DF, Spicer JA, et al. Radionuclide therapy of intractable bone pain: emphasis on strontium-89. Semin Nucl Med 1992;22:28-32.

[35] Kirkbride P, Aslanidis J. Single fraction radiation therapy for bone metastases—a pilot study using a dose of 12 Gy [Abstract581]. Clin Invest Med 1996;19:S87.

[36] Loblaw DA, Wu JSY, Warde P, et al. Pain flare in patients with bone metastases after palliative radiotherapy: A nested randomized controlled trial. Sup Care Cancer 2007;15:451-5.

[37] Chow E, Ling A, Davis L, et al. Pain flare following external beam radiotherapy and meaningful change in pain scores in the treatment of bone metastases. Radiother Oncol 2005;75:64-9.

[38] Hird A, Chow E, Zhang L, et al. Determining the incidence of pain flare following palliative radiotherapy for symptomatic bone metastases: results from three Canadian cancer centres. Int J Rad Onc Biol Phys 2009 (in press).

[39] Hird A, Wong R, Flynn C, et al. Impact of pain flare on patients treated with palliative radiotherapy for symptomatic bone metastases. J Pain Manage, in press.

[40] Hempen C, Weiss E, Hess CF. Dexamethasone treatment in patients with brain metastases and primary brain tumors: Do the benefits outweigh the side-effects? Sup Care Canc 2002;10:322-8.

[41] Weissman DE, Dufer D, Vogel V, Abeloff D. Corticosteriod toxicity in neuro-oncology patients. J Neur Enter 1987;5:125-8.

[42] Kirkbride PA, Bezjak A, Pater J, et al. Dexamethasone for the prophylaxis for radiation-induced emesis: a National Cancer Institute of Canada Clinical Trials Group phase III study. J Clin Oncol 2000;18:1960-6.

[43] Chow E, Loblaw DA, Harris K, et al. Dexamethasone for the prophylaxis of radiation-induced pain flare after palliative radiotherapy for bone metastases—a pilot study. Support Care Cancer 2007;15:643-64.

[44] Foro P, Algara M, Reig A, et al. Randomized prospective trial comparing three schedules of palliative radiotherapy. Preliminary results [Spanish]. Oncologia 1998;21:55-60.

[45] Roos DE, Turner SL, O'Brien PC, et al. Randomized trial of 8 Gy in 1

[46] versus 20 Gy in 5 fractions of radiotherapy for neuropathic pain due to bone metastases (Trans-Tasman Radiation Oncology Group, TROG 96.05). Radiother Oncol 2005;75:54-63.

[47] McCune JS, Hawke RL, LeCluyse EL, et al. In vivo and in vitro induction of human cytochrome P4503A4 by dexamethasone. Clin Pharmacol Ther 2000;68:356-66.

[48] Sirera R, Salvador A, Roldan I, Talens R, Gonzalez-Molina A et al. Quantification of proinflammatory cytokines in the urine of congestive heart failure patients. Its relationship with plasma levels. Eur J Heart Failure 2003:5:27-31

[49] Erickson DR, Xie SX, Bhavanandan VP, et al. A Comparison of Multiple Urine Markers for Interstitial Cystits. J Urology:2002:167: 2461-9

[50] Zurbonsen K, Bressolle F, Solassol I, Aragon P.J., Culine S, Pinguet F. Simultaneous determination of dexamethasone and 6bhydroxydexamethasome in urine using solid-phase extraction and liquid chromatography: applications to in vivo measurement of cytochrome P450 3A4 activity. J Chromatography B 2004;804: 421-9.

[51] Puisset F, Chatelut E, Dalenc F, Busi F, Cresteil T, Azema J, Poublanc M, Hennebelle I, Lafont T, Chevreau C, Roche H. Dexamethasone as a probe for docetaxel clearance. Cancer Chemother Pharmacol 2004;54:265-72.

[52] English J, Chakraborty J, Marks V, Parke A. A radioimmunoassay procedure for dexamethasone plasma and urine levels in man. Eur J Clin Pharmacol 1975;9:239-44.

[53] Minagawa K, Kasuya Y, Baba S, KnappG, Skelly JP. Identification and quantification of 6B-hydroxydexamethasone as a major urinary metabolite of dexamethasone in man. Steroids 1986;47(2-3):175-88.

[54] Gentile DM, Tomlinson ES, Maggs JL, Park BK, Back DJ. Dexamethasone metabolism by human liver in vitro. Metabolite identification and inhibition of 6-hydroxylation. J Pharmacol Exp Ther 1996;277:105-12.

[55] Rodchenkov GM, Uralets VP, Semenov VA, Leclercq PA. Analysis of dexamethasone, triamcinolone, and their metabolites in human urine by microcolumn liquid and capillary gas chromatography mass spectrometry. J High Resolut Chromatogr 1988;11:283-8.

[56] Jewell CM, Cidlowski JA. Molecular evidence for a link between the N363S glucocorticoid receptor polymorphism and altered gene expression. J Clin Endocrinol Metab 2007;92(8):3268-77.

In: Advanced Cancer   ISBN: 978-1-62808-239-5
Editors: N. Thavarajah, N. Pulenzas, B. Lechner et al.   © 2013 Nova Science Publishers, Inc.

Chapter 37

Bone metastases and quality of life

Roseanna Presutti, BSc (C)[1], Janet Nguyen, BSc (C)[1],
Amanda Hird, BSc (C)[1], Alysa Fairchild, MD[2],
Mark Clemons, MD[3], Marc Kerba, MD[4], Arjun Sahgal, MD[1]
*and Edward Chow, MBBS[*1]*

[1]Rapid Response Radiotherapy Program, Department of Radiation Oncology,
Odette Cancer Centre, Sunnybrook Health Sciences Centre, University of Toronto,
Toronto, Ontario, Canada
[2]Rapid Access Palliative Radiotherapy Program, Department of Radiation Oncology,
Cross Cancer Centre Institute, Edmonton, Alberta, Canada
[3]Division of Medical Oncology, Princess Margaret Hospital, Toronto, Ontario, Canada
[4]Tom Baker Cancer Centre, University of Calgary, Calgary, Alberta, Canada

Bone metastases are a common consequence of many malignancies.Few clinical trials have evaluated quality of life (QOL) as an endpoint in studies directed to medical or radiotherapy interventions for bone metastases. Given the lack of well-developed bone metastases specific QOL instruments, our group initiated the development of a bone metastases questionnaire in accordance with the European Organization for Research and Treatment of Cancer's (EORTC) module development guidelines. The module is currently in the final stage of development (international field testing) and is available for clinical use through the EORTC. This chapter addresses previous clinical trials in patients with bone metastases receiving palliative RT, and describes the QOL assessments completed. The development of the EORTC bone metastases module and future research directions are also discussed.

[*] Correspondence: Edward Chow, MBBS, PhD, FRCPC, Department of Radiation Oncology, Odette Cancer Centre, Sunnybrook Health Sciences Centre, 2075 Bayview Avenue, Toronto, ON M4N 3M5, Canada. E-mail: Edward.Chow@sunnybrook.ca.

Introduction

With effective anti-cancer systemic treatments, survival of patients with bone metastases has substantially improved. For example, patients with metastatic breast and prostate cancer, with predominately bone or bone-only spread, have life expectancies that can now range from 2-5 years (1). As a result of prolonged survival, the prevalence of patients with bone metastases is now estimated to be double the incidence (2), and requires proper study to ensure that we treat our patients effectively and kindly.

Management of symptoms from bone metastases during these years is essential for reducing skeletal complications and for maximizing quality of life (QOL), because (3):

- Pain arising from bone metastases is the most common symptom requiring palliative radiotherapy (RT) in cancer patients. Fifty to 75% of patients with bone metastases suffer from severe pain (4).
- The symptoms of bone metastases can be severe, and may develop early in the clinical course of their disease than symptoms from visceral metastases.
- Complications from skeletal metastases can seriously impair mobility in 65-75% of patients, fractures of weight-bearing long bones occur in 10-20% of patients; hypercalcaemia occurs in 10-15% of patients; and spinal cord or nerve root compression occurs in 5% of patients
- The care of this group of patients is frequently poorly integrated.

The World Health Organization describes palliative care as "an approach that improves the quality of life of patients, and their families facing the problem associated with life-threatening illness" (5). In palliative intervention trials, QOL should be a major endpoint as the goal of therapy is not to improve survival but to improve the patients symptomatic state at the end of life. In particular for patients with bone metastases, the treatment of cancer pain commonly involves multiple care providers including medical and radiation oncologists, pain specialists, surgeons and other health care professionals. Therefore, it becomes increasingly complex to determine the benefit from bone specific treatment on a patients pain control and overall state of being. Therefore, QOL measures are important as a major endpoint for studies given that they take into account the patients' state as a whole. QOL measures are subjective and multidimensional and, therefore, reflect functional status, psychosocial well-being and disease- and treatment-related symptoms. It also incorporates many aspects of a patient's life including expectations, satisfaction, and their value system (6). This paper addresses the evaluation of QOL as an endpoint in bone metastases RT trials, and the development of a bone metastases specific QOL assessment tool. Previous and future research into QOL for patients with bone metastases is also discussed.

Our study

Traditionally, clinical trials have largely focused on objective endpoints such as analgesic consumption and skeletal related events endpoints such as hypercalcaemia, pathological fractures, spinal cord compression and requirement for surgery or radiation (3). As palliative interventions are unlikely to lead to survival prolongation or tumor regression, QOL is probably a more meaningful endpoint and has been a major focus of research at the University of Toronto (7).

Our group prospectively evaluated change in common symptoms and QOL after external beam RT for bone metastases using the Edmonton Symptom Assessment System (ESAS) (7). The ESAS is a validated patient-based assessment that evaluates 10 symptoms: global pain, index pain (pain at the irradiated site), fatigue, nausea, depression, anxiety, drowsiness, appetite, sense of well-being, and shortness of breath on a numerical rating scale of 0 to 10 (0 = absence of symptom; 10 = worst possible symptom) (8). Assessments including analgesic intake were conducted at baseline and at 1, 2, 4, 8, and 12 weeks in 518 patients. Statistically significant improvements were observed for the following ESAS domains (the range of the mean difference from the baseline): global pain (–0.9 to –1.4), index pain (–2.1 to –2.9), anxiety (–0.6 to –0.8), sense of wellbeing (–0.7 to –0.8), and shortness of breath (–0.5) in at least one follow-up interval. However, in the first two weeks after RT there was slight worsening of fatigue (0.5 to 0.8) experienced by all patients (7).

Developing a bone metastases quality of life module

In light of the great need to assess the benefits and side effects of bone metastases specific interventions, our group carried out an extensive literature search on MEDLINE, PSYCHINFO and all relevant databases to identify the relevant QOL issues for bone metastases patients (3,9). All relevant QOL questionnaires, including general QOL and disease-specific questionnaires on bone metastases were reviewed.

We found that most trials reporting QOL used the European Organization of Research and Treatment of Cancer (EORTC) QLQ-C30. Others used the Brief Pain Inventory, Functional Living Index-Cancer (FLIC), Functional Assessment of Cancer Therapy tools (FACT), Short Form-36, social support list, global QOL, or performance status score (9). We determined that most bone metastases trials have measured QOL by the EORTC QLQ-C30, version 3. This tool was developed with the principle to assess key general QOL issues, and is the most frequently used measure in cancer clinical trial research (10,11), however, it was not designed with the intent to cover the key QOL issues relevant for patients with bone metastases. It was our conclusion that well-developed bone metastases specific QOL instruments were lacking.

Our group previously administered the EORTC QLQ-C30 to patients in the Bone Metastases Clinic at the Odette Cancer Centre, Sunnybrook Health Sciences Center, Toronto, Ontario, Canada for patient feedback (7). Our patients uniformly expressed that the instrument was not relevant to their own situations. Specifically, the EORTC QLQ-C30 did not assess QOL issues related to the complications of bone metastases such as hypercalcaemia, pathological fracture, spinal cord compression, mobility, functional impairment nor the side effects of treatments such as bisphosphonates, orthopaedic surgery or RT. The International Bone Metastases Consensus Working Party then recommended in 2002 the development of a bone-metastases-specific QOL instrument tool (12).

In response to this need for a comprehensive bone metastases specific QOL instrument, our group initiated the development of the Bone Metastases Module (EORTC QLQ-BM22) to supplement the EORTC-QLQ-C30. According to the module development guidelines of the

EORTC Quality of Life Group (QLG), four phases must be completed: phase I—generation of relevant QOL issues; II—operationalization of the QOL issues into a set of items; III—pre-testing the module questionnaire; and IV—large-scale international field-testing (13). The following section discusses our progress to date.

Table 1. List of 61 QOL issues from the literature and qualitative interviews grouped

	Symptom
1	Long-term (or chronic) pain
2	Short-term (or acute), severe pain
3	Paint at rest (i.e. when sitting)
4	Pain with activity (i.e. when walking)
5	Pain aggravation with movement or weight-bearing
6	Uncontrolled, unmanageable pain
7	Pain at night preventing sleep
8	Aches and stiffness
9	*Lack of energy*
10	Numbness
11	Tingling
12	Burning sensation
13	Postural problems
	Function
14	Limited movement due to pain
15	Difficulty planning activities outside the home
16	Difficulty travelling outside the home (i.e. using public transportation, driving, sitting in a car)
17	Difficulty in carrying out meaningful activity (including employment)
18	*Able to perform self-care*
19	Able to return to work promptly
20	*Difficulty carrying out usual daily tasks (i.e. grocery shopping, work outside the home, housework)*
21	Difficulty bending
22	Difficulty lifting
23	Difficulty standing up
24	Difficulty climbing stairs
25	Difficulty sitting
26	Difficulty lying in bed
27	Difficulty lying flat
28	Ability to have sex
	Side Effect from Treatment of Bone Metastases
29	Drowsiness
30	Confusion
31	Dizziness
	Psychosocial
32	*Able to perform role functioning (including domestic and family roles)*
33	*Feeling socially isolated*
34	Strengthened relationships with family/ friends
35	*Have a clear, alert mind*
36	Feel in control, positive, and confident
37	Hope to live as long as possible
38	Reluctance to pain medication
39	Fear of addiction to pain medication
40	*Anxiety*

Psychosocial	
41	Frustration
42	*Mood changes*
43	Emotional stress of diagnosis of advanced, incurable cancer
44	Increased focus on spiritual issues
45	Loss of interest in activities you normally enjoy
46	Loss of interest in sex
47	Worry about pain
48	Worry about suffering
49	Worry about loss of mobility compromising independence
50	Worry about becoming dependent on others
51	Worry about current health status
52	Worry about the future
53	Worry about becoming bed-bound
54	Worry about disease progression, deterioration in condition, and future complications
55	Worry about running out of medical treatments
56	Worry about hospitalization
57	Worry about ending days in a hospital or nursing home
58	Worry about death
Treatment Expectation	
59	Hope for sustained pain relief (reduce pain for as long as possible)
60	Hope treatment will reduce pain as much as possible
Other issue	
61	*Financial burden due to the illness*

Italicized issues are included in the EORTC QLQ-C30.

EORTC QLQ-BM22 development: Phase I

In the first phase, relevant QOL issues for patients with bone metastases were identified through an extensive literature and qualitative interviews with patients and health care professionals (HCP). The literature search was conducted using Medline (1966-2005) and Psychinfo (1966-2005) databases. A list of possible issues was compiled and presented to Canadian, Australian and German HCPs experienced in treating patients with bone metastases. The HCPs were asked to rate the issues from 1 – 'not relevant' to 4 – 'very relevant', to select 5–10 core issues to be definitely included in the questionnaire and to provide suggestions as to any missing items they thought relevant. The list of issues was also presented to patients from five cancer centres (three in Canada, one in Australia and one in Germany). Patients were asked to indicate the degree to which they had experienced each issue during the past week, to select which 5–10 issues they considered as the most important, and to list any additional issues which they felt were missing from the questionnaire (14,15).

Preliminary interviews were conducted with 61 patients and 58 HCPs, generating a list of 61 relevant symptoms summarized in the following domains (see table 1): symptoms (13 issues); function (15 issues); side-effects from treatment of bone metastases (3 issues); psychosocial (27 issues); treatment expectation (2 issues); and financial (1 issue). This list was formatted into a questionnaire and distributed to a new cohort of bone metastases patients and HCPs.

Table 2. Patient and health care professional demographics for phase I interviews

Patient Demographics (N=413)*.	Number (%)
Centre/Country	
PMH/Canada	132 (32.0%)
OCC/Canada	131 (31.7%)
TBCC/Canada	67 (16.2%)
Liverpool/Australia	42 (10.2%)
Charité/Germany	41 (9.9%)
Sex	
Female	239 (57.9%)
Male	174 (42.1%)
Age (years) (n=409)	
Mean ± SD	63.4 ± 11.8
Median (range)	64 (30 – 93)
Primary Cancer Site (n=412)	
Breast	160 (38.8%)
Prostate	71 (17.2%)
Multiple myeloma	61 (14.8%)
Lung	57 (13.8%)
Renal	20 (4.9%)
Gastrointestinal	16 (3.4%)
Colorectal	9 (2.2%)
Unknown	5 (1.2%)
Others	22 (5.3%)
Treatment (current/past)	
Chemotherapy (n=329)	231 (70.2%)
Radiation (n=348)	242 (69.5%)
Hormonal therapy (n=314)	175 (55.7%)
Bisphosphonates (n=322)	177 (55.0%)
Surgery (n=372)	20 (5.4%)
Skeletal Related Event	
Pathological fracture (n=371)	29 (7.8%)
Spinal cord compression (n=372)	21 (5.6%)
Hypercalcaemia (n=372)	16 (4.3%)
Health Care Professional Demographics (N=152)*	**Number (%)**
Centre/Country	
PMH/Canada	47 (30.9%)
OCC/Canada	45 (29.6%)
Liverpool/Australia	26 (17.1%)
TBCC/Canada	23 (15.1%)
Charité/Germany	11 (7.2%)
Specialty	
Radiation Oncologists	46 (30.3%)
Medical Oncologists	40 (26.3%)
Nurses	33 (21.7%)
Palliative Care Physicians	18 (11.8%)
Surgeons	7 (4.6%)
Social Workers	5 (3.3%)
Others	3 (2.0%)

*The n value differs depending on the item evaluated because of missing data.

A total of 413 patients (174 males and 239 females) and 152 HCPs were then interviewed across five cancer centres in Canada, Australia, and Germany (see table 2). Patients had a median age of 64 years (range 30–93 years). The most common primary cancer sites were breast (39%), prostate (17%) and multiple myeloma (15%). At the time of interview, most patients had received chemotherapy (70%), RT (70%), hormonal therapy (56%) or bisphosphonates (55%). Few patients had experienced pathological fractures (8%), spinal cord compression (6%) or hypercalcaemia (4%). Of the 152 HCPs interviewed, the majority were radiation oncologists (30%), medical oncologists (26%) or nurses (22%) (14,15).

The results from Phase I interviews were analysed using descriptive statistics: 1) mean score for each item; 2) range of responses; 3) prevalence ratios (number of patients who experienced each complaint, i.e. who scored 2, 3 or 4, divided by the total number of patients who completed that item, multiplied by 100) and 4) the proportion of patients or professionals prioritising the issue. Items were selected according to the following criteria: a mean score of at least 2.5; range of responses of at least two points, i.e. 1–3 or 2–4; a prevalence ratio of at least 30%; and at least 33% of patients or health care professionals prioritizing the item. Items were retained if they met at least three of four of the above criteria. After analysis of the Phase I interviews for both patients and HCPs, 39 issues were removed (15).

Differences in perspectives

The extent to which patients experienced each of the 61 issues during the course of his or her illness was compared to how relevant HCPs felt each item was in terms of QOL scores. Patients and HCPs reported significantly different mean scores for all 61 items (p < 0.0055) except for the item "feel in control, positive and confident" where the mean scores were 3.07 and 3.10 respectively (p = 0.2215). In addition, the mean scores reported by HCPs were almost always higher than that of patients (14,15).

Both patients and HCPs agreed that the four items which affected bone metastases patients most profoundly were: "long-term (chronic) pain", "difficulty carrying out usual daily tasks", "able to perform self-care" and "able to perform role-functioning" (see table 3). However, the difference in ranking between the two groups was substantial with respect to the somatic and psychosocial issues. Patients focused more on psychosocial items (4 of 10 items) and included three "worry" issues within their top 10 ("worry about becoming dependent on others, "worry about lost of mobility compromising independence" and "worry about disease progression, deterioration in condition and future complications"). These issues ranked 20th, 22nd and 16th respectively by HCPs. Instead, HCPs focused more on items related to symptoms (7 of 10 items) with an emphasis on issues relating to pain (7 of 10 items). Somatic issues were ranked lower by patients than by HCPs (14,15).

Cancer pain is undoubtedly a significant problem in the bone metastases population and many of the HCPs interviewed are actively involved in its treatment (4). Unrelieved cancer pain can have a negative impact on patient QOL (17-23), but may not be the sole or the most significant factor. RustØen et al. found that pain only had a small impact on QOL, explaining 8.6% of the variance of QOL scores (24). When physical and social functioning were added to the analysis, the explained variance increased to 28.4%; however, depression seemed to have the most significant impact with an absolute increase of 28.4% explained variance (23).

Therefore, pain is a problem for patients with bone metastases, but there may be additional and/or more important issues influencing QOL, such as psychosocial issues (24).

Table 3. Top ten issues patient of health care professionals

Rank	Issue	% Patients	Issue	% HCP
1	**Long-term (or chronic)** *pain*	41.4	**Able to perform self-care**	62.1
2	**Difficulty carrying out usual daily tasks (grocery shopping work outside the home housework)**	39.7	Uncontrolled unmanageable *pain* not relieved by pain killers	61.0
3	*Worry* about becoming dependent on others	38.7	**Long-term (or chronic)** *pain*	54.2
7	*Worry* about loss of mobility compromising independence	37.3	Short-term (or acute) severe *pain*	52.4
5	*Worry* about disease progression deterioration in condition and future complications	32.9	*Pain* at night preventing sleep	50.0
6	**Able to perform self-care**	32.6	Limited movement due to *pain*	46.9
7	Difficulty in carrying out meaningful activity (including employment)	32.1	*Pain* at rest (when sitting)	45.1
8	**Able to perform role functioning (including domestic and family roles)**	32.0	*Pain* with activity (when walking)	41.0
9	Financial burden due to the illness	24.3	**Able to perform role functioning (including domestic and family roles)**	39.3
10	Hope treatment will reduce *pain* as much as possible	23.6	**Difficulty carrying out usual daily tasks (grocery shopping work outside the home housework)**	35.9

Boldface represents items that patients and HCPs agree should be included.

Patient self-report of symptoms is considered the gold standard (25,26). Patients therefore should be the primary source regarding what issues are included in a QOL assessment tool (27). The relevance of each domain may vary according to stage of illness, treatment, age or cultural backgrounds which make it important that a wide range of patients are interviewed in the development of any instrument (27). If we are able to understand the patient's perspective of their illness, management strategies appropriate to their individual needs can be developed (14).

Alternatively, HCPs may provide a more objective evaluation of the patients' problems and symptoms (26). Therefore, the HCPs' perspective is also important in the development of QOL instruments as they are responsible for incorporation of these tools into everyday practice. In 1996, 7% of HCPs formally collected and used QOL information (28). The following year, Bezjak et al reported that although 74% of physicians felt QOL research findings should be incorporated into clinical practice, 48% believed existing QOL instruments do not provide clinically relevant results (29). Many felt that current QOL instruments are too complicated, time consuming or costly to incorporate into clinical practice (30). It is also unlikely HCPs will accept an instrument which they feel is inadequate (31, 32). Therefore, it is important that HCPs contribute to questionnaire development in terms of its content and structure to increase the likelihood of acceptance.

QOL research has significantly contributed to the approval of new chemotherapeutic agents and supportive care measures (33,34). The next step is application to everyday clinical practice (35). Ideally, physicians would determine QOL scores at each clinic visit and identify the changes and reasons for their changes since the last visit. This would facilitate discussion and help HCPs understand the patient's total environment (36). In a study by Detmar et al. physicians who utilized patient QOL scores identified a greater percentage of patients with moderate-to-severe health problems than those who did not (36). It is important to help the patient interpret the data and suggest how they can employ this information into their daily life, just as we do with their disease and treatment information (14). Ongoing development of QOL instruments should aim at identifying issues that most affect patients' illness experience and provide an objective assessment tool for HCPs to adopt into everyday practice.

Operationalization of a provisional questionnaire: Phase II

In Phase II of module development, the remaining 22 issues from Phase I were constructed into items according to the following criteria: a) questions should be compatible with EORTC QLQ-C30 response categories 'not at all', 'a little', quite a bit' and 'very much'; b) questions compatible to the 1-week time frame of EORTC QLQ-C30 wherever possible and c) questions should refer to ongoing states rather than to changes. Existing questionnaire items were harmonized to ensure comparability of items across modules using the EORTC QOL Item Bank (37). The Item Bank includes all existing EORTC QOL questionnaire items with their appropriate translations. The Item Bank is organized by themes, with identification of the original module and all other modules containing each item. Items were constructed from the 22 retained issues. Wording was modified based on structure of the items available in the Item Bank. The draft module was reviewed for the clarity wording and repetition by two members of the EORTC QLG and was subsequently translated to German, Chinese, Spanish, Greek and Dutch according to EORTC QLG guidelines (15).

Pretesting the questionnaire: Phase III

The third phase of module development involved testing the provisional questionnaire for acceptability and relevance. This phase identified problems relating to the wording and clarity of items, and determined the need for adding or deleting items. The provisional module was tested in a separate patient cohort from participating countries. This phase was critical as well to determine whether the set of module items are comparable cross-culturally, particularly among non-English speaking countries. Patients completed the EORTC QLQ-C30 and the bone metastases module (EORTC QLQ-BM22) indicating if they found any questions annoying, confusing, upsetting or intrusive, and if so, they were asked to suggest alternative phrasings. Patients were also asked whether any questions were irrelevant or whether there were additional issues that were not included (15).

The EORTC QLQ-C30 and the provisional bone metastases module were pretested on 170 patients from nine countries (see table 4). The majority (68%) were non-English speaking. Overall, 83 patients were male (49%) and 87 were female (51%). Median time from primary cancer diagnosis to diagnosis of bone metastases was one year (range: 0–21 years). The prevalence ratio of all additional EORTC QLQ-BM22 items exceeded 30% with the exception of items 3, 4, 5 and 8 (which are all pain-related items).

If the EORTC QLQ-BM22 is to be used as a QOL questionnaire in a clinical setting, it is essential to include pain items. The assessment of characteristics of pain (i.e. questions 6–8 & 15) and the gradient that assesses pain during various movements (i.e. questions 9–14) will enable clinicians to assess changes in functional status over time (15).

Table 4. Phase III patient demographics

Country	N=170
Canada	35 (21%)
Greece	29 (17%)
The Netherlands	22 (13%)
China (Hong Kong)	20 (12%)
Germany	20 (12%)
Australia	16 (9%)
Argentina	14 (8%)
Spain	10 (6%)
United Kingdom	4 (2%)
Gender (n=170)	
Female	87 (51%)
Male	83 (49%)
Age (n=146) in years	
Median (range)	60 (29-92)
Primary Cancer Site (n=170)	
Breast	52 (31%)
Multiple Myeloma	33 (19%)
Lung	22 (13%)
Prostate	20 (12%)
Colorectal	19 (11%)
Renal Cell	8 (5%)
Others	16 (9%)

Bone metastases frequently affect more than one region of the bone. Successful localized treatment of one specific bony metastatic site may 'unmask' pain in other bone lesions. Therefore, questions that specify the exact location of pain (i.e. questions 1–5) can enable HCPs to differentiate pain affecting multiple metastatic sites and to accurately assess if treatment impacts locally or systemically. Although the prevalence ratio was lower for items 3 (14%), 4 (15%), 5 (15%) and 8 (23%), the mean scores of all pain-related items were >1.5. It is necessary to include both location of pain and functional interference to assist in accurately assessing changes over time. For these reasons, all pain items have been included in the final EORTC QLQ-BM22 QOL questionnaire (15).

The original questionnaire asked if there were problems in either sitting or lying down. This item was subsequently split into two questions at the request of patients in several countries. The question 'have you been thinking about your illness? was deleted after Phase III feedback suggested that the question is self-evident, upsetting and depressing. We compared the responses of patients with bone metastases from solid cancers to those in our study with multiple myeloma. There was no significant difference in mean score and prevalence ratio in the two groups. Therefore, the inclusion of patients with multiple myeloma in the validation of the EORTC QLQ-BM22 did not alter our results. The development process and the final questionnaire were reviewed and approved by the executive members of the EORTC QOL Module Development Committee (see appendix I) (15).

International validation of the BM22: Phase IV

The final phase of module development, international field testing, is currently underway to test the reliability, clinical, and psychometric validity of the EORTC QLQ-BM22 across languages and cultures. At present, collaborators from Germany, Greece, Hong Kong, the Netherlands, Spain, Argentina, Australia, the UK, and Canada are participating. All patients will prospectively complete the EORTC QLQ-BM22 (see appendixI) and EORTC QLQ C15-PAL. The EORTC QLQ-C15-PAL palliative core questionnaire is used in place of the EORTC QLQ-C30 since bone metastases patients are palliative and often demonstrate rapid deterioration and it can be too great of a burden for a patient to provide self-reported data for a QOL questionnaire. Using the EORTC QLQ-C15-PAL alongside the EORTC QLQ-BM22 reduces the total number of questionnaire items from 52 to 37, easing patient burden. Furthermore, this reduction allows for the potential to increase heterogeneity of our study population as it may allow an increased number of patients to complete study requirements.

The EORTC QLQ-C15-PAL was developed using the same metric scale and is compatible with the scores from the original scales of the QLQ C30-item questionnaire allowing for the maintenance of the original version and the already collected data from previous studies. By careful reduction of the number of EORTC QLQ-C30-items, the developers aimed at addressing the problems that make the EORTC QLQ-C30 unsuitable for use in palliative care settings: length and inappropriate or irrelevant content for patients receiving palliative care (38). The resulting 15-item EORTC QLQ-C15-PAL can be considered a 'core questionnaire' for palliative cancer patients. It can be supplemented by additional items, modules or questionnaires. The developers concluded that this new questionnaire "…has good content validity as a 'core palliative care questionnaire' assessing the symptoms and problems for which patients are frequently treated."

In Phase IV, patients are grouped into seven categories (groups A-G) according to their active treatment(s) and reason for visit to the cancer centre (Table 5). Patients undergoing active treatment complete the EORTC QLQ-BM22 and EORTC QLQ-C15-PAL prior to the given treatment (i.e. prior to radiotherapy, bisphosphonate treatment, or surgical intervention) and one month following bone metastases specific treatment. Patients in Group G complete the assessment during the clinic visit and one week after the initial interview to assess the test-retest reproducibility of the questionnaire since these patients have stable disease and are not receiving any new bone metastases-specific treatments.

Table 5. Phase IV patient groups

Group	Description
A	Patients receiving palliative radiotherapy or radiosurgery (RS)
B	Patients receiving a new bisphosphonate (e.g. pamidronate/clondronate/zoledronic acid) within the previous two weeks
C	Patients receiving a new systemic therapy (e.g. chemotherapy/hormone therapy) within the previous two weeks
D	Patients undergoing orthopaedic stabilization (impending or pathological fracture/spinal cord compression)
E	Patients undergoing minimally invasive procedures (e.g. vertebroplasty/cementoplasty/kyphoplasty)
F	Patients undergoing analgesic adjustments in pain and symptom management clinic
G	Patients with stable bone metastases not undergoing new treatment for at least two weeks (e.g. breast or prostate cancer patients with bone metastases)

* If the patient has received two of the above mentioned treatments for the first time within the previous two weeks, the patient will be classified based on which treatment was the most recent.

Upon completion of this final phase, we hope to accrue 350 patients, with approximately 50 patients in each of the seven patient groups. Progress will be reported at the EORTC Semi-Annual Meeting for feedback to ensure our methodology is consistent with the EORTC QLG standards for module development.

Discussion related to international literature

Advances in research and treatment published and presented from other institutions

In the palliative care setting, QOL as an outcome measure is increasingly being incorporated into trials (7). The following section outlines several trials for bony metastases that have examined QOL as an endpoint (7,39-43).

Gaze et al assessed QOL and emotional status in a randomized trial comparing two fractionation schedules (10 Gy in a single fraction versus 22.5 Gy in five fractions) in 280 patients (39). The physicians completed the Spitzer QOL index (44) according to the verbal description most closely reflecting the patient's status. The Spitzer index contains five items relating to activity, daily living, health, support and outlook, each rated from zero to two. Patients also completed a Hospital Anxiety and Depression (HAD) questionnaire to assess clinically significant levels of anxiety and depression (45). Assessments were completed at baseline, one-week, three to four weeks after completion of RT and then at two-month intervals. Of 216 patients assessed post-RT, the Spitzer QOL and HAD scores were available for 209 and 200, respectively (39). No significant differences were observed.

The study found no association between initial QOL parameters and the likelihood of achieving pain control (39). However, the prevalence of both anxiety and depression, was reduced following RT, from a median score of six before treatment to five. The prevalence of definite (HAD score = 11) and borderline (HAD score 7-10) anxiety was 49% and 39% for depression at baseline. After treatment, this was reduced to 35% and 32%, respectively. The

Spitzer Index improved from a median pre-treatment score of 6 (range, 0-10) to 7 (range, 0-10) post-RT. As QOL was assessed by non-blinded physicians in this study, the possibility of over-estimation of post-treatment Spitzer scores exist. Nevertheless, a trend in improvement of patient self-rated anxiety and depression was observed (39).

Nielsen et al examined global QOL using a visual analogue scale (VAS) in a trial of a single 8Gy versus 20Gy in 4 fractions (40). Two hundred and forty-one patients were enrolled in this trial. Patients completed a pain and global QOL evaluation on the first day of RT and at 4-, 8-, 12- and 20-weeks after the beginning of treatment. With the exception of the initial and final visits, two clinic visits could be replaced by written correspondence. The authors reported no difference in the relative change of QOL at any point between the two treatment arms. At 4- weeks, approximately 34%, 20% and 11% of patients in each arm achieved increases of >25%, >50%, and >75% respectively in their VAS QOL scores when compared to baseline. However, the proportion of patients achieving complete well-being was only 7% in each arm (40).

In the largest reported randomized trial for the palliation of bone metastases (N=1,157) conducted by Steenland et al, QOL was evaluated using the Rotterdam Symptom Checklist (41,46) and the EORTC QLQ-C30 questionnaires (10). Overall QOL was also measured using five EuroQOL questions on mobility, self-care, usual activities, pain/discomfort and anxiety/depression. The questionnaire (containing almost 60 questions) was filled out by the patients at baseline, then weekly for three months, and monthly for up to two years. No statistically significant differences in overall QOL were observed between the two fractionation schedules. Further details of the more specific domains of QOL, the assessment of the various QOL instruments and the impact of RT on QOL in this study are yet to be published (41).

A prospective cohort study by Fossa et al specifically examined QOL after palliative RT for men with hormone refractory prostate cancer (24, 42). In this trial, 31 patients were treated with the radioisotope 89Sr (Strontium) and 106 received external beam RT. Of the latter group, 24 patients with poor performance status were treated with single fraction hemi-body irradiation, and the remainder with fractionated treatments to localized fields. Only 19 of 31 men treated with strontium and 54/106 men receiving external beam RT completed a planned 3-month questionnaire. The 73 patients who completed the questionnaire reported slight pain relief, with mean scores decreasing from 51 to 44. Three-months after RT, however, 20/57 evaluable patients had reduced their analgesic intake. Global QOL was virtually unchanged, with a mean of 54 pre-treatment and 52 at 3-months.

More recently, Broom et al developed a 16-item Functional Assessment of Cancer Therapy-Bone Pain (FACT-BP) scale to assess cancer-related bone pain using a Likert-type scale of 0 (not at all) to 4 (very much) for each questionnaire item. A higher aggregate score is indicative of a higher QOL and lesser bone pain. The performance of the FACT-BP was evaluated using combined data from two prospective trials in which patients with metastatic breast cancer receiving clodronate or pamidronate with disease progression or with an SRE were switched to a third-generation bisphosponate (zoledronic acid or ibandronate). The FACT-BP, FACT-G (general), Brief Pain Inventory (BPI), and Karnofsky Performance Scale (KPS) were evaluated at baseline, weekly for four weeks and at weeks 8 and 12 (43).

The FACT-BP scale showed high internal consistency at each assessment (Cronbach's a's 0.93-0.96), and was closely correlated with the pain intensity scales of the BPI ($|r|$=0.69-0.73; $p<0.01$) but modestly related to KPS (r=0.32, $p<0.05$). Changes in PWB, FACT-G and

FACT-BP when compared to changes in the BPI (worst pain in past three days) were significant (p=0.002, 0.045, and <0.001, respectively). At week 8, patients rating themselves as worse on the BPI, as compared to baseline, had decreased PWB (subscale score), FACT-G and FACT-BP scores. Broom et al. found the 16-item FACT-BP to be a robust and consice tool for assessing cancer-related bone pain, and it is now ready for use in cross-sectional and longitidual studies on metastatic bone pain (43).

It is vitally important to document the impact of QOL of palliative interventions. Though external beam RT is a local treatment, previous clinical trials have shown it can improve QOL in patients with symptomatic bone metastases as well as provide pain relief (7).

Future research and directions

Easing patient burden

Timely and complete assessment of patients' subjective symptomatology in a palliative care setting is important to ensure good quality of care. However, patients with advanced disease may have low performance status as well as a limited life expectancy. There is a need to reduce responder burden when assessing QOL in these patients (38,47). In view of this, a preliminary analysis was conducted by our group to determine if the 22-item EORTC QLQ-BM22 (original version prior to the completion of Phase III) could be shortened to reduce patient burden and increase the duration by which patients are able to continue the QOL follow-up assessment in a routine clinical or clinical trial setting was conducted by our group. Differential item functioning (DIF) analyses with regard to different translations will be used. Several methods of analysis of DIF have been used (48-51), which include contingency tables, logistic regression and item response theory (IRT). IRT seeks to make scores from a shortened questionnaire compatible with the scores from the original questionnaire (47). IRT will be used to attempt to shorten the BM22.

Conclusion

In addition to investigating traditional endpoints (such as survival or local control), QOL is a valuable endpoint in clinical trials determining the worth of an intervention for bone metastases. Given the lack of a comprehensive QOL instrument specific to patients with bone metastases, our group initiated the development of a bone metastases module, the BM22, according to EORTC module development guidelines. At present, the BM22 is available for use through the EORTC website, and we are currently in the final phase of validation.

The BM22 is a consistent and valid module questionnaire, and the aim is for HCPs to use this tool to reliably follow patients' QOL. This will generate relevant information as to the patients state to guide treatment choice and eventually assess the cost effectiveness of various treatment options. Research into shortening the BM22 may be necessary to reduce patient burden in completing these lenghty tools, and allow for the assessment of QOL in a more heterogeneous population of bone metastases patients.

References

[1]   Harrington KD. Prophylactic management of impending fractures. In: Harrington KD, ed. Orthopedic management of metastatic bone disease. St Louis, MO: Mosby 1988;283-307.

[2]   Harrington KD. The management of acetabular insufficiency secondary to metastatic malignant disease. J Bone Joint Surg 1981;63:653-4.

[3]   Patrick DL, Ferketich SL, Frame PS, et al. National Institutes of Health State-of-the-Science Conference Statement: Symptom management in cancer: Pain, depression, and fatigue, July 15-17, 2002. J Natl Cancer Inst 2003;95(15):110-7.

[4]   Pain palliation of bone metastases. Overview. InSightec.com. 1 April 2005. InSightec Image Guided Treatment Ltd. Retrieved 1 October 2009. <http://www.insightec.com/135-en-r10/BoneMetastases.aspx>.

[5]   Palliative care" Who.com. 2009. The World Health Organization. Retrieved 29 May 2009. <http://www.who.int/cancer/palliative/en/>.

[6]   Soni MK, Cella D. Quality of life and symptom measures in oncology: an overview. Am J Manag Care 2002;8(18):S560-73.

[7]   Chow E, Hruby G, Davis L, et al. Quality of life after local external beam radiation therapy for symptomatic bone metastases: a prospective evaluation. Support Cancer Ther 2004;1(3):179-84.

[8]   Bruera E, Kuehn N, Miller MJ, et al. The Edmonton Symptom Assessment System (ESAS): a simple method for the assessment of palliative care patients. J Palliat Care 1991;7:6-9.

[9]   Chow E, Hoskin P, van der Linden, et al. Quality of life and symptom endpoints in palliative bone metastases trials. Clin Oncol 2006; 18:67-69.

[10]   Aaronson NK, Ahmedzai S, Bergman B, et al. The European Organization for Research and Treatment of Cancer QLQ-C30: a quality- of-life instrument for use in international clinical trials in oncology. J Natl Cancer Inst 1993;85:365-76.

[11]   "EORTC QLQ-C30". European Organisation for Research and Treatment of Cancer. Quality of life. Retrieved 25 April 2009.

[12]   < http://www.eortc.be/home/qol>

[13]   Chow E, Wu JS, Hoskin P, et al. International consensus on palliative radiotherapy endpoints for future clinical trials in bone metastases. Radiother Oncol 2002;64:275-80.

[14]   Blazeby J, Sprangers M, Cull A, et al. EORTC Quality of Life Group: guidelines for developing questionnaire modules. Third edition revised. http://groups.eortc.be/qol/downloads/200208module_development_guidelines.pdf. Cited 25 April 2009.

[15]   Chow E, Harris K, Tharmalingam S, et al. Early phase in the development of a bone metastases quality of life module. Clin Oncol (R Coll Radiol) 2007;19(3 Suppl):S26.

[16]   Chow E, Hird A, Velikova G, et al. The European Organisation for Research and Treatment of Cancer Quality of Life Questionnaire for patients with bone metastases: the EORTC QLQ-BM22. Eur J Cancer 2009 ;45(7):1146-52.

[17]   Ferrell B, Grant M, Padilla G, et al. The experience of pain and perceptions of quality of life: validation of a conceptual model. Hosp J 1991;7:9-24.

[18]   Miaskowski C, Dibble SL. The problem of pain in outpatients with breast cancer. Oncol Nurs Forum 1995;22:791-87.

[19]   Rummans TA, Frost M, Suman VJ, et al. Quality of life and pain in patients with recurrent breast and gynecological cancer. Psychosomatics 1998;39:437-45.

[20]   Strang P, Qvarner H. Cancer-related pain and its influence on quality of life. Anticancer Res 1990;10:109-12.

[21]   Sandblom G, Carlsson P, Sigsjo P, Varenhorst E. Pain and health-related quality of life in a geographically defined population of men with prostate cancer. Br J Cancer 2001;85:497-503.

[22]   Burrows M, Dibble SL, Miaskowski C. Differences in outcomes among patient experiencing different types of cancer-related pain. Oncol Nurs Forum 1998;25:4361-7.

[23]   Esnaola NF, Cantor SB, Johnson ML, et al. Pain and quality of life after treatment in patients with locally recurrent rectal cancer. J Clin Oncol 2002;20:4361-7.

[24]   Rustøen T, Moum T, Padilla G, et al. Predictors of quality of life in oncology outpatients with pain from bone metastasis. J Pain Symp Manage 2005;30(3):234-42.

[25]   Fossa SD, Aaronson NK, Newling D, et al. Quality of life and treatment of hormone resistant prostate cancer. The EORTC Genito-Urinary Group. Eur J Cancer Clin Oncol 1990;26:1133-6.

[26]   Higginson IJ. Can professionals improve their assessment? [commentary] J Pain Symptom Manag 1998;15:149-50.

[27]   Petersen MA, Larsen H, Pedersen L, et al. Assessing health-related quality of life in palliative care: comparing patient and physician assessments. Eur J Cancer 2006;42:1159-66.

[28]   Constantini M, Mencaglia E, Giulio PD, et al. Cancer patient as "experts" in defining quality of life domains. A multicentre survey by the Italian Group for the Evaluation of Outcomes in Oncology (IGEO). Qual Life Res 2000;9:151-9.

[29]   Taylor KM, Macdonald KG, Bezjak A, et al. Physician's perspective on quality of life: an exploratory study of oncologists. Qual Life Res 1996;5:5-14.

[30]   Bezak A, Ng P, Taylor KM, et al. A preliminary survey of oncologists' perceptions of quality of life information. Psychooncology 1997;6:107-13.

[31]   Movsas B. Quality of life in oncology trials: a clinical guide. Rad Oncol 2003;13(3):235-47.

[32]   Taylor KM, Feldstein ML, Skeel RT, et al. Fundamental dilemmas on the randomized clinical trial process. Results of the 1737 Eastern Cooperative Group Investigators. J Clin Oncol 1994;12:1796-1805.

[33]   Bradley NM, Husted J, Sey MS, et al. Review of patterns of practice and patient's preferences in the treatment of bone metastases with palliative radiotherapy. Support Care Cancer 2006;4:373-85.

[34]   Hortobagyl GN, Theriault RL, Porter L, et al. Efficacy of pamidronate in reducing skeletal complications in patients with breast cancer and lytic bone metastases. Protocol 19 Aredia Breast Cancer Study Group. New Engl J Med 1996;335:1785-91.

[35]   Tannock IF, Osoba D, Stockley MR, et al. Chemotherapy with mitoxantrone plus prednisone or prednisone alone for symptomatic hormone resistant prostate cancer: a Canadian randomized trial with palliative end points. J Clin Oncol 1996;14:1756-64.

[36]   Anonymous. Quality of life from a patient's perspective: can we believe the patient? Curr Probl Cancer 2005;29:326-31.

[37]   Detmar SB, Muller MJ, Schornagei JH, et al. Health-related quality-of-life assessments and patient-physician communication: a randomized controlled trial. JAMA 2002;288(23):3027-34.

[38]   Hirabayashi H, Ebara S, Kinoshita T, Yuzawa Y, Nakamura I, Takahashi J, et al. Clinical outcome and survival after palliative surgery for spinal metastases. Cancer 2003;97:476-84.

[39]   Groenvold M, Petersen MA, Aaronson N, et al. The development of the EORTC QLQ-C15-PAL: a shortened questionnaire for cancer patients in palliative care. Eur J Cancer 2006;42:55-64.

[40]   Gaze MN, Kelly CG, Kerr GR, et al. Pain relief and quality of life following radiotherapy for bone metastases: a randomised trial of two fractionation schedules. Radiother Oncol 1997;45:109-16.

[41]   Nielsen OS, Bentzen SM, Sandberg E, et al. Randomized trial of single dose versus fractionated palliative radiotherapy of bone metastases. Radiother Oncol 1998;47:233-40.

[42]   Steenland E, Leer JW, van Houwelingen H, et al. The effect of a single fraction compared to multiple fractions on painful bone metastases: a global analysis of the Dutch Bone Metastasis Study. Radiother Oncol 1999;52:101-9.

[43]   Fossa SD. Quality of life after palliative radiotherapy in patients with hormone-resistant prostate cancer: single institution experience. Br J Urol 1994;74:345-51.

[44]   Broom R, Hongyan D, Clemons M, Eton D, Dranitsaris G, Simmons C, Ooi W, Cella D. Switching breast cancer patients with progressive bone metastases to third-generation bishphosphonates: measuring impact using the functional assessment of cancer therapy-bone pain. J Pain Symptom Manag 2009, in press.

[45]   Spitzer WO, Dobson AJ, Hall J, et al. Measuring the quality of life of cancer patients: a concise QL-index for use by physicians. J Chronic Dis 1981;34:585-97.

[46]   Zigmond AS, Snaith RP. The hospital anxiety and depression scale. Acta Psychiat Scand 1983;67:361-70.

[47] de Haes JC, Olschewski M, Fayers P. Measuring the quality of life of cancer patients with the Rotterdam Symptom Checklist (RSCL): a manual. Groningen: North Centre Healthcare Res series 9, 1996.

[48] Petersen MA, Groenvold M, Aaronson N, Blazeby J, Brandberg Y, de Graeff A, et al. Item response theory was used to shorten EORTC QLQ-C30 scales for use in palliative care. J Clin Epidemiol 2006; 59(1):36-44.

[49] Holland PW, Wainer H. Differential Item Functioning. Hilsdale, NJ: Lawrence Erlbaum, 1993.

[50] French AW, Miller TR. Logistic regression and its use in detecting differential item functioning in polytomous items. J Educ Meas 1996; 33: 315-32.

[51] Swaminathan H, Rogers HJ. Detecting differential item functioning using logistic-regrssion procedures. J Educ Meas 1990;27:361-70.

[52] Teresi JA, Kleinman M, Ocepek-Welikson K. Modern psychometric methods for detection of differential item functioning: Application to cognitive assessment measures. Stat Med 2000;19: 1651-83.

Appendix I

BM22 after the phase III (Subject to modification after phase IV)

Patients sometimes report that they have the following symptoms or problems. Please indicate the extent to which you have experienced these symptoms or problems during the **past week**. Please answer by circling the number that best applies to you.

During the *past week* have you had *pain* in any of the following parts of your body?	Not at All	A Little	Quite a Bit	Very Much
in your back?	1	2	3	4
in your leg(s) or hip(s)?	1	2	3	4
in your arm(s) or shoulder(s)?	1	2	3	4
in your chest or rib(s)?	1	2	3	4
in your buttock(s)?	1	2	3	4
During the *past week*:				
Have you had constant pain?	1	2	3	4
Have you had intermittent pain?	1	2	3	4
Have you had pain not relieved by pain medications?	1	2	3	4
Have you had pain while lying down?	1	2	3	4
Have you had pain while sitting?	1	2	3	4
Have you had pain when trying to stand up?	1	2	3	4
Have you had pain while walking?	1	2	3	4
Have you had pain with activities such as bending or climbing stairs?	1	2	3	4
Have you had pain with strenuous activity (e.g. exercise, lifting)?	1	2	3	4
Has pain interfered with your sleeping at night?	1	2	3	4
Have you had to modify your daily activities because of your illness?	1	2	3	4
Have you felt isolated from those close to you (e.g. family, friends)?	1	2	3	4
Have you worried about loss of mobility because of your illness?	1	2	3	4
Have you worried about becoming dependent on others because of your illness?	1	2	3	4
Have you worried about your health in the future?	1	2	3	4
Have you felt hopeful your pain will get better?	1	2	3	4
Have you felt positive about your health?	1	2	3	4

In: Advanced Cancer
Editors: N. Thavarajah, N. Pulenzas, B. Lechner et al.

ISBN: 978-1-62808-239-5
© 2013 Nova Science Publishers, Inc.

Chapter 38

Positron Emission Tomography and bone metastases

*Gillian Bedard, BSc(C), Liang Zeng, MD(C), Henry Lam, MLS,
Natalie Lauzon, MRT(T), Katharine Hicks, BSc(C)
and Edward Chow, MBBS*[*]*

Rapid Response Radiotherapy Program, Department of Radiation Oncology,
Odette Cancer Centre, Sunnybrook Health Sciences Centre, University of Toronto,
Toronto, Ontario, Canada

Positron Emission Tomography (PET) is increasingly being used to diagnose bone metastases. In this chapter we review the literature to determine the accuracy, specificity, and sensitivity of PET scans used in this diagnosis. A literature search was conducted in the Medline database (1946 to February week 5 2012). Articles describing the sensitivity, specificity, accuracy and usage of PET scans in the diagnosis of bone metastases were included in this review. Studies discussing primary cancers in terms of bone metastases other than lung, breast, prostate and thyroid were excluded, along with studies not describing the pharmacokinetics of radioactive tracers. A total of forty-four publications were identified. Primary cancers of the breast, prostate, thyroid, and lung were studied in relation to PET scan results for each type of osseous lesion. Different tracers for PET scan were also explored, along with the determination of which tracer would be best for each primary cancer. Choline tracers worked best for sclerotic metastases, while tracers that focused on glucose metabolism visualized lytic metastases. Mixed metastases may be best imaged with a mix of 18F-flouride and fluorodeoxyglucose. All studies, but one, have demonstrated that PET scan is superior to bone scan, with the usage of fluorodeoxyglucose (FDG), which is currently the main radioactive tracer used. FDG detects osteolytic lesions with great accuracy, but is unsuccessful in detecting osteoblastic lesions. Tracers such as 68Ga-bisphosphonates are superior to FDG for diagnosis of osteoblastic lesions.

[*] Correspondence: Professor Edward Chow MBBS, MSc, PhD, FRCPC, Department of Radiation Oncology, Odette Cancer Centre, Sunnybrook Health Sciences Centre, 2075 Bayview Avenue, Toronto, ON, Canada M4N 3M5. E-mail: Edward.Chow@sunnybrook.ca.

Introduction

Metastases to the bone are a common complication of cancer, occurring in about 70% of the advanced cancer population (1). Many of these patients are asymptomatic, and often times when symptoms do arise, there is significant disease progression (2). There are three types of bone metastases; osteolytic lesions, sclerotic or osteoblastic lesions, and mixed lesions that include both lytic and sclerotic components. When metastasizing to bone, cancer cells release cytokines and growth factors that lead to lysis or sclerosis. Some cells secrete factors that stimulate osteoclasts such as parathyroid hormone-related protein, tumor factor alpha or beta, and interleukin-1 and -6 (3). The osteoclasts then work to break down the bone, causing a destructive or lytic lesion. Other cells secrete factors that stimulate osteoblast activity, such as epidermal factor, transforming growth factor alpha and beta, and insulin-like growth factor. Osteoblasts then work to form new bone, developing a sclerotic lesion that is characterized by abnormal increased bone growth (3). The occurrence of one type of lesion over the other is often influenced by the primary cancer that spreads to the bone.

Bone metastases are the cause of skeletal related events such as pathological fracture, bone pain, need for surgery of bone, radiotherapy required for pain relief, and hypercalcemia. The burden of skeletal related events, and bone pain in particular results in a decrease in patient quality of life. In order to treat these symptoms of bone metastases, they must first be diagnosed.

For many years bone scan has been the primary radiographic technique used to determine the presence of bone metastases in cancer patients. Recently, there have been many studies to validate the usage of PET and PET/CT in the diagnosis of bone metastases. Bone scans have proven effective in detecting metastases from prostate and breast cancer, both of which display sclerotic type lesions. The major disadvantage of bone scan however is its insensitivity in detecting lytic metastases from primary cancers such as renal cell, thyroid, lung, and multiple myeloma (4). Due to their higher sensitivity in detecting lytic metastases PET scans are being more commonly used in the cancer setting (5).

PET or Positron Emission Tomography is a nuclear imaging technique which produces images via emission of high-energy photons that are able to capture the high-resolution image during positron decay of radioisotopes (1). This type of scan is very sensitive to malignancies; however it has poor spatial resolution which limits the anatomical localization of the disease. The addition of Computed Tomography (CT) to the PET scan is able to overcome this problem, and thus PET/CT is being more commonly used in the diagnosis of bone metastases (6).

The purpose of this review was to determine the degree of success of the PET scan in diagnosing lytic, sclerotic and mixed metastases. Successfulness of the PET or PET/CT was determined by the sensitivity, specificity, and accuracy of the scan. Different types of radioactive tracers were also identified, and the pharmacokinetics of each tracer, along with which type of lesion they have the largest uptake in is also discussed.

Literature review

A literature review was conducted using the OvidSP platform on the Medline (1946 to February week 5 2012) database. Subject headings and keywords "PET" or "Positron Emission Tomography" were coupled with "cancer", "neoplasms:, "bone metastases", "bone neoplasms/sc", and "radioactive tracers" to elicit relevant literature.

Articles that pertained to studies in which the specificity, accuracy, and sensitivity of PET scans were determined in relation to the detection and diagnosis of bone metastases in cancer patients were included in this review. Those that discussed the primary cancers of lung, breast, prostate, and thyroid were included and articles that pertained primarily to any other primary cancers were excluded as these cancers are less common to metastasize to bone. Articles that discussed the pharmacokinetics of radioactive tracers used in PET scans for cancer patients were also included in this review.

Findings

Forty-four papers that discussed primary breast, lung, prostate, and thyroid cancer in relevance to the diagnosis of bone metastases on a PET or PET/CT scan met the eligibility criteria and were included in this review. These articles ranged in publication date from 1991 – 2011. Eight papers discussed lung cancer alone, 10 discussed prostate cancer, 8 discussed breast, 2 discussed thyroid, 11 pertained to many different cancers, and 5 discussed different radioactive tracers.

Breast

Breast cancer, when metastasizing to bone, most often causes a combination of osteolytic and osteosclerotic lesions (7-9) (see figure 1). Langsteger et al. determined the rate of metastases in their patient population to be mostly lytic, but 15-20% sclerotic (10). The majority of studies that determined the presence of bone metastases utilized fluorodeoxyglucose as the radioactive tracer in PET scan alone (8) or PET combined with CT (5,9).

Yang et al. utilized FDG for the diagnosis of bone metastases in 40 breast cancer patients. This study compared PET scan with bone scan, and determined the sensitivity of PET to be 95.2%, and the accuracy to be 94.5% with 5 of 127 lesions being false positive. The sensitivity and accuracy of PET was greater than that of the bone scan, and the bone scan had more false positive results. A separate study by Abe et al. determined the sensitivity of PET scan to be 100% with the use of FDG, however other studies with the use of PET/CT determine sensitivity to be lower, only 96% (5,7). It is currently believed that the use of CT leads to higher detection rate of metastases (5). Further study with FDG PET concludes a much lower sensitivity rate of only 83.3% per patient (11).

Article	Number of subjects	Primary Cancer	Type of Lesion	Type of Scan	Specificity	Sensitivity	Accuracy	PPV	PPN	False positive	False negative	Tracer
Comparing whole body 18F-2-deoxyglucose positron emission tomography and technetium-99m methylene diphosphonate bone scan to detect bone metastases in patients with breast cancer (8)	40	Breast	Mixed (sclerotic and lytic)	FDG PET	N/A	95.2%	94.5%	N/A	N/A	5/127 lesions	N/A	18F-2 deoxyglucose
Comparison of FDG-PET with 99mTc-HMDP scintigraphy for the detection of bone metastasis in patients with breast cancer (7)	44	Breast	Mixed (sclerotic and lytic) "Many bone metastasis from breast cancer form osteoblastic laesions"	FDG PET	N/A	100%	N/A	N/A	N/A	N/A	N/A	18F-2 deoxyglucose
18F-fluoride PET/CT for assessing bone involvement in prostate and breast cancers (12)	34	Breast or Prostate	N/A	PET/CT	Breast: 79.3 Prostate: 94.7 Overall: 84.2	Breast: 73.9 Prostate: 100 Overall: 76%	Breast: 0.76 Prostate: 0.96 Overall: 80%	Breast: 86.1 Prostate: 85.7	Breast: 63.7 Prostate: 100	1/33	4/33	18F-fluoride
Comparison of FDG-PET/CT and bone scintigraphy for detection of bone metastases in breast cancer (5)	29	Breast	Majority was mixed metastases (69%)	FDG PET/CT	92	96	N/A	N/A	N/A	N/A	N/A	FDG
A meta-analysis of 18FDG-PET, MRI and bone scintigraphy for diagnosis of bone metastases in patients with breast cancer (11)	N/A	Breast	N/A	N/A	94.5 per patients 99.6 per lesion	83.3 per patient 52.7 per lesion	N/A	N/A	N/A	N/A	N/A	N/A

Figure 1. PET scan for the diagnosis of bone metastases in breast cancer patients.

18F-fluoride is another tracer commonly used to diagnose bone metastases. Withofs et al. determined the accuracy, specificity and sensitivity of PET/CT to be 76%, 79.3% and 73.9% respectively. In this study, the positive predictive value was 86.1 and the negative predictive value was 63.7 (12). The authors concluded that fluoride displays much lower sensitivity, specificity and accuracy than when using FDG as the radioactive tracer.

Langsteger et al. concluded that FDG has an advantage over 18F-fluoride which could potentially be due to the fact that FDG is sensitive to altered tumor glucose metabolism, while 18F – fluoride is associated with the coating of fluoroapatite on the bone which is detected by the PET scan (10). The majority of lytic and mixed-pattern lesions show increased uptake with FDG, but few sclerotic lesions do, as these lesions do not have an increased rate of glycolysis (9).

Conclusions were unanimous throughout the mentioned studies that PET scans are superior to bone scans in detecting bone metastases, however the higher sensitivity of PET scan on a per lesion basis may have little impact on overall patient staging as most patients have multiple bone metastases (5). Although PET scan appears to be superior to the bone scan, there is a decreased accuracy and specificity in which they are able to detect sclerotic lesions. The CT component of these scans, however, is able to increase the detection rate (5).

Prostate

When metastasizing to bone, prostate cancer causes sclerotic lesions, which are characterized by abnormal bone growth. Tiwari et al. included 16 prostate cancer patients to assess the role of FDG use with PET in diagnosing bone metastases. Patients were required to fast for at least six hours prior to intravenous administration of FDG, and imaging occurred 60 minutes post administration. The results of this study concluded that FDG is readily able to detect soft tissue involvement, but there was low sensitivity in detection of sclerotic metastases (see figure 2). Recommendations of this study were to potentially combine 18F –fluoride with FDG in order to accurately image both types of metastases (13). Another study utilizing FDG as the tracer also concluded that when used for prostate cancer, many false negatives appear as FDG has poor performance in detecting sclerotic metastases. This is possibly due to the smaller tumor volume relative to the size of the metastasis, thus it may be less likely to view the lesion on the scan (14).

Evan-Sapir et al. determined the usage of 18F-fluoride for bone metastases detection with PET and PET/CT in prostate patients. 18F-fluoride is believed to clearly demonstrate the involvement of osteosclerotic activity (15). In this study, for PET scan alone, the sensitivity was 62%, specificity 100%, and positive predictive value 74%. When combined with CT, all previous values increased to 100% (16).

Choline is a component of radioactive tracers such as 18F –fluorocholine (FCH), and 11C-choline, commonly used to diagnose bone metastases in prostate cancer patients (15,17-19). Choline has been determined to be more sensitive and specific than FDG, as choline uptake appears to be a marker of cell proliferation in prostate cancer cells, where as FDG relies on glucose metabolism (15,19). Behesti et al. determined the accuracy of PET/CT with FCH to be 84%, sensitivity to be 97% and specificity to be 79% (17). This group completed a similar study and confirmed these finding with values of 99%, 74%, and 85% for sensitivity, specificity and accuracy respectively (20). Although choline appears to be an improvement over FDG, Beheshti et al. discovered that in their study of 70 prostate patients, those who had a Hounsfield unit (unit of density) greater than 825 had an absence of FCH uptake. Most of these patients were currently undergoing hormone therapy. It may be possible that because of the hormone therapy, these lesions may no longer take up choline (17). Fuccio et al. also concluded that follow-up of bone metastases may not be possible with this tracer due to the low uptake while on hormone therapy (18).

Article	Number of subjects	Primary Cancer	Type of Lesion	Type of Scan	Specificity	Sensitivity	Accuracy	PPV	PPN	Tracer
Detection of bone metastases in patients with prostate cancer by 18F fluorocholine and 18F fluoride PET–CT: a comparative study (20)	38	Prostate	Sclerotic	PET/CT	18F : 93 FCH 99	18F: 81 FCH: 74	18F: 86 FCH: 85	N/A	N/A	18F-fluro-choline and 18F fluoride
Diagnosis of Bone Metastases in Urological Malignancies— An Update(3)	N/A	Prostate	Sclerotic	PET	96-100%	62-100%	N/A	N/A	N/A	N/A
The Detection of Bone Metastases in Patients with High-Risk Prostate Cancer: 99mTc-MDP Planar Bone Scintigraphy, Single- and Multi-Field-of-View SPECT, 18F-Fluoride PET, and 18F-Fluoride PET/CT(16)	44	Prostate		PET/CT	PET: 62 PET/CT 100	PET: 100 PET/CT 100	N/A	PET:74 PET/CT 100	PET:100 PET/CT 100	18F-fluoride
The Use of F-18 Choline PET in the Assessment of Bone Metastases in Prostate Cancer: Correlation with Morphological Changes on CT(17)	70	Prostate	Sclerotic	PET	79	97	84	N/A	N/A	F-18 choline

Figure 2. PET scan for the diagnosis of bone metastasis in prostate cancer patients.

Acetate is another type of radioactive tracer that has been proven to be more accurate in the detection of bone metastases in prostate patients. Acetate, like choline is involved in imaging lipid metabolism. It is now thought that lipid metabolism may be a more accurate process to target when scanning a patient with primary prostate cancer. Yu et al. confirmed this hypothesis when they compared FDG and C11 – acetate in the detection of bone metastasis in 8 prostate cancer patients. In this study, 83% of lesions were detected with acetate, while only 75% were detected with FDG (21).

Lung cancer

Unlike breast and prostate cancer, primary lung cancer results in lytic bone metastases (22-25). Because these lesions are lytic or destructive in nature, different radioactive tracers will be of more use than the ones previously described for prostate cancer (see figure 3). Takenaka et al. displaced good results for PET/CT in a group of non-small cell lung cancer patients. This study, comprised of 115 patients, resulted in a specificity of 95.4%, sensitivity of 97%, and accuracy of 95.5% on a per lesion basis using FDG as the tracer (26). Song et al. displayed similar results in their study of 1000 non-small cell lung cancer patients, again utilizing FDG as the radioactive tracer. Values obtained for specificity, sensitivity and accuracy were 98.8%, 94.3%, and 90% respectively (6). Other studies by Bury et al., Cheran et al., Liu et al. and Min et al. displayed very similar values with the usage of FDG and PET/CT (22,23,25,27,28).

    Kruger et al. compared 18F-fluoride PET with 18F—FDG PET/CT, in a study of 126 non-small cell lung cancer patients. In the data obtained, FDG PET/CT detected 14 true-positive lesions, 50 true-negative lesions and 4 false-negative lesions, while 18F PET detected 17 true-positive lesions, 50 true-negative lesions and 1 false-negative lesion. FDG PET/CT missed 4 lesions that were detected on 18F PET, thus it was concluded that 18F-fluoride may be superior to FDG for the detection of lytic lung metastases (24).

Thyroid cancer

Differentiated thyroid cancer (DTC) often causes mixed osseous lesions (29) (see figure 4). Ito et al. studied 47 DTC patients using PET and found a sensitivity rate of 84.7% and an accuracy rate of 97.8%. They concluded that PET scanning with the utilization of FDG was limited in detection of osseous lesions (30). Due to this limitation, Phan et al. concluded in their study of 24 DTC patients that FDG PET cannot replace the bone scan in this population of cancer patients. This conclusion was drawn after the data obtained showed that 38% of bone metastases were missed on the PET scan and were identified on the bone scan, with most of these osseous metastases being osteosclerotic in nature (29).

Radioactive tracers and pharmacokinetics

Radionucleotides are often organic compounds that can be labeled by substituting radioactive elements without disturbing the body's biological pathways (31) (see figure 5). In cancer patients, areas of increased metabolism are targeted since cancerous cells are known for their abnormal cell growth. Cellular processes such as glycolysis, angiogenesis, apoptosis and hypoxia are often the main targets for radioactive tracers as these are the processes that malfunction or are increased within a cancerous cell (32).

Article	Number of subjects	Primary Cancer	Type of Lesion	Type of Scan	Specificity	Sensitivity	Accuracy	PPV	NPV	False positive	False negative	Tracer
Detection of Bone Metastases in Non-Small Cell Lung Cancer Patients: Comparison of Whole-Body Diffusion-Weighted Imaging (DWI), Whole-Body MR Imaging Without and With DWI, Whole-Body FDGPET/CT, and Bone Scintigraphy (26)	115	NSCLC	N/A	PET/CT	95.4 Pt based: 85.6	97% Pt. based: 96.0	95.5 Pt. based: 87.8	59.6 Pt. based 64.9	99.8 Pt. based 98.7	N/A	N/A	FDG
Efficacy comparison between 18F-FDG PET/CT and bone scintigraphy in detecting bony metastases of non-small-cell lung cancer (6)	1000	NSCLC	N/A	PET/CT	98.8	94.3	98.3	90	99.3	1.2	5.7	FDG
The Role of Whole-Body FDG PET/CT, Tc 99m MDP Bone Scintigraphy, and Serum Alkaline Phosphatase in Detecting Bone Metastasis in Patients with Newly Diagnosed Lung Cancer (27)	30	Lung	N/A	Pet/CT	94.1	93.3	93.4	75.5	95.6	9	0	N/A
Bone metastasis in patients with non-small cell lung cancer: The diagnostic role of F-18 FDG PET/CT(22)	362	NSCLC	Lytic	PET/CT	98.9%	93.9%	97.8%	N/A	N/A	N/A	N/A	18F-2 deoxyglucose FDG
Comparison of FDG-PET/CT and bone scintigraphy for detection metastases in patients with a new diagnosis of lung cancer(23)	257	NSCLC	Lytic	PET	96%	91%	94%	85%	97%	9/257 pts	5/257 pts	2-deoxy-2-[18F]fluoro-d-glucose FDG

Figure 3. (Continued)

Article	Number of subjects	Primary Cancer	Type of Lesion	Type of Scan	Specificity	Sensitivity	Accuracy	PPV	NPV	False positive	False negative	Tracer
Detection of bone metastases in patients with lung cancer: 99mTc-MDP planar bone scintigraphy, 18F-fluoride PET or 18F-FDG PET/CT(24)	126	NSCLC	Lytic	PET/CT PET	PET/CT more specific then PET alone	N/A	N/A	N/A	N/A	0%	FDG PET/CT missed 4 lesions that 18F PET found – potential that 18F is superior to FDG for detection of mets from NSCLC PET/CT: 17.7 % PET: 0%	18F-2 deoxyglucose 18F-fluoride
Fluorine-18 deoxyglucose positron emission tomography for the detection of bone metastases in patients with non-small cell lung cancer(25)	110	NSCLC	Lytic	N/A	98%	90%	96%	90%	98%	N/A	2	2-deoxy-2-[18F]fluoro-d-glucose FDG

Figure 3. PET scan for lung cancer metastasis diagnosis statistics.

Article	Number of subjects	Primary Cancer	Type of Lesion	Type of Scan	Specificity	Sensitivity	Accuracy	PPV	PPN	Tracer
Comparison of 18F-FDG-PET/CT with 99mTc-MDP bone scintigraphy for the detection of bone metastases in cancer patients(4)	70	Breast, unknown, lung, naropharynx, non-hodgkin lymphoma, rectum, prostate, thyroid, pancrease, bladder, gastric, kidney, liver, larynx, malignant mesenchymal tumor	Breast and lung: sclerotic	PET/CT	N/A	97.1	N/A	N/A	N/A	F-FDG
Screening for bone metastases: whole-body MRI using a 32-channel system versus dual-modality PET-CT(33)	30	Breast, GI, melanoma, hepatocellular, non-Hodgkin lymphoma, rhabdomyosarcoma	N/A	PET/CT	100	91	78	94	47	N/A
One-stop-shop staging should we prefer FDG-PETCT or MRI for the detection of bone metastases (28)	109	NSCLC, melanoma	N/A	PET/CT	99	45	94	89	94	N/A

Figure 4. PET scan for the diagnosis of bone metastases in various cancers.

Article	Tracer	Mechanism	Comments
Beyond 18F-fluorodeoxyglucose: making the next generation of PET radiotracers available for oncology research in the UK (40)	FDG	Tumor has high glycolytic rate and glucose metabolism is regulated by many pathways, changed in FDG uptake can be biomarker for many process	First used to study CNS disorders New tracers: cell proliferation: 18F-fluorothymidine (FLT), apoptosis: 18F-ML-10, angiogenesis (18F-GE135, hypoxia (18F-fluromisonidazole, 64Cu-diactely-bis(N4-methylthiosemicarbazone) and 18F-HX4
Molecular Mechanisms of Bone 18F-NaF Deposition (34)	18F-NaF	Uptake in blood flow and most is retained in bone after first pass metabolism Diffusable across membranes, Cleared from plasma and excreted in kidneys 18F ions pass from plama through ECF Absortion onto hydroxyapatite, 18F exchanges with OH on hydroxyapatite matrix to form fluoroapatite Uptake depends on area of bone surface with is larger in bone disorders Relationship between osteoblasts and clasts determines incorporation of 18F-NaF into bone matrix	Initial high uptake in lytic lesions Low uptake in mixed lesions Good uptake in blastic lesions
Non FDG PET(32)	11C-choline 18F-choline (prostae) 1C-methionine (brain) 118F-DOPA (18F-deoxiphenilalanine) 68Ga-DOTANOC (neuroendocrine), 11C-acetate (prostate) 18F-FLT	11C-choline – prostate, integrated into cell membrane as phophatidilcholine, high affinitiy in malignant prostate cells 18F-choline - longer half life for prostate patients, also used for hepatocellular carcinoma 11C-methionine – amino acid that does not accumulate in normal brain 18F-DOPA – amino acid precursor to dopamine 11C-acetate – liver 18F-FLT -thymidine, follows salvage pathway of DNA synthesis, but not incorporated into DNA , uptake is correlated with cell proliferation , may show uptake in liver that is not malignant 18F-fluoride – good for blastic bone mets, more sensitive than choline	Hypoxia - 18F-misonidazole, 64Cu-ATSM, 18F- EF5 Angiogenesis - 64Cu-DOTA or 18F galacto Apoptosis – cells express phosphatidylserine on cell membrane,annexin – V is a protein with high calcium dependant affinity for phosphatidylserine on cell membrane annexin-V can be labeled with radionuclide and used in apoptosis imaging
PET/CT imaging of osteoblastic bone metastases with 68Ga-bisphosphonates: first human study (39)	68Ga-bisphonates	Bisphosphonates work well for BS and SPECT and now good for PET Taken up by osteoclasts that have famesyl diphosphate synthase enzyme in HMG-CoA reductase pathway	N/A
S-11C-Methyl-L-Cysteine: A New Amino Acid PET Tracer for Cancer Imaging (37)	S-11C-methyl-L-cysteine	Good for amino acid PET tracer Good for solid tumors	Tumor uptake reflects increased active transport and protein synthesis Amino acids taken up by sodium-independent L-type amino acid transporter system and sodium-dependent transporter system 11C-MCYS non-protein-composition amino acid tracer, not incorporated into proteins

Figure 5. PET scan radioactive tracer characteristics.

Fluorodeoxyglucose (FDG)

First used to study central nervous system disorders, FDG relies upon the high glycolytic rate of tumors and glucose metabolism. FDG enters cells via the GLUT 1 and GLUT 5 transporters where it is then converted to FDG-6-phosphate by hexokinase and is trapped within the tumor. FDG then accumulates inside the cell in proportion to the rate of glycolysis and glucose uptake. Due to the high rate of glycolysis in cancerous cells, this is a tracer that is widely used to detect bone, visceral and lymph node lesions. FDG is able to detect the soft tissue component of metastases along with the bone component. Lytic lesions in particular have a high glycolytic rate, while sclerotic metastases do not as they are acellular (31).

Hypoxia in cells may also prove to be a reason for increased FDG uptake due to the fact that these cells will rely solely on glycolysis as opposed to the Krebs cycle, to create ATP, thus utilizing no oxygen (14). In addition, cells utilizing glycolysis as their only energy source often have increased uptake of glucose.

With this tracer, patients are often asked to fast for at least 6 hours prior to the examination to ensure that blood glucose levels are below 150mg/dL. Buscopan is sometimes applied intravenously along with FDG to avoid first-pass uptake of FDG into smooth muscle. Additionally, 20mg of furosemide may be given to increase renal excretion of the tracer and avoid accumulation in non-malignant cells. At least an hour after the injection of FDG, the scan takes place (33).

18F- fluoride

18F-Fluoride is able to diffuse through capillary and bone with extracelluar fluid promoting the exchange of fluoride ions with hydroxyapatite crystals. This exchange forms fluoroapatite which is stored at the surface of bone after remodeling and turnover. First pass extraction is almost 100% and the clearance from plasma to the bone is three times higher in metastatic lesions than in benign tissue. This tracer has a high level of accumulation in sclerotic lesions, however lytic lesions have poor uptake as they have no blastic reaction. Often, 18F is overly sensitive to degenerative changes, which can cause false positives to appear on PET scans (10).

18F-NaF

18F-NaF is a tracer very similar to 18F-fluoride in that it is retained in the bone after first pass metabolism. This tracer is diffusible across membranes, and the ions pass from blood plasma through the extracelluar fluid where they are exchanged with the hydroxide ions on the hydroxyapatite matrix to form fluoroapatite. Uptake depends on the area of the bone surface and the relationship between osteoblasts and osteoclasts to determine the incorporation of 18F-NaF into the bone matrix (34). Uptake of 18F-NaF is initially high in lytic lesions and good in sclerotic lesions. For mixed lesions, uptake is low (34). This tracer is effective at detecting early sclerotic changes and in turn is better for slow growing tumor detection (35).

Choline tracers

There are various types of choline tracers such as 11C-choline and 18F-choline. Choline is a natural element present in the cell membrane. It is transported into cells, phosphorylated and trapped in the membrane to be used for synthesis of phospholipids. These tracers are integrated in the cell membrane as phosphatidylcholine, and often there is a high affinity for this in malignant prostate cancer cells. Due to the increased cell proliferation in tumors and up regulation of choline kinase in cancer cells, choline is more readily taken up by these cells than by normal cells (20). 18F-choline has a longer half-life than 11C-choline and can detect both bone and lymph node metastases, thus it is more readily used in PET scans (32,36).

Acetate tracers

Similar to the choline tracers, C-11 acetate is a tracer that is involved in the lipid metabolism pathway. Acetate uptake is completed by fatty acid synthase, where it is then distributed into biosynthetic pathways for phospholipid membrane synthesis. Fatty acid synthase expression occurs early in metabolism and it may result in an increase of acetate. This increase will become a marker for tumor activity and lipid metabolism, and thus for increased cell proliferation (21). This tracer is also good for imaging of hepatic cancer cells (32).

Amino acid tracers

Amino acid tracers are often used to image metastases or cancer of the brain, and currently their usage in the bone metastases population is unclear. 11C-methionine is one of these tracers, along with S-11C-methyl-L-cysteine (32). S-11C when taken up in tumors is reflective of the increased transport and protein synthesis in those tumors. Amino acid tracers are taken up by sodium-independent L-type amino acid transport systems and sodium-dependent transporter systems. S-11C is a non-protein-composition amino acid tracer that is not incorporated into proteins, but is still effective in imaging this pathway (37). Patients who are imaged with this tracer are instructed to fast for at least six hours prior to examination.

18F-DOPA is an amino acid precursor to dopamine that is often seen as uptake in abnormal brain cells. 18F-FLT is another tracer that contains thymidine. It follows the salvage pathway of DNA synthesis, but is not incorporated into DNA. Uptake of this tracer is correlated with cell proliferation, however the disadvantage of this tracer is that it may show uptake in the liver cells that are not malignant.

Bisphosphonates

Often used to manage bone symptoms, whether metastases or osteoporosis, bisphosphonates bind to hydroxyapatite crystals and inhibit their formation and dissolution in order to correct hypercalcaemia, hypercalciuria, reduce pain and limit fracture risk (38).

Bisphosphonates have been proven to work effectively for bone scan and SPECT, and through a study by Fellner et al. have now been validated for use in PET scans. DOTA-based bisphosphonate has been labeled using the 68Ge/Ga generator-derived positron emitter, and the result is a tracer that works effectively in PET scans. This tracer is taken up by osteoclasts that have the famesyl diphosphate synthase enzyme in the HMG-CoA reductase pathway (39). The tracer appears to be superior at imaging sclerotic lesions and may be the ideal tracer for planning and monitoring bisphosphonate therapy for bone metastases, multiple myeloma, and osteoporosis.

Discussion

In patients with advanced cancer, imaging modalities that are able to detect osseous changes at a relatively early stage are crucial. It is important to know if there are metastases and where these metastases are. Physicians require these scans in order to effectively plan treatment for their patients. Depending on the extent and location of metastases, physicians have different treatment options that can be offered to the patient such as radiation therapy, chemotherapy, surgery, or simply palliative care.

Positron Emission Tomography is progressively becoming the standard imaging modality for cancer patients with suspected bone metastases. The incorporation of computed tomography with PET leads to increased sensitivity, accuracy and specificity of the scan. PET alone is able to image the body in regards to tracer uptake however it is limited in anatomical localization. The addition of CT allows for this localization and a more accurate image of the bone metastases is produced. In almost every study reviewed here, PET/CT has been the modality in which the highest rates of accuracy and specificity have been obtained. A single study in thyroid cancer patients concluded that PET could not replace the bone scan in that population. This study used FDG as the radioactive tracer, which may be the reason behind why the scan showed such little uptake in the mixed lesions of thyroid cancer (29).

Each primary cancer has its own type of osseous lesion. Metastatic bone lesions are classified as lytic, sclerotic or mixed. It can be concluded from the literature that breast cancer metastasizes to bone in a mixed lesion fashion along with thyroid cancer. Prostate cancer has a high occurrence of sclerotic lesions, while lung cancer produces lytic lesions. Each of these lesion types can be imaged using PET/CT, but the use of one radioactive tracer over another plays a large part in the sensitivity, specificity, accuracy and false-positive/negative outcomes of the scan.

Tracers that focus on the glycolytic rate of cell growth have been proven to be effective in imaging lytic osseous lesions, since lytic lesions are characterized as having increased glycolytic rates. Fluorodeoxyglucose is a tracer in which uptake directly reflects glycolytic rates, as it accumulates within the cell and can be easily viewed on a PET/CT. In turn, FDG has been proven to be effective in the imaging of lung cancer bone metastases, as these metastases are lytic in nature (2,6,11,22,23,25-27). FDG is also sometimes effective in the imaging of breast cancer metastases as this cancer produces mixed lesions, some of which are lytic (8).

Prostate cancer produces sclerotic bone metastases, of which FDG shows poor uptake. Numerous studies have demonstrated that FDG has poor uptake in sclerotic lesions, but high uptake in lytic lesions, thus different radioactive tracers have been found to better image prostate metastases. Tracers that are comprised of choline such as 18F-fluorocholine and 11C-choline have been proven to be more sensitive and specific than FDG in this part of the cancer population (19). These tracers work best with sclerotic lesions due to the fact that this type of lesion has a high choline kinase activity rate (20). This patient population, while on hormone therapy has been found to have a decreased level of tracer uptake, especially if the patient's HU level is above 825. This was demonstrated in a study, where FCH was utilized as the radioactive tracer (17).

Cancers that metastasize to bone with mixed lesions such as breast and thyroid are difficult to image on PET/CT due to the fact that many tracers are unable to show both lytic and sclerotic metastases. In the studies discussed, FDG has been the tracer of choice; however this has resulted in lower than appreciable values for specificity, sensitivity and accuracy of the scan. A combination of different tracers such as FDG and F-18 may be an option in the future for this group of cancer patients, in hopes that FDG will have uptake in lytic lesions and F-18 in sclerotic lesions (13).

Throughout the literature there are discrepancies as to which tracer is best for which type of cancer. Even while utilizing the same tracer, different results have been obtained in regards to sensitivity, specificity and accuracy of the scan. In order to accurately determine these values, future studies should incorporate a large patient population segregating for each primary cancer or each type of lesion. Currently the pooling of data for patients with different types of primary cancer and metastases may be altering results.

A common limitation to these studies is combining patients who have different primary cancers which result in different types of bone metastases. This will alter results as it has been proven that tracers that have high uptake in lytic lesions often have low uptake in sclerotic lesions and vice versa.

In the future, studies should be done that compare two different tracers in the same primary cancer population as there are currently few studies comparing tracers. In addition more studies should be conducted utilizing new radioactive tracers, such as ones that are currently used to image the brain. These tracers that result in uptake in cells with increased amino acid metabolism may prove to be viable for the imaging of bone metastases. Future studies should also work to find a biological pathway that lytic and sclerotic lesions have in common that a radioactive tracer could target. This pathway would have to be one that has increased activity or is altered when the cell becomes cancerous. Future research into radioactive tracers and their effect and incorporation into biological pathways is needed to find a tracer that would be effect in mixed lesion patients in order to effectively diagnose bone metastases in breast and thyroid cancer patients.

Acknowledgments

We thank Stacy Yuen for the secretarial support and the generous support of Bratty Family Fund, Michael and Karyn Goldstein Cancer Research Fund, Joseph and Silvana Melara Cancer Research Fund, and Ofelia Cancer Research Fund.

References

[1]   Costelloe CM, Rohren EM, Madewell JE, Hamaoka T, Theriault RL, Yu TK, et al. Imaging bone metastases in breast cancer: techniques and recommendations for diagnosis. Lancet Oncol 2009;10:606-14.

[2]   Portilla-Quattrociocchi H, Banzo I, Martinez-Rodriguez I, Quirce R, Jimenez-Bonilla J, de Arcocha Torres M, et al. Evaluation of bone scintigraphy and (18)F-FDG PET/CT in bone metastases of lung cancer patients. Rev Esp Med Nucl 2011;30:2-7.

[3]   Rajarubendra N, Bolton D, Lawrentschuk N. Diagnosis of bone metastases in urological malignancies--an update. Urology 2010;76:782-90.

[4]   Ozulker T, Kucukoz Uzun A, Ozulker F, Ozpacac T. Comparison of (18)F-FDG-PET/CT with (99m)Tc-MDP bone scintigraphy for the detection of bone metastases in cancer patients. Nucl Med Commun 2010;31:597-603.

[5]   Hahn S, Heusner T, Kummel S, Koninger A, Nagarajah J, Muller S, et al. Comparison of FDG-PET/CT and bone scintigraphy for detection of bone metastases in breast cancer. Acta Radiol 2011;52:1009-14.

[6]   Song JW, Oh YM, Shim TS, Kim WS, Ryu JS, Choi CM. Efficacy comparison between (18)F-FDG PET/CT and bone scintigraphy in detecting bony metastases of non-small-cell lung cancer. Lung Cancer 2009;65:333-8.

[7]   Abe K, Sasaki M, Kuwabara Y, Koga H, Baba S, Hayashi K, et al. Comparison of 18FDG-PET with 99mTc-HMDP scintigraphy for the detection of bone metastases in patients with breast cancer. Ann Nucl Med 2005;19:573-9.

[8]   Yang SN, Liang JA, Lin FJ, Kao CH, Lin CC, Lee CC. Comparing whole body (18)F-2-deoxyglucose positron emission tomography and technetium-99m methylene diphosphonate bone scan to detect bone metastases in patients with breast cancer. J Cancer Res Clin Oncol 2002;128:325-8.

[9]   Du Y, Cullum I, Illidge TM, Ell PJ. Fusion of metabolic function and morphology: sequential [18F]fluorodeoxyglucose positron-emission tomography/computed tomography studies yield new insights into the natural history of bone metastases in breast cancer. J Clin Oncol 2007;25:3440-7.

[10]   Langsteger W, Heinisch M, Fogelman I. The role of fluorodeoxyglucose, 18F-dihydroxyphenylalanine, 18F-choline, and 18F-fluoride in bone imaging with emphasis on prostate and breast. Semin Nucl Med 2006;36:73-92.

[11]   Liu T, Cheng T, Xu W, Yan WL, Liu J, Yang HL. A meta-analysis of 18FDG-PET, MRI and bone scintigraphy for diagnosis of bone metastases in patients with breast cancer. Skeletal Radiol 2011;40:523-31.

[12]   Withofs N, Grayet B, Tancredi T, Rorive A, Mella C, Giacomelli F, et al. (18)F-fluoride PET/CT for assessing bone involvement in prostate and breast cancers. Nucl Med Commun 2011;32:168-76.

[13]   Tiwari BP, Jangra S, Nair N, Tongaonkar HB, Basu S. Complimentary role of FDG-PET imaging and skeletal scintigraphy in the evaluation of patients of prostate carcinoma. Indian J Cancer 2010;47:385-90.

[14]   Fogelman I, Cook G, Israel O, Van der Wall H. Positron emission tomography and bone metastases. Semin Nucl Med 2005;35:135-42.

[15]   Beheshti M, Langsteger W, Fogelman I. Prostate cancer: role of SPECT and PET in imaging bone metastases. Semin Nucl Med 2009;39:396-407.

[16]   Even-Sapir E, Metser U, Mishani E, Lievshitz G, Lerman H, Leibovitch I. The detection of bone metastases in patients with high-risk prostate cancer: 99mTc-MDP Planar bone scintigraphy, single- and multi-field-of-view SPECT, 18F-fluoride PET, and 18F-fluoride PET/CT. J Nucl Med 2006;47:287-97.

[17]   Beheshti M, Vali R, Waldenberger P, Fitz F, Nader M, Hammer J, et al. The use of F-18 choline PET in the assessment of bone metastases in prostate cancer: correlation with morphological changes on CT. Mol Imaging Biol 2010;12:98-107.

[18] Fuccio C, Castellucci P, Schiavina R, Santi I, Allegri V, Pettinato V, et al. Role of 11C-choline PET/CT in the restaging of prostate cancer patients showing a single lesion on bone scintigraphy. Ann Nucl Med 2010;24:485-92.

[19] Luboldt W, Kufer R, Blumstein N, Toussaint TL, Kluge A, Seemann MD, et al. Prostate carcinoma: diffusion-weighted imaging as potential alternative to conventional MR and 11C-choline PET/CT for detection of bone metastases. Radiology 2008;249:1017-25.

[20] Beheshti M, Vali R, Waldenberger P, Fitz F, Nader M, Loidl W, et al. Detection of bone metastases in patients with prostate cancer by 18F fluorocholine and 18F fluoride PET-CT: a comparative study. Eur J Nucl Med Mol Imaging 2008;35:1766-74.

[21] Yu EY, Muzi M, Hackenbracht JA, Rezvani BB, Link JM, Montgomery RB, et al. C11-acetate and F-18 FDG PET for men with prostate cancer bone metastases: relative findings and response to therapy. Clin Nucl Med 2011;36:192-8.

[22] Liu N, Ma L, Zhou W, Pang Q, Hu M, Shi F, et al. Bone metastasis in patients with non-small cell lung cancer: the diagnostic role of F-18 FDG PET/CT. Eur J Radiol 2010;74:231-5.

[23] Cheran SK, Herndon JE,2nd, Patz EF,Jr. Comparison of whole-body FDG-PET to bone scan for detection of bone metastases in patients with a new diagnosis of lung cancer. Lung Cancer 2004;44:317-25.

[24] Kruger S, Buck AK, Mottaghy FM, Hasenkamp E, Pauls S, Schumann C, et al. Detection of bone metastases in patients with lung cancer: 99mTc-MDP planar bone scintigraphy, 18F-fluoride PET or 18F-FDG PET/CT. Eur J Nucl Med Mol Imaging 2009;36:1807-12.

[25] Bury T, Barreto A, Daenen F, Barthelemy N, Ghaye B, Rigo P. Fluorine-18 deoxyglucose positron emission tomography for the detection of bone metastases in patients with non-small cell lung cancer. Eur J Nucl Med 1998;25:1244-7.

[26] Takenaka D, Ohno Y, Matsumoto K, Aoyama N, Onishi Y, Koyama H, et al. Detection of bone metastases in non-small cell lung cancer patients: comparison of whole-body diffusion-weighted imaging (DWI), whole-body MR imaging without and with DWI, whole-body FDG-PET/CT, and bone scintigraphy. J Magn Reson Imaging 2009;30:298-308.

[27] Min JW, Um SW, Yim JJ, Yoo CG, Han SK, Shim YS, et al. The role of whole-body FDG PET/CT, Tc 99m MDP bone scintigraphy, and serum alkaline phosphatase in detecting bone metastasis in patients with newly diagnosed lung cancer. J Korean Med Sci 2009;24:275-80.

[28] Heusner T, Golitz P, Hamami M, Eberhardt W, Esser S, Forsting M, et al. "One-stop-shop" staging: should we prefer FDG-PET/CT or MRI for the detection of bone metastases? Eur J Radiol 2011;78:430-5.

[29] Phan HT, Jager PL, Plukker JT, Wolffenbuttel BH, Dierckx RA, Links TP. Detection of bone metastases in thyroid cancer patients: bone scintigraphy or 18F-FDG PET? Nucl Med Commun 2007;28:597-602.

[30] Ito S, Kato K, Ikeda M, Iwano S, Makino N, Tadokoro M, et al. Comparison of 18F-FDG PET and bone scintigraphy in detection of bone metastases of thyroid cancer. J Nucl Med 2007;48:889-95.

[31] Cook GJ. Skeletal metastases: what is the future role for nuclear medicine? Eur J Nucl Med Mol Imaging 2009;36:1803-6.

[32] Nanni C, Fantini L, Nicolini S, Fanti S. Non FDG PET. Clin Radiol 2010;65:536-548.

[33] Schmidt GP, Schoenberg SO, Schmid R, Stahl R, Tiling R, Becker CR, et al. Screening for bone metastases: whole-body MRI using a 32-channel system versus dual-modality PET-CT. Eur Radiol 2007;17:939-49.

[34] Czernin J, Satyamurthy N, Schiepers C. Molecular mechanisms of bone 18F-NaF deposition. J Nucl Med 2010;51:1826-9.

[35] Chua S, Gnanasegaran G, Cook GJ. Miscellaneous cancers (lung, thyroid, renal cancer, myeloma, and neuroendocrine tumors): role of SPECT and PET in imaging bone metastases. Semin Nucl Med 2009;39:416-30.

[36] Palmedo H, Grohe C, Ko Y, Tasci S. PET and PET/CT with F-18 fluoride in bone metastases. Recent Results Cancer Res 2008;170:213-24.

[37] Deng H, Tang X, Wang H, Tang G, Wen F, Shi X, et al. S-11C-methyl-L-cysteine: a new amino acid PET tracer for cancer imaging. J Nucl Med 2011;52:287-93.

[38]   Fleisch H. Bisphosphonates. Pharmacology and use in the treatment of tumour-induced hypercalcaemic and metastatic bone disease. Drugs 1991;42:919-44.

[39]   Fellner M, Baum RP, Kubicek V, Hermann P, Lukes I, Prasad V, et al. PET/CT imaging of osteoblastic bone metastases with (68)Ga-bisphosphonates: first human study. Eur J Nucl Med Mol Imaging 2010;37:834.

[40]   Gilbert FJ, Fleming IN, Marsden PK. Beyond 18F-fluorodeoxyglucose: making the next generation of PET radiotracers available for oncology research in the UK. Nucl Med Commun 2011;32:1-3.

SECTION SIX:
ADVANCED LUNG DISEASE

In: Advanced Cancer ISBN: 978-1-62808-239-5
Editors: N. Thavarajah, N. Pulenzas, B. Lechner et al. © 2013 Nova Science Publishers, Inc.

Chapter 39

A review of the impact of oxygen therapy in patients with advanced lung disease

Kaitlin Koo, BSc (C), Justin Kwong, MD (C),
Janet Nguyen, MD (C), Florencia Jon, MRT(T),
Liang Zeng, MD (C), Kristopher Dennis, MD,
Lori Holden, MRT(T), Shaelyn Culleton, MD (C),
Luluel Khan, MD, Amanda Caissie, MD PhD
and Edward Chow, MBBS[*]

Rapid Response Radiotherapy Program, Department of Radiation Oncology,
Odette Cancer Centre, Sunnybrook Health Sciences Centre, University of Toronto,
Toronto, Ontario, Canada

Due to the poor prognosis associated with cancerous and non-cancerous advanced lung disease, the main intention of treatment is to improve the patient's quality of life (QOL). A treatment option that may achieve this goal is oxygen therapy. Currently, there is little literature analyzing the QOL of patients with advanced lung cancer receiving oxygen therapy for dyspnea. However, research has been conducted on patients with chronic obstructive pulmonary disease (COPD) suffering from dyspnea. The similarities of symptoms and underlying pulmonary function between patients with advanced lung cancer and COPD suggest that these populations could be similarly impacted by oxygen therapy. A systematic, computerized literature search was performed using the Ovid search engine for the following databases: MEDLINE® (1950 to September Week 1, 2010), EMBASE (1980 to 2010 Week 37) and PsychINFO (1967 to September Week 2, 2010). Search strands were designed to retrieve articles on patients with advanced lung cancer or COPD, oxygen therapy, QOL and survival. Based on the 12 articles reviewed,

[*] Correspondence: Professor Edward Chow MBBS, MSc, PhD, FRCPC, Department of Radiation Oncology, Odette Cancer Centre, Sunnybrook Health Sciences Centre, 2075 Bayview Avenue, Toronto, ON M4N 3M5, Canada. E-mail: Edward.Chow@sunnybrook.ca.

studies have contrasting conclusions with regards to the patients' QOL when using oxygen therapy. Further research is suggested to explore the impact of oxygen therapy on patients with advanced lung disease.

Introduction

As defined by the American Thoracic Society, dyspnea is the subjective experience of breathing discomfort that consists of qualitatively distinct sensations that vary in intensity (1). The prevalence of severe dyspnea has been reported in palliative patients with heart failure (65%), lung cancer (70%) and chronic obstructive pulmonary disorder (90%) (2). Some of the etiologies of dyspnea include: muscle weakness, anemia, restrictive and obstructive lung changes, brochospasm, anxiety and hypoxia (3). Dyspnea often intensifies during the dying process thereby eroding one's quality of life, psychological well-being and social functioning (4). Dyspnea is a common symptom that accompanies a diagnosis of chronic obstructive pulmonary disorder (COPD) and often interferes with the patient's health-related quality of life (QOL) (4). More specifically, COPD is a devastating respiratory disease common amongst the elderly that causes significant morbidity and mortality (5). It is the fourth leading cause of death worldwide and is predicted to be the third leading cause of death worldwide by 2020 (6). Patients with COPD also commonly suffer from co-morbid conditions that produce a variety of symptoms. Therefore, the symptoms of COPD can vary greatly between patients; however, some of the common symptoms of COPD include cough, dyspnea and sputum production (7). Similarly, patients with advanced malignant lung disease (patients with primary lung cancer or metastatic lung cancer) often exhibit dyspnea, which can reduce their QOL (8). Due to the poor prognosis associated with advanced lung disease, the main intention of treatment is to improve the patient's QOL. Improving dyspnea may be a means to achieve this goal. A treatment option that may reduce dyspnea would be the use of oxygen therapy. The proposed benefit of oxygen therapy is the provision of supplementary oxygen to the patient as room air consists of about 21% oxygen (9). Oxygen is transported into our tissues via binding to hemoglobin (97%) and dissolving in plasma (3%) (9). Oxygen therapy may relieve dyspnea by depressing the hypoxic drive mediated by peripheral chemoreceptor, improving respiratory musculature function, altering the level of awareness of oxygen uptake or by stimulating non-specific nasal receptors (10). Currently, there is little literature analyzing the QOL of patients with advanced lung cancer receiving oxygen therapy for dyspnea. However, research has been conducted on patients with COPD suffering from dyspnea. The similarities of symptoms and underlying pulmonary function between patients with advanced lung cancer and patients with COPD suggest that these populations could be similarly impacted by oxygen therapy, and that the influence of therapy on the QOL of one group may be of reference to the other.

Literature review

A systematic, computerized literature search was performed using the Ovid search engine for the following databases: MEDLINE® (1950 to September Week 1, 2010), EMBASE (1980 to

2010 Week 37) and PsychINFO (1967 to September Week 2, 2010). Search strands were designed to retrieve articles on patients with advanced lung cancer or COPD, oxygen therapy, quality of life and survival. To search for article abstracts pertaining to the quality of life in patients with advanced lung cancer using oxygen therapy, the following strand of subject headings was used: *("lung neoplasms" OR "advanced lung cancer" OR "lung metastases") AND ("oxygen inhalation therapy" OR "oxygen therapy") AND ("quality of life" or "survival").* To search for articles assessing quality of life in COPD patients receiving oxygen therapy, the following search strand was used: *("chronic obstructive pulmonary disease" OR "chronic obstructive lung disease" OR "chronic obstructive airway disease" OR "chronic airflow limitation" OR "chronic obstructive respiratory disease" or "COPD") AND ("oxygen inhalation therapy" OR "oxygen therapy") AND ("quality of life" OR "survival").*

The abstracts from the references produced by these literature searches were read by two independent authors (KK and JK), to select full articles for subsequent review according to the predetermined criteria that the abstract must contain detailed assessments of quality of life in patients with COPD or advanced lung cancer receiving oxygen therapy.

Inclusion criteria

Inclusion criteria included published journal articles and review articles. Abstracts from articles within the reference lists of articles meeting the inclusion criteria were searched according to the same criteria.

Exclusion criteria

Exclusion criteria included duplicate articles, articles not written in English and articles without published abstracts.

Findings

Overview of the results

A total of 925 article references were identified by the literature searches. Three hundred and fifteen citations were reviewed in detail to determine which articles were related to the question of interest. Editorials and articles unrelated to quality of life in COPD patients receiving oxygen therapy, based on their respective abstracts, were excluded. Upon further investigation, these articles were assessed and further exclusions were made based on the relevance of the article to the systematic review. At the end, 10 of the most relevant articles were included in the review.

When the literature search was conducted regarding: patients with advanced lung cancer, oxygen therapy and quality of life, 15 papers were identified and 13 articles were excluded as they were unrelated to oxygen therapy in patients with advanced lung cancer. Overall, 2 papers were retrieved and analyzed. All of the studies reviewed are listed in Table 1.

Table 1. outlines all of the studies reviewed in this paper. The authors, year, country, title, number in the sample, age, sex, design interventions and findings are presented in this table

Author, Year, Country, Title	Number in Sample, Age, Sex	Design Interventions	Findings	
			Positive Improvements	No Improvements/ Worse Outcome
Crockett et al., 2001 Australia Survival on long-term oxygen therapy in chronic airflow limitation: from evidence to outcomes in the routine clinical setting	N=505 Age mean: Male-69.9± 9.1 years Female-71.0± 9.4 years 249 males and 256 females	A list of patients prescribed domiciliary oxygen therapy for Chronic Airway Limitation was generated from Respiratory Unit records and hospital financial records for the supply of this therapy. Survival was compared with that reported for the original randomized control trials, and for Swedish and Belgian COPD patients. Factors influencing survival were studied.	Improvements in QOL and survival greater in female patients with hypoxia and oxygen therapy compared to males.	
Lai et al., 2007 Hong Kong China Perceptions of dyspnea and helpful interventions during the advanced stages of lung cancer: Chinese patients' perspective	N=11 51-80 years 3 women and 8 men	Semi-structured and open-ended interactive interviews (20-35 minutes) conducted in Cantonese. Interviews were: Transcribed verbatim Transcripts were read again to acquire overall feeling of what participants were recounting Significant phrases and sentences were extracted Coding was assigned and grouped	All 11 participants were on oxygen therapy. Most participants verbalized that oxygen therapy was essential for them.	5 participants expressed that oxygen therapy was a burden and caused inconveniences as they could not move freely without oxygen therapy
Jaturapatporn et al., 2010 Canada Patients' experience of oxygen therapy and dyspnea: a qualitative study in home palliative care.	N=8	8 patients from a specialty home Palliative program were approached. A qualitative in-depth interview, using an interview guide, was conducted with each participant in their respective homes in Toronto, Canada from January to June 2008. A framework approach was used for qualitative data analysis as follows: Familiarization Identifying a thematic framework Indexing and charting Mapping and interpretation	In 4 out of 8 patients, shortness of breath persisted but was improved on oxygen. The other four patients reported that using oxygen therapy completely reversed their shortness of breath.	
Bruera et al., 1992 Canada Symptomatic benefit of supplemental oxygen in hypoxemic patients with terminal cancer: the use N of 1 randomized controlled trial.	N=1 Age=53 years Female	A before and after study was conducted on an advanced ovarian cancer patient. Double blind crossover, six randomized trials of 6-minute trials of oxygen or air by mask. Measurements were taken at rest and then after the intervention. Patient rated dyspnea by Dyspnea VAS (0-100). The difference between interventions was also rated on a scale of: 1 (not important) to 6 (great importance).	VAS: Baseline versus Air p<0.01 VAS: Baseline versus oxygen p<0.01 VAS: Air versus oxygen p<0.01 Patient chose oxygen over air p=0.09 Patient rating effect of 4.8/6	Baseline versus air was not statistically significant.

Author, Year, Country, Title	Number in Sample, Age, Sex	Design Interventions	Findings	
			Positive Improvements	No Improvements/ Worse Outcome
Swinburn et al., 1993 United Kingdom Symptomatic benefit of supplemental oxygen in hypoxemic patients with chronic lung disease.	N=22 Age Mean=58 years 13 Males & 9 Females	A before and after, prospective, two double blind random trial period of oxygen and air involving 10 interstitial lung disease and 12 patients with COPD. Measurements were taken at rest and post- intervention. Patient rated dyspnea using VAS (0-100).	Based on the VAS, oxygen was better than air for ILD, COPD $p<0.05$ Both air and oxygen were reported as helpful but oxygen was more consistent and frequent than air $p<0.01$	Not all significant differences for patients with ILD and COPD were observed.
Bruera et al., 1993 Canada Effects of oxygen on dyspnea in hypoxic terminal cancer patients.	N=14 Age mean=64 years 8 Males & 6 Females	Before and after, crossover trial, prospective, double blind of patients with advanced cancer-lung primary and metastatic, no COPD. 2 trials each of oxygen or air by mask. Then cross over to the other intervention. 2 blinded trials of more effective treatment	Baseline to oxygen, and air to oxygen, statistical significance for all measures. Patient chose oxygen as most effective gas twice in 12 cases. The investigator chose oxygen as most effective gas twice for same 12 patients.	Baseline to air-no statistical significance in any measures.
Currows and Agar, 2009 Australia Does palliative home oxygen improve dyspnoea?	N=413	A 4-year consecutive cohort from a regional community palliative care service was used to compare baseline breathlessness before oxygen therapy with dyspnea sub-scales on the symptom assessment scores (SAS; 0-10) 1 week and 2 weeks after the introduction of oxygen.	150 out of 413 people had more than a 20% improvement in mean dyspnea scores.	There were no significant differences overall 1 or 2 weeks ($p=0.28$) nor for any sub-groups.
Okubadejo et al., 1996 UK Does long-term oxygen therapy affect quality of life in patients with chronic obstructive pulmonary disease and sever hypoxaemia?	N=23 47-82 years 15 females and 8 males	Patients were selected from out-patient chest clinics. Used the SGRQ, the SIP and the Hospital Anxiety and Depression Scale (HADS) to evaluate QOL. Patients were prescribed oxygen concentrators and assessed at baseline. Patients were reassessed after 2 weeks, 3 and 6 months.	After six months of treatment, the study group had small improvements that were not significant. ($p=0.69$)	Start of the study, the study group with more severe hypoxaemia had a significantly worse quality of life (SGRQ and SIP). Two weeks, the study group had a mean improvement in SGRQ Total score of 6.8 compared to an improvement of 4.0 in the control group. The improvement was not significant ($p=0.48$). Therefore, significant correlations between changes in oxygen use and quality of life scores were not observed.

Table 1. (Continued)

Author, Year, Country, Title	Number in Sample, Age, Sex	Design Interventions	Findings	
			Positive Improvements	No Improvements/ Worse Outcome
Abernethy et al., 2010 Australia, USA and UK Effect of palliative oxygen versus room air in relief of breathlessness in patients with refractory dyspnoea: a double-blind, randomized controlled trial	N=239	Double-blind randomized control. Patients with life-limiting illness, refractory dyspnoea, and partial pressure of oxygen in arterial blood. Patients were randomly assigned to receive oxygen or room air and were instructed to use for 15h/day. Breathlessness was measured twice a day (morning and evening) on a numerical rating scale of 0-10.		Breathlessness did not differ between groups at any time during the study period. 58 (52%) of 112 patients assigned to oxygen and 40 (40%) of 101 patients assigned to room air responded to interventions. QOL did not differ between groups. 43(18%) of participants did not want to receive oxygen after the study. 63 (26%) said that they derived no benefit from the intervention. 41 (17%) requested and received unblended oxygen after the study. 74 (31%) requested oxygen but did not receive it.
Eaton et al., 2006 New Zealand Short-burst oxygen therapy for COPD patients: a 6-month randomised, controlled study	N=78 subject available for rando-mization 36 males and 42 females	A 6-month randomised, double-blind, placebo-controlled, parallel study group of cylinder oxygen versus cylinder air versus usual care was performed. Health-related questionnaires use for this study include: Chronic respiratory questionnaire (CRQ), Medical Outcomes Study 36-item Short-Form Health Survey (SF-36) and the Hospital Anxiety and Depression (HAD) scale		There were no significant differences between patients groups in any of the HRQOL measures (CRQ, SF-36, HAD) over the 6-month period.
Booth et al., 1996 United Kingdom Does oxygen help dyspnea in patients with cancer?	N=38 Age mean=71 years 16 Males & 22 Females	Study was conducted on patients with advanced cancer (20-lung, 2-mesothelioma, 16-lung metastases, 13-COPD and 4-CHF). Before and after, single blind random trial, one trial of each oxygen and airflow. Measures were taken at rest and post intervention using VAS (0-100), Modified Borg Scale and Arterial O_2 saturation & pulse oximetry.		VAS & Borg revealed no significant difference between oxygen and air effect. No difference in sequencing of intervention. No correlation between baseline saturation and change in VAS after O_2. No difference in benefits between cancer and cardiopulmonary disease. No significant difference in initial levels of dyspnea between any subgroups.
Tsara et al., 2008 Greece Quality of life and social-economic characteristics of Greek male patients on long-term oxygen therapy	N=85 Age means: LTOT Group-70.7± 8.4 years Control Group-63.5± 10.6 years All male subjects, no female subjects	Quality of life was evaluated with the 36-question Medical Outcomes Study Short Form (SF-36). The SF-36 HRQOL data from the study subjects was compared to published SF-36 assessments of normal Greek persons.		The HRQOL measurements were low in most SF-36 domains compared to the normal Greek subjects. Patients with COPD using LTOT experience marked impairments of HRQOL and psychological status. Suggest that patients with COPD perceive dyspnea as the leading symptom of the disease that affects their QOL.

Quality of life assessment tools

Amongst the 12 articles reviewed, some of the assessment tools used to assess the patient's quality of life included: the St. George's Respiratory Questionnaire (SGRQ), the Sickness Impact Profile (SIP), Hospital Anxiety and Depression Scale (HADS), EORTC QLQ-C30, Chronic Respiratory Questionnaire (CRQ) and the Medical Outcomes Study 36-item Short-Form Health Survey (SF-36).

Articles showing benefit with the use of oxygen therapy

The aim of the Crockett et al. study was to determine whether the survival of chronic airflow limitation (CAL) patients prescribed long-term oxygen therapy (LTOT) at Flinders Medical Centre (FMC) was gender-and-age related, and equivalent to that reported in randomized trials. A total of 505 participants (249 males and 256 females) were prescribed LTOT for CAL in this study. Concentrator oxygen information was obtained from the 3 to 6 monthly service reports to estimate compliance with the therapy. The amount of continuous oxygen therapy received was compared to the patients' survival rates. The authors concluded that improvements in survival were greater in female patients with hypoxia and oxygen therapy compared to males (11).

A qualitative descriptive design was used in Lai et al.'s study to explore, describe, interpret and understand the perceptions of dyspnea in patients with advanced lung cancer. Eleven patients (8 men and 3 women) with a medical diagnosis of terminal lung cancer were studied. The participants were interviewed in Cantonese using semi-structured and open-ended interactive interviews that were 20-35 minutes in duration. The interviews were all tape-recorded, transcribed verbatim, reviewed for overall feeling of the patients' accounts, significant phrases and sentences were extracted from the transcripts and then coded into categories. Based on the results, most of the participants verbalized that oxygen therapy was essential for their management of dyspnea. However, five out of the eleven participants expressed that oxygen therapy was a burden to them and caused inconveniences (12).

A recent study by Jaturapatporn et al (13) reported the prevalence and described the experiences of dyspnea, pattern of oxygen use and burdens of oxygen therapy in home palliative care patients receiving oxygen. Qualitative in-depth interviews were conducted using an interview guide on eight participants from a specialty home palliative program. Qualitative data analysis included: familiarization, identifying a thematic framework, indexing and charting, and mapping and interpretation. Conclusions from this study indicated that 5 out of 8 participants perceived oxygen therapy was a tool that increased their functional capacity and was a life-saving intervention. Some of the disadvantages mentioned in this study included: decreased mobility, discomfort in the nasal and ear cavity due to the nasal prongs and the noise related to the equipment. The authors concluded that the participants identified more advantages than disadvantages of oxygen therapy use (13).

Moreover, Bruera et al (14) conducted a before and after, double blind crossover clinical trial to determine the symptomatic effects of supplementary oxygen by mask in one hypoxic, dyspneic patient with cancer. The clinical trial compared two interventions by administering the two conditions (airflow and oxygen use) in a random order. The subjects' rating of dyspnea by Visual Analogue Scale (VAS) using a scale of 0-100mm, after six randomized trials of oxygen versus airflow, showed a significant difference. This paper concluded that the benefits demonstrated by oxygen use were significantly better than air flow in this patient (14).

Swinburn et al(15) investigated 22 hypoxic patients with chronic obstructive and interstitial lung disease with dyspnea at rest. A before and after, prospective, double blind random trial of oxygen and air was measured at rest and post intervention. Patients rated their dyspnea using the VAS (0-100mm). After two trial of both airflow and oxygen by mask, patients revealed that oxygen relieved their dyspnea to a greater degree and more consistently than air (15).

Finally, in 1993, a study by Bruera et al (16) was conducted with a sample of 14 hypoxic patients with advanced cancer involving the lung with dyspnea at rest. A before and after, double blind, crossover prospective trial concluded that there was no significant improvement in dyspnea from baseline to intervention with airflow. However, significant improvements were demonstrated in relief with oxygen by mask (16).

Studies that revealed no effect on QOL when using oxygen therapy

Currow and Agar (17) conducted a four-year consecutive cohort study from a regional community palliative care service in Western Australia. They defined any symptomatic benefit of the provision of home oxygen by recording baseline breathlessness before oxygen therapy; dyspnea sub-scales in the symptom assessment scores 1 and 2 weeks after the introduction of oxygen were also analyzed. Currow and Agar concluded that oxygen prescribed, on the basis of breathlessness alone, across a population predominantly with cancer does not improve breathlessness for the majority of people (17).

Okubadejo et al (18) studied a group of 23 patients (15 males and 8 females) with a diagnosis of COPD from an out-patient chest clinic in the East London area. The SGRQ, SIP, and the Hospital Anxiety and Depression Scale (HADS) were used to evaluate patient QOL. The patients were assessed at baseline and were then prescribed oxygen concentrators for the provision of LTOT for at least 15 hours per day. At the start of the study, the study group with more severe hypoxemia had a significantly worse quality of life (SGRQ and SIP). At the two week data collection, the study group had a mean improvement in SGRQ total score of 6.8 compared to an improvement of 4.0 in the control group. The improvement was not significant (p=0.48). After six months of treatment, the study group had small improvements that were not significant (p=0.69). This study suggests that LTOT provided by an oxygen concentrator does not adversely affect quality of life, but provides little benefit (18).

In the Abernethy et al study (19), 239 participants were randomly assigned by a central computer-generated system to receive oxygen or room air via a concentrator (oxygen, n=120; room, n=119) as well as complete seven dates of assessment. "Breathlessness right now" was recorded by the patient twice a day (morning and evening) in a diary with a scale of 0 (not breathless at all) to 10 (breathlessness as bad as you can imagine). The patients' QOL was assessed everyday using the McGill quality of life questionnaire. Their findings suggested that breathlessness did not differ between groups at any time (morning or evening) during the study period. In addition, the change in quality of life did not differ between the control and study group. The distribution of preferences was similar between the two groups since: 43(18%) of participants did not want to receive oxygen after the study, 63 (26%) stated that they derived no benefit from the intervention, 41 (17%) requested and received unblended oxygen after the study, 74 (31%) requested oxygen but did not receive it. Therefore, oxygen did not provide any additional symptomatic benefit for relief of refractory breathlessness as both groups (oxygen and room air) did not demonstrate any significant changes in breathlessness or QOL (19).

One of the objectives of Eaton et al (20) study was to determine whether short-burst oxygen therapy improved health-related quality of life. They conducted a 6-month randomized, double-blind, placebo-controlled parallel study group of cylinder oxygen versus cylinder air versus usual care with a sample size of 78 patients. Health-related quality of life questionnaires used included: the Chronic Respiratory Questionnaire (CRQ), Medical Outcome Study 36-item Short-Form Health Survey and the Hospital Anxiety and Depression Scale. There were no significant differences between patient groups in any of the HRQOL measures over the 6-month period except for the CRQ emotion domain occurring in the usual care group. The availability of short-burst oxygen did not improve health-related QOL nor did it reduce acute healthcare utilization (20).

Booth et al (21) conducted a before and after, single-blind random trial with 38 dyspneic subjects with advanced cancer. Measurements of patients' dyspnea were taken at rest and post intervention using the VAS (0-100). This study concluded that there was no correlation between baseline oxygen saturation and change in dyspnea score by VAS after administration of oxygen (21).

Negative effect on QOL when using oxygen therapy as a treatment for COPD

Tsara et al. investigated health-related QOL in Greek male patients with COPD using LTOT. A group of 85 patients with COPD and hypoxemia on LTOT, and a control group of 48 patients with stable COPD but without hypoxemia were analyzed. The quality of life was evaluated using the 36-question Medical Outcomes Study Short Form (SF-36) and psychological status was evaluated using the Greek version of the 30-question General Health Questionnaire for mental status. Eighty percent of the LTOT group had severe COPD, and 20% had moderate COPD. In the control group, 30% had severe COPD, 36% had moderate COPD and 34% had mild COPD. Results from the SF-36 indicated that patients with COPD using LTOT experienced noticeable impairment of HRQOL and psychological status (22).

Discussion

Based on the articles reviewed, studies have demonstrated a range of varying effects in the patients' QOL when using oxygen therapy. Crockett et al., Jaturapatpron et al., Bruera et al., Swinbrun et al., and Lai et al. studies demonstrated an increase in quality of life when oxygen therapy was used (11-16). Patients involved with these studies included: CAL patients, palliative care patients, dyspneic patient with cancer, patients with chronic obstructive and interstitial lung disease and patients with advanced stage lung cancer. Several studies by Currow & Agar, Okubadejo et al., Eaton et al., Abernethy et al., and Booth et al., concluded that oxygen did not affect the patients' QOL nor did it cause any adverse effects (17-21). One study conducted in Greece by Tsara et al. concluded that oxygen therapy had a negative impact on the patients' QOL (22).

Based on the articles reviewed, patients' quality of life in several of the studies demonstrated an increase in overall quality of life. In the study by Okubadejo et al., significant correlations between changes in oxygen use and quality of life scores were not observed (18). However, patients receiving LTOT had a slightly greater improvement in their quality of life compared to the control group; this was not statistically significant during the study period. It was suggested that the questionnaires used were not appropriate for the population of interest. Therefore, selection of an appropriate QOL questionnaire is crucial to the success of any successive study analyzing the effects of oxygen therapy in patients.

Patients receiving oxygen therapy often have chronic obstructive pulmonary disease, hypoxemia, advanced lung cancer or a condition that limits the uptake of oxygen. Greater than 80% of patients with lung cancer die within a year and fewer than 15% achieve long-term survival (8). Therefore due to the poor prognosis associated with these patients, potential benefits in treatment are often short-lived and only aid in ensuring that the patient is comfortable during the terminal stages of their disease.

Oxygen therapy is a central component of the routine treatment of COPD patients with chronic severe hypoxemia (18, 19). Many of the symptoms experienced by COPD patients such as cough, dyspnea and sputum production (7) are also experienced by patients with advanced lung cancer. Therefore, the possible impact associated with the use of oxygen therapy in COPD patients could be applied to patients with advanced lung disease due to the similar characteristics of both conditions.

As suggested, the use of oxygen therapy in patients with advanced lung cancer should be further investigated to determine the potential effects of patients' QOL. Lai et al.'s study regarding advanced lung patients receiving home oxygen therapy is limited due to the small sample size and lack of standardized assessment tools to evaluate quality of life. It was the first study to investigate the benefit of oxygen in patients with cancer; therefore there is lack of information regarding these patients and further investigation is required specific to this patient population

Although there is some evidence that supports the benefits of using oxygen therapy, it becomes difficult to distinguish the sources of improvement. Abernethy et al. randomly assigned patients to receive room air or oxygen by concentrator and nasal cannula. Their results demonstrated that there was no change in quality of life between the two groups. Therefore, benefits may be observed due to: the movement of gas across the nasal passage which affects the sensation of dyspnea, the mere presence of intervention which may alleviate the patient's anxiety, the concentrator as a placebo thereby inducing the expectation of some benefit, and finally the additional attention may improve psychological status thereby reducing breathlessness (19). Hence, these factors should be considered when analyzing the benefits and effects that oxygen therapy has on QOL in patients with advanced lung disease.

One of the problems with comparing quality of life for patients with advanced lung cancer was the numerous variations of QOL questionnaires used; this created inconsistent methods of comparing patients' quality of life. Patients requiring oxygen therapy may be on other medications which can affect the outcomes of oxygen therapy as well as the patient's QOL. Some patients may be sedated failing to potentially benefit from this treatment. The only study by Lai et al. which analyzed patients with cancer had a sample size of 11 participants. This study may be biased due to the limited number of participants and collection of data from one care unit in Hong Kong (12).

It is suggested that the use of an appropriate assessment tool to analyze the population of interest and obtain a comprehensive idea of the patients' QOL is required to properly analyze the benefits associated with oxygen therapy. To accurately measure the benefit associated with the use of oxygen therapy in patients with advanced lung cancer, follow-ups should be conducted soon after the initial administration of oxygen therapy. Based on the current literature for patients with COPD and the wide-ranging effects of using oxygen therapy, further research is suggested regarding the possible benefits of oxygen therapy use in patients with advanced lung cancer.

The benefits of oxygen therapy are unknown and could possibly decrease patients' quality of life due to the additional limitations of being confined to a portable oxygen machine. This may present additional problems as the patients may be limited in activities they would normally carry out on a day-to-day basis. Moreover, the additional oxygen could possibly increase tumor growth as more oxygen is being provided in the blood allowing for an increase in uptake of oxygen in the tissues. Therefore, further research is suggested to explore if oxygen therapy may help in providing the patient with more comfort and an increased quality of life when living with advanced lung cancer. Their QOL should also be evaluated since these patients often have a poor prognosis. The main objective of treatment at this stage of their disease is to improve their quality of life. Therefore, further investigation into the effects of oxygen therapy in patients with advanced lung cancer on quality of life would be urgently needed.

Acknowledgments

This study was supported by the Michael and Karyn Goldstein Cancer Research Fund and we thank Mrs. Stacy Yuen for her administrative assistance.

References

[1]   American Thoracic Society Board Of Directors. Dyspnea. Mechanisms, Assessment, And Management: A Consensus Statement. American Thoracic Society. Am J Respir Crit Care Med 1999;159(1):321-40.

[2]   Lynn J, Teno JM, Phillips RS et al. Perceptions By Family Members Of The Dying Experience Of Older And Seriously Ill Patients. SUPPORT Investigators. Study To Understand Prognoses And Preferences For Outcomes And Risks Of Treatments. Ann Intern Med 1997;126(2):97-106.

[3]   Gallagher R, Roberts D. A Systematic Review Of Oxygen And Airflow Effect On Relief Of Dyspnea At Rest In Patients With Advanced Disease Of Any Cause. J Pain Palliat Care Pharmacother 2004;18(4):3-15.

[4]   Tanaka K, Akechi T, Okuyama T, et al. Prevalence And Screening Of Dyspnea Interfering With Daily Life Activities In Ambulatory Patients With Advanced Lung Cancer. J Pain Symptom Manage 2002;23(6):484-9.

[5]   Nazir SA, Redland ML. Chronic Obstructive Pulmonary Disease: An Update On Diagnosis And Management Issues In Older Adults. Drugs Aging 2009;26(10):813-31.

[6]   Rocker G, Horton R, Currow D, et al. Palliation Of Dyspnoea In Advanced COPD: Revisiting A Role For Opioids. Thorax 2009;64(10):910-5.

[7]   Jablonski A, Gift A, Cook K. Symptom Assessment Of Patients With Chronic Obstructive Pulmonary Disease. West J Nurs Res 2007;29(7):845-63.

[8]   Ozturk A, Sarihan S, Ercan I, et al. Evaluating Quality Of Life And Pulmonary Function Of Long-Term Survivors Of Non-Small Cell Lung Cancer Treated With Radical Or Postoperative Radiotherapy. J Clin Oncol 2009;32(1):65-72.

[9]   Pruitt WC, Jacobs M. Breathing Lessons: Basics Of Oxygen Therapy. Nursing 2003; 33(10):43-5.

[10]   Spector N, Connolly MA, Carlson KK. Dyspnea: Applying Research To Bedside Practice. AACN Adc Crit Care 2007;18(1):45-58.

[11]   Crockett AJ, Cranston JM, Moss JR, et al. Survival On Long-Term Oxygen Therapy In Chronic Airflow Limitation: From Evidence To Outcomes In The Routine Clinical Setting. Intern Med J 2001;31(8):448-54.

[12]   Lai YL, Chan CW, Lopez V. Perceptions Of Dyspnea And Helpful Interventions During The Advanced Stage Of Lung Cancer: Chinese Patients' Perspectives. Cancer Nurs 2007;30(2):E1-8.

[13]   Jaturapatporn D, Moran E, Obwanga C, et al. Patients' Experience Of Oxygen Therapy And Dyspnea: A Qualitative Study In Home Palliative Care. Support Care Cancer 2010;18:765-70.

[14]   Bruera E, Schoeller T, Maceachern T. Symptomatic Benefit Of Supplemental Oxygen In Hypoxemic Patients With Terminal Cancer: The Use Of N Of 1 Randomized Controlled Trial. J Pain Symptom Manage 1992;7(6): 365-8.

[15]   Swinburn C, Mould H, Stone T, et al. Symptomatic Benefit Of Supplemental Oxygen In Hypoxemic Patients With Chronic Lung Disease. Am Rev Respir Dis 1991;143: 913-5.

[16]   Bruera E, De Stoutz N, Velasco-Leiva A, et al. Effects Of Oxygen On Dyspnea In Hypoxaemic Terminal-Cancer Patients. Lancet 1993;342:13-4.

[17]   Currow DC, Agar M, Smith J, et al. Does Palliative Home Oxygen Improve Dyspnoea? A Consecutive Cohort Study. Palliat Med 2009;23(4):309-16.

[18]   Okubadejo AA, Paul EA, Jones PW, et al. D And Severe Hypoxaemia? Eur Respir J 1996; 9(11):2335-9.

[19]   Abernethy AP, Mcdonald CF, Frith PA et al. Effect Of Palliative Oxygen Versus Room Air In Relief Of Breathlessness In Patients With Refractory Dyspnea: A Double-Blind Randomized Controlled Trial. Lancet 2010:376:784-93.

[20]   Eaton T, Fergusson W, Kolbe J, et al. Short-Burst Oxygen Therapy For COPD Patients: A 6-Month Randomised, Controlled Study. Eur Respir J 2006;27(4):697-704.

[21]   Booth S, Kelly M, Cox N, et al. Does Oxygen Help Dyspnea In Patients With Cancer? Am J Respir Crit Care Med 1996;153:1515-8.

[22]   Tsara V, Serasli E, Katsarou Z, et al. Quality Of Life And Social-Economic Characteristics Of Greek Male Patients On Long-Term Oxygen Therapy. Respir Care 2008;53(8):1048-53.

[23]   Plywaczewski R, Sliwinski P, Nowinski A, et al. Incidence Of Nocturnal Desaturation While Breathing Oxygen In COPD Patients Undergoing Long-Term Oxygen Therapy. Chest 2000; 117(3):679-83.

[24]   Stoller JK, Panos RJ, Krachman S, et al. Long-Term Oxygen Treatment Trial Research, Group. Oxygen Therapy For Patients With COPD: Current Evidence And The Long-Term Oxygen Treatment Trial. Chest 2010;138(1):179-87.

In: Advanced Cancer
Editors: N. Thavarajah, N. Pulenzas, B. Lechner et al.
ISBN: 978-1-62808-239-5
© 2013 Nova Science Publishers, Inc.

Chapter 40

Long-term survival in patients with brain metastases from non small cell lung carcinoma

Rehana Jamani, BSc(C), Kristopher Dennis, MD,
Florencia Jon, MRT(T), Nemica Thavarajah, BSc(C),
Alex Mingay, BSc(C), Emily Chen, BSc(C), Janet Nguyen, BSc(C),
Natalie Lauzon, MRT(T) and Edward Chow, MBBS[*]

Rapid Response Radiotherapy Program, Department of Radiation Oncology,
Odette Cancer Centre, Sunnybrook Health Sciences Centre, University of Toronto,
Toronto, Canada

This chapter describes a cohort of patients with brain metastases from non-small cell lung carcinoma experiencing long-term survival. A prospectively-gathered database from an outpatient palliative radiotherapy clinic was retrospectively searched for patients referred between January 2005 and July 2009 who experienced long-term survival after a diagnosis of brain metastases from non-small cell lung carcinoma. Demographic, treatment, and survival data were reviewed. From 748 patients referred with symptomatic brain metastases, 5 with non-small cell lung carcinoma had survived ≥ 12 months after brain metastases had been diagnosed. Patient #1 was RPA class 2, GPA score 1.5 at the time of referral and survived 22 months from the time of brain metastases diagnosis. Patient #2 was RPA class 2, GPA score 1.0 and survived 36 months, Patient #3 was RPA class 2, GPA class 1.5 and survived 13 months, Patient #4 was RPA class 3, GPA score 2.0 and survived 23 months, and Patient #5 was RPA class 1, GPA score 3.0 and survived 23 months. Three patients received surgery and radiotherapy and two patients received radiotherapy alone for brain metastases treatment. Long-term survival with brain metastases from non-small cell lung carcinoma is rare, but possible. Treatments should be customized according to patient, tumor and treatment-related factors.

[*] Correspondence: Edward Chow, MBBS, PhD, FRCPC, Department of Radiation Oncology, Odette Cancer Centre, Sunnybrook Health Sciences Centre, 2075 Bayview Avenue, Toronto, ON M4N 3M5, Canada. E-mail: Edward.Chow@sunnybrook.ca.

Introduction

Brain metastases occur in 30% of patients with cancer, making it the most prevalent neurologic complication of malignancy (1). One third to one half of affected patients die as a direct result of their brain metastases (2). The average survival of patients with untreated brain metastases is one month. When treated with corticosteroids or palliative whole brain radiotherapy (WBRT), patients survive on average two to six months respectively (3). Despite improvements in systemic therapies and aggressive surgical and radiotherapeutic approaches to intracranial disease, long-term survival for patients with brain metastases from lung cancer is still guarded due to the aggressive nature of the disease, and reports of long-term survival are uncommon (4). We present here a case series of five patients with brain metastases from non-small cell lung carcinoma (NSCLC) who achieved long-term survival, and interpret their clinical characteristics through common prognostic assessment systems for patients with brain metastases (2,5).

Our study

A prospectively gathered database from an outpatient palliative radiotherapy clinic was reviewed retrospectively to identify all NSCLC patients with brain metastases and long-term survival. Long-term survival was defined as ≥ 12 months from the time brain metastases were first diagnosed. All patients had received palliative cranial radiotherapy between January 2005 and July 2009. Other information extracted included date of birth, gender, age at diagnosis of primary cancer, primary cancer treatments, the degree of intracranial disease (single vs. multiple metastases), age at diagnosis of brain metastases, brain metastases treatments, the presence of extracranial metastases, the most recent cranial imaging results, the date of most recent follow-up, and date of death. Patients were also categorized according to two prognostic assessment systems: the Recursive Partitioning Analysis (RPA) system and the Graded Prognostic Assessment (GPA) system.

The RPA system is based on data from three Radiation Therapy Oncology Group (RTOG) brain metastases studies [2]. RPA Class 1 includes patients with a Karnofsky Performance Status (KPS) of 70 or more and controlled primary disease, age under 65 years, and no extracranial metastases. RPA Class 2 patients also have a KPS ≥ 70 but have uncontrolled primary disease, are aged 65 years or more, and/or have extracranial metastases. RPA Class 3 represents the patients with a KPS<70. RPA Class 1, 2, and 3 patients have estimated median survival times of 7.1 months, 4.2 months, and 2.3 months respectively (Table 1).

The newer GPA system includes primary cancer- specific classifications based on a brain metastases database study completed by the RTOG [5]. The important prognostic factors for patients with lung cancer include age, KPS, the presence of extracranial metastases, and the number of brain metastases when they are first diagnosed. Patients are allocated between 0 and 4 points depending on their characteristics (see table 2). Higher scores imply an improved prognosis. The overall median survival for NSCLC patients within this system is 7 months.

Table 1. The Recursive Partitioning Analysis (RPA) scoring system

Class 1	Class 2	Class 3
-KPS* ≥ 70 -controlled primary disease -age < 65 -no ECM†	-KPS ≥ 70 AND at least one of the following: -uncontrolled primary -age ≥ 65 -ECM	-KPS < 70
Median survival time: 7.1 months	Median survival time: 4.2 months	Median survival time: 2.3 months

*KPS: Karnofsky Performance Status
†ECM: extracranial metastases

Table 2. The Graded Prognostic Assessment (GPA) scoring allocation method

Factor	0 points	0.5 points	1.0 points
Age	>60	50-60	<50
KPS*	<70	70-80	90-100
ECM†	Present	-------	Absent
# BM‡	>3	2-3	1

*KPS: Karnofsky Performance Status
†ECM: extracranial metastases
‡BM: brain metastases

Our findings

The database contained 748 patients with brain metastases and 5 with non-small cell lung carcinoma met our long-term survival inclusion criteria with survival ≥ 12 months after brain metastases had been diagnosed. Their clinical characteristics are summarized in Table 3. At the time of referral, patients ranged from RPA class 1-3 and GPA scores 1.0-3.0. Patient #1 was RPA class 2, GPA score 1.5 at the time of referral and survived 22 months from the time of brain metastases diagnosis. Patient #2 was RPA class 2, GPA score 1.0 and survived 36 months, Patient #3 was RPA class 2, GPA class 1.5 and survived 13 months, Patient #4 was RPA class 3, GPA score 2.0 and survived 23 months, and Patient #5 was RPA class 1, GPA score 3.0 and survived 23 months.

Three patients received surgery and radiotherapy and two patients radiotherapy alone for brain metastases treatment. Three patients initially had single brain metastases but all later developed multiple lesions. Survival times from the time of diagnosis of brain metastases ranged from 13 months to 36 months.

Table 3. Clinical and treatment characteristics for patients with brain metastases from non-small cell lung carcinoma

Baseline characteristics at time of brain mets diagnosis	Brain Metastases treatments & disease course	Intracranial progression at last follow-up?	Alive at last follow-up?	Survival from time of first brain metastases diagnosis
-80yo female - KPS* 80 - Single brain metastasis - No extracranial metastases - RPA[†] Class 2 - GPA[‡] Score 1.5	- SRS[§] - WBRT[‖] for new multiple brain metastases 12 months post SRS - Extracranial metastases (liver, lung, bone)	No	No	22 months
-50yo male -KPS 80 -Multiple brain metastases -No extracranial metastases -RPA Class 2 -GPA Score 1.0	-WBRT -Repeat RT[¶] for new brain metastases 20 months post WBRT -Extracranial metastasis (spine)	No	Yes	36 months (last F/U**)
-age unknown -KPS 70 -Single brain metastasis -No extracranial metastases -RPA Class 2 -GPA Score 1.5	-Brain metastasis resected -Post-op WBRT 1 month post craniotomy -to be seen by neurosurgery at last follow-up -extracranial metastasis (bone)	Yes (recurrence of brain mets)	Yes	13 months (last F/U)
-67yo male -KPS 60 -Single brain metastasis -No extracranial metastases -RPA Class 3 -GPA Score 2.0	-Brain metastasis resected -WBRT 2 months after operation -Localized RT for recurrence of brain metastases 13 months post WBRT -No extracranial metastases	Yes (tumour progression, RT treatment not possible)	Yes	23 months (last F/U)
-53yo female -KPS 90 -Multiple brain metastases -No extracranial metastases -RPA Class 1 -GPA Score 3.0	-WBRT -SRS 6 months post WBRT due to growth of lesions -Brain metastasis resected 9 months later -RT 4 months after operation -Patient on chemotherapy 4 months after last radiation treatment -No extracranial metastases	No	Yes	23 months (last F/U)

* KPS: Karnofsky Performance Status.
[†] RPA: Recursive Partitioning Analysis.
[‡] GPA: Graded Prognostic Assessment.
[§] SRS: Stereotactic Radiosurgery.
[‖] WBRT: Whole Brain Radiotherapy.
[¶] RT: Radiotherapy.
** F/U: Follow-up.

Discussion

We have shown here that patients with brain metastases from NSCLC can indeed experience long-term survival. Chao and colleagues reported 32 patients with brain metastases who survived 5 or more years after being treated with whole-brain radiation therapy (WBRT), surgery, stereotactic radiosurgery, salvage chemotherapy, and/or implant therapy [1]. Survival time was measured from the date of the MRI or CT scan documenting metastases and the median survival of the group was 9.3 years, much longer than the 23 months from our series. Factors contributing to longer survival were age under 65 years, a controlled primary tumor, a lack of systemic disease, a higher RPA class, and a single brain metastasis at diagnosis. Only 17 of the 32 patients had NSCLC, however.

Similarly, Yuile and colleagues reviewed a cohort of patients with brain metastases that received radiotherapy. Their overall median survival was 3 months, with survival measured from the time of completion of radiotherapy [3]. Only 15% of patients with a lung cancer primary survived beyond 12 months (the median survival was 6 months), comparatively shorter than our figure of 23 months. For the whole cohort, patients undergoing resection or receiving higher doses of radiotherapy had improved survival.

Luterbach and colleagues published a paper regarding long-term survival of patients with brain metastases undergoing WBRT [4]. Long-term survival was defined as two or more years after WBRT initiation. The median survival was 3.4 months with 5.6%, 2.9%, 1.8%, and <1% of patients alive at two years, three years, five years, and ten years respectively. Survival times for patients with NSCLC primaries were higher than these figures with 5.8%, 3.5%, 2.3%, and 0% alive at two years, three years, five years, and ten years respectively. It was stated that aggressive therapy in RPA Class 1 and Class 2 patients with single brain metastases could have accounted for longer survival times.

Our patients all had longer survival times than would have been predicted by their RPA classes (Table 3). Four of five patients also exceeded their predicted GPA survival estimates (Table 3). The RPA and GPA systems both state that the presence of extracranial metastases has a negative impact on survival, yet three of our five patients with extracranial disease still lived longer than expected. This may suggest that systemic treatments available now are able to better prolong life than were the available therapies at the time the RTOG databases were created. We must be mindful of this in patients with brain metastases, and that the potential for long-term survival exists, even for patients with lung cancer primaries. Sperduto et al. stated that all forms of treatments were better than WBRT alone for NSCLC patients with brain metastases [5]. Our long-term survivors indeed received a variety of surgical and radiotherapeutic interventions, but interestingly one of them received only WBRT alone.

It is important to have an understanding of systems such as the RPA and GPA, as well as the surgical, radiotherapeutic and systemic treatment options available for patients with brain metastases. As many management approaches are available for patients, it is important to tailor them appropriately on a case-to-case basis, to follow and report their outcomes, and to remember that long-term survival is possible even in patients with lung cancer primaries.

Acknowledgments

We thank the generous support of Bratty Family Fund, Michael and Karyn Goldstein Cancer Research Fund, Joseph and Silvana Melara Cancer Research Fund, and Ofelia Cancer Research Fund.

References

[1]　　Chao ST, Barnett GH, Liu SW, Reuther AM, Toms SA, Vogelbaum MA, et al. Five-year survivors of brain metastases: a single-institution report of 32 patients. Int J Radiat Oncol Bio Phys 2006;66(3):801-9.

[2]　　Gaspar L, Scott C, Rotman M, Asbell S, Phillips T, Wasserman T, et al. Recursive partitioning analysis (RPA) of prognostic factors in three radiation therapy oncology group (RTOG) brain metastases trials. Int J Radiat Oncol Biol Phys 1997;37(4):645-51.

[3]　　Yuile PG, Tran MH. Survival with brain metastases following radiation therapy. Australasian Radiol 2002;46:390-5.

[4]　　Lutterbach J, Bartelt S, Ostertag C. Long-term survival in patients with brain metastases. J Cancer Res Clin Oncol 2002;128:417-25.

[5]　　Sperduto PW, Chao ST, Sneed PK, Luo X, Suh J, Roberge D, et al. Diagnosis-specific prognostic factors, indexes, and treatment outcomes for patients with newly diagnosed brain metastases: a multi-institutional analysis of 4,259 patients. Int J Radiat Oncol Biol Phys 2010;77(3): 655-61.

Chapter 41

Palliative radiotherapy in the treatment of lung metastases or advanced lung cancer

Jasmine Nguyen, MBBCh(C), Dominic Chu, MBBCh(C),
Gillian Bedard, BSc(C), Erin Wong, BSC(C), Flo Jon, MRTT,
Cyril Danjoux, MD, Elizabeth Barnes, MD, May Tsao, MD,
Lori Holden, MRTT, Edward Chow, MBBS
and Natalie Lauzon, MRTT[*]

Rapid Response Radiotherapy Program, Department of Radiation Oncology,
Odette Cancer Centre, Sunnybrook Health Sciences Centre, University of Toronto,
Toronto, Ontario, Canada

External beam radiotherapy (EBRT) given to advanced lung cancer patients undergoing palliative care is intended to relieve the symptoms that disrupt a patient's overall Quality of Life (QOL). This treatment, however, may also pose unwanted toxicities and side effects. This report presents five cases in which patients have been diagnosed with advanced lung cancer or lung metastases and were subsequently treated with external beam radiotherapy. In an attempt to assess the efficacy of the treatment, diaries were given to the patients to fill out at baseline, during treatment and 10 days after treatment. The diary collected data on the medications taken by the patient and evaluated the perceived severity of the following acute toxicity symptoms: coughing, hemoptysis, dysphagia, chest pain and dyspnea. In addition, the patients completed QOL questionnaires, the EORTC QLQ-C15-PAL as well as the EORTC QLQ-LC13. Four of the patients generally had an improved or stabilized QOL, while one felt intensified symptoms and a worsened QOL. The information gathered from these assessments can

---

[*] Correspondence: Ms. Natalie Lauzon BSc, MRTT Department of Radiation Therapy, Odette Cancer Centre, Sunnybrook Health Sciences Centre, 2075 Bayview Avenue, Toronto, ON Canada. Email: Natalie.Lauzon@Sunnybrook.ca.

give clinicians a greater understanding of the experience of EBRT through the patients' perspective.

Introduction

Lung cancer often presents itself as an incurable and non-resectable disease as it is usually identified in its advanced stages or has metastasized to other regions of the body (1). Patients usually face numerous and debilitating symptoms such as anxiety, fatigue, weakness, loss of appetite, dyspnea, cough, and hemoptysis (2). In order to help these patients, we provide palliation of these symptoms through chemotherapy, surgery, or radiotherapy. This report examines specifically external beam radiotherapy (EBRT), which is effective in controlling some of the symptoms (2), however, the effects of the treatment itself need to be examined.

This case series examines five patients with advanced lung cancer who were treated with EBRT. The referrals were made to a palliative outpatient radiotherapy clinic. In this report, we attempt to decipher whether or not the benefits of such a treatment outweigh the toxicities of five advanced lung cancer patients with the use of an acute toxicity symptoms evaluation diary and the European Organization for Research and Treatment of Cancer (EORTC) Quality of Life Questionnaire Core 15 Palliative (QLQ-C15-PAL) in conjunction with the EORTC QLQ-Lung Cancer (QLQ-LC13).

Case report

Case #1

The first patient is an eighty-year old female who was diagnosed with primary bladder cancer metastatic to the lungs and was referred due to dyspnea and hemoptysis. Consequently, the patient was treated with palliative EBRT with 20Gy/5fr. At the baseline point prior to treatment, the patient took neither medications nor oxygen for her lung symptoms. However, she experienced slight hemoptysis and mild shortness of breath, which she found to moderately interfere with her daily activities. According to the EORTC QLQ-C15-PAL and the EORTC QLQ-LC13, she noticed nausea, trouble sleeping, fatigue, mild tension, tingling on her hands/feet and slight depression.

During treatment, she no longer experienced hemoptysis. She briefly experienced dyspnea and chest pain, but for the last 2 days of treatment, the patient was symptom free. Over the course of the treatment, her diary entries suggested that she found that her symptoms were in a better state than at baseline and did not interfere with her daily activities. On the last day of treatment, the patient was re-administered the EORTC QLQ-C15-PAL along with the EORTC QLQ-LC13 surveys, which showed that her fatigue and dyspnea had increased during the prior week, however she no longer experienced tingling on her hands/feet, hemoptysis and had lessened nausea. All other evaluated symptoms remained the same.

After treatment, the patient did not take any pain medication. She had encountered slight coughing and reacquired her slight dyspnea until both symptoms went away 5 days post-treatment. She was briefly symptom free, but later encountered dysphagia until the last assessment. Within those 10 days, the patient noted that her symptoms had improved and had not been interfering with her daily activities.

Case #2

The second patient is a sixty-nine year old male who was diagnosed with primary lung cancer that metastasized to the brain. He was referred to the clinic for chest pain. Subsequently, the patient was treated with palliative EBRT with 20Gy/5fr. At baseline, the patient noted on the diary that he took neither medications nor oxygen and noticed no acute toxicity symptoms (coughing, hemoptysis, dysphagia, chest pain and dyspnea); however, on the first day of treatment, he took the EORTC QLQ-C-15-PAL and the EORTC QLQ-LC-13 and noted that he had experienced slight coughing and slight hemoptysis. He also claimed he had an excellent QOL (7/7).

Out of the four consecutive days of treatment, the patient did not take any pain medications. The patient experienced a sustained cough and a brief, mild hemoptysis. Overall, none of the symptoms seemed to have interfered with his daily activities.

For the 10 days after the radiation treatment that were followed-up on the diary, the patient did not take any pain medications and felt only slight coughing urges. The patient was re-assessed a month later, only noting a slight cough. During that time, the patient, again, ranked his QOL as excellent.

Case #3

The third patient is a forty-eight year old female who was diagnosed with primary lung cancer metastatic to bone and was referred due to her superior vena cava obstruction. The patient was treated with EBRT with 20Gy/5fr. At baseline, the patient noted in her diary that she did not take any oxygen but took Advil as a pain medication. She also felt slight coughing as well as slight dyspnea; however, the symptoms did not interfere with her daily activities. A day before the treatment, the patient noted that she also had had slight pain and severe depression on the EORTC QLQ-C15-PAL, and graded her quality of life at a 4/7. According to the EORTC QLQ-LC13, she also seemed to notice slight coughing and a little pain in her arms/shoulders and neck.

During treatment, she noticed slight dyspnea, mild chest pain, nausea, tiredness, and cough. She also still claimed that her symptoms were in a better state than before treatment. On the last day of treatment, she noted her much-worsened dyspnea, increased fatigue, and nausea; however, she no longer noticed any pain on her body and she felt no depression.

After treatment, the patient started taking Dexamethasone alongside Advil. She experienced a brief cough, intensified dyspnea, dysphagia, and increased chest pain. On all 10 days, the patient noted that her symptoms post-treatment were worse than before treatment and that all the symptoms strongly interfered with her daily activities. She completed the EORTC QLQ-C15-PAL and the EORTC QLQ-LC13 again which showed that all the symptoms remained the same since she last completed the questionnaires, except for her worsened lack of appetite, pain in her neck, trouble swallowing, and sore throat/tongue. In addition, the pain in her arms/shoulders, chest and the tingling in her hands and feet seemed to have disappeared. At that time, she also graded her quality life to be 3/7, which was slightly worse than at baseline.

Approximately a month after the treatment started, the patient again took the C15 and the LC13 and noted that her dyspnea, coughing and soreness in her mouth/tongue had improved, while her nausea, tension, fatigue, dysphagia, and chest pain had worsened. The pain in her neck seemed to have moved to her back and she felt slightly depressed. In the same entry, the patient also claimed that she took Tylenol 3 as a pain medication. Finally, she considered her quality of life to be at a 1/7, implying that it was much worse than it was at baseline.

Case #4

The fourth patient is a sixty-year old female who was diagnosed with primary ovarian cancer metastatic to the lung, was referred for mild coughing and slight hemoptysis. She was thereby treated by EBRT with dosage of 30 Gy/10 fr.

At baseline, the patient was experiencing moderate coughing which required only non-narcotic medication and slight hemoptysis. She did not use any pain medications nor did she take oxygen, and her symptoms only slightly affected her daily activities. At baseline, she also completed the *EORTC QLQ*-C15-PAL, which conveyed that she had slight fatigue, trouble sleeping, quite a bit of pain, slight constipation, mild tension and little depression. Lastly before her treatment, she completed the *EORTC QLQ*-LC13, which additionally showed that she had slight hair loss and a noticeable amount of pain in her groin.

Over the course of the treatment, the patient did not take any pain medications. Her hemoptysis became slightly worse at the start of treatment, but improved back to baseline (as measured by her diary) by the 3rd day. Her coughing also improved by the 3rd day. Throughout her treatment, the patient notes that her symptoms did not interfere with her daily activities at all except for the days in which her hemoptysis worsened. On the last day of treatment, The EORTC QLQ-LC13 showed that the pain that was in her groin moved to her abdomen but to a lesser extent, while other complaints had not exacerbated except for nausea, constipation, tension, and depression, all of which improved. Overall, she ranked her quality of life 1 grade higher on this test than the one at baseline point for a score of 7/7.

By the third day post-treatment, the hemoptysis stopped as recorded in her diary. Only by the 6th day after treatment did the patient start noticing an improvement in her acute toxicity symptoms compared to the start of treatment. Approximately a week after the radiation treatment ended, the patient again took the *EORTC QLQ*-C15-PAL, which revealed that there was an improvement in all complaints except for fatigue. She also re-took the *EORTC QLQ*-LC13 as well, which showed a great progression in her abdominal/groin pain, while the hair loss and coughing still persisted. She also maintained her abstinence from pain medications.

Case #5

The fifth patient is a 78 year-old male who was diagnosed with primary lung cancer, metastatic to other parts of the lung and was referred due to coughing and hemoptysis. He was treated with EBRT with dosage of 20 Gy/5 fr to the lower lobes of the lung. At the baseline, his diary entry showed that he had slight coughing accompanied by slight hemoptysis. He also took the *EORTC QLQ*-C15-PAL, which showed that this patient was very weak and fatigued, had much trouble with short walks, lacked appetite, had constipation and was quite depressed. He graded his quality of life a 4/7. Lastly before treatment, he took the *EORTC QLQ*-LC13, which only showed that he was experiencing a large amount of coughing.

Over the entire course of treatment, coughing was apparent and the patient took neither medication nor oxygen. He developed hemoptysis and slight dyspnea, which both went away near the end of treatment. During the days that he felt hemoptysis and slight dyspnea, he noted that his symptoms were in a worse state than at baseline, however after both of the symptoms subsided, he claimed that his symptoms were in the same state as before treatment. On the last day, the patient repeated the *EORTC QLQ*-C15-PAL and the *EORTC QLQ*-LC13 surveys, which presented an improvement in his cough and hemoptysis. However, the tests also displayed a slight regression in his dyspnea and the emergence of slight dysphagia. In addition, the patient considered his quality of life to be the same as it was at baseline point.

After treatment, he still abstained from pain medications and initially felt better with no symptoms. However, he experienced a brief cough and dyspnea in the first few days post-treatment, as well as significant dysphagia near the end of the diary entries.

Approximately a month after the treatment had ended, the patient repeated the *EORTC QLQ*-C15-PAL and the *EORTC QLQ*-LC13, which showed that he became slightly tense and quite depressed. He also perceived his cough to be much worse however; his dyspnea and dysphagia seemed to both have improved. Again, the patient saw no change in his quality of life.

Discussion

Emphasis on palliation is imperative in the treatment of advanced lung cancer patients in light of the incurable nature of the disease as well as the symptom burden it carries. Keeping that in mind, all treatments should ideally foster benefits and lighten that burden and should therefore have no acute toxicities. This report focuses on solely EBRT as the treatment of choice, which functions by prompting tumor regression and thus alleviating most of the patients' lung symptoms (3). However, EBRT is also known to bear acute toxicities, the most common being: coughing, hemoptysis, dysphagia, chest pain and dyspnea, all of which can potentially introduce a diminished QOL post-treatment as they may often conflict with the lung cancer patients' pre-treatment symptoms, which most commonly consist of: fatigue, pain, appetite loss, dyspnea and chest pain (4).

Out of the common pre-treatment symptoms mentioned above, coughing and fatigue were found to be the most prominent, both affecting four out of five patients. The two symptoms were followed by dyspnea and pain, which were apparent in three of five patients. Lastly, appetite loss seemed to have been a pre-treatment symptom for only one patient. These findings are consistent with those of Langendijk et al, who found that the most common pre-treatment symptom is fatigue, followed by cough, dyspnea, pain, and appetite loss respectively (4).

A notable trend was found when assessing the patients while they received their treatment. Coughing was apparent as a pre-treatment symptom in the third, fourth and fifth patient, and persisted as an acute treatment toxicity as well. It had also slightly developed within the first and second patient who had no initial complaints of coughing. These findings are coherent with those of Sundstrom et al who discovered that a mere 20% of patients with advanced non-small-cell lung carcinoma (NSCLC) found that their cough progressed after receiving radiotherapy (5), implying that only a small percentage of patients find radiotherapy to be effective in improving their cough. However, Sundstrom et al. also contrasts this idea in the same study as they discovered that clinicians found that cough was improved amongst 40-55% of NSCLC patients within their sample size (5). This contrast presents the highly scrutinized discrepancy between patient-assessed and clinician-assessed symptoms – thus, the fact that all assessments were subjective to the five patients may have presented a limitation to this report.

The second most common acute toxicity during treatment was hemoptysis, which was present in four of the five patients. However, hemoptysis was found to be temporary and merely lasted for a maximum of three days during treatment time. Hemoptysis was followed by dyspnea and dysphagia, the latter of which both affected three patients. Dyspnea was shown to disappear eventually in two of its three cases. Dysphagia, on the other hand, persisted in all three of its cases, which is in parallel with the findings of Falk et al. who found that dysphagia was the most common adverse effect amongst patients over a time span of over a year post-treatment (6).

Furthermore, post treatment assessments showed that in general, overall symptoms had subsided, while overall QOL had increased; three of five cases showed symptom palliation, one displayed no change in QOL but the emergence of a slight cough and lastly, another case showed an actual decline with the appearance of many acute toxicities post-treatment. All patients who experienced hemoptysis during treatment did not experience it within the ten days post-treatment and symptoms such as coughing, dyspnea, pain, and lack of appetite tended to improve or disappear completely. An exception was the third patient, who had a slight improvement in some symptoms, such as dyspnea, cough, and soreness in the throat, but symptoms such as nausea, fatigue, dysphagia, chest and back pain, and depression exacerbated. The extent of her pain post-treatment led her to replace her use of Advil and Dexamethasone with Tylenol 3. The significance of these findings is still controversial, in that different studies have found that patients have taken to EBRT in different ways. Sundstrom et al (5) found that up to 90% of patients will benefit from the effects of EBRT in reducing cough and hemoptysis, while Falk et al (6) found no statistically significant evidence that palliative thoracic radiotherapy had any beneficial effect to thoracic symptoms such as cough, hemoptysis, or dyspnea. However, the post-treatment symptoms found in this case study cannot be considered definitive as they were only assessed over the course of ten days. A longer analysis of the patients' symptoms post-treatment may have yielded different results, which is justified by Auchter et al (7) who have shown that overall toxicity scores in patients with advanced NSCLC have been seen to initially reduce post-treatment, but then increase past baseline thereafter, implying that EBRT benefits may only be temporary.

Within this case series, we found that it could not be concluded that the change in the patients' symptom burden was a direct product of the EBRT as our sample size was far too small thus; a conclusion could not be drawn regarding the actual effects of EBRT within this patient population. In addition, EBRT specifically targets local pulmonary symptom control. With this, we could not surmise that the persistence or alleviation of systemic symptoms such as nausea, fatigue, loss of appetite or constipation was a consequence of the treatment but rather, it could be hypothesized that it may have been due to the extra-thoracic spread of their disease. Ultimately, this case report highlights the necessity for further, more rigorous clinical trials to provide more in-depth and accurate evaluation of the toxicities and effects of EBRT within this patient population.

Acknowledgments

We thank the generous support of Bratty Family Fund, Michael and Karyn Goldstein Cancer Research Fund, Joseph and Silvana Melara Cancer Research Fund, and Ofelia Cancer Research Fund.

References

[1]   Mallick I, Sharma SC, Behera D. Endobronchial brachytherapy for symptom palliation in non-small cell lung cancer-Analysis of symptom response, endoscopic improvement and quality of life. Lung Cancer 2007;55(3):313-8.

[2]   Bezjak A. Palliative therapy for lung cancer. Semin Surg Oncol 2003;21(2):138-47.

[3]   Janjan NA. Radiation for bone metastases. Cancer 1997;80:1628-45.

[4]   Langendijk JA, Ten Velde GPM, Aaronson NK, De Jong JMA, Muller MJ, Wouters EFM. Quality of life after palliative radiotherapy in non-small cell lung cancer: A prospective study. Int J Radiat Oncol Biol Phys 2000;47(1):149-55.

[5]   Sundstrom S, Bremnes R, Aasebo U, et al. Hypofractionated palliative radiotherapy (17 Gy per two fractions) in advanced non-small-cell lung carcinoma is comparable to standard fractionation for symptom control and survival: a national phase III trial. Am J Clin Oncol 2004;22(5):801-10.

[6]   Falk SJ, Girling DJ, White RJ, et al. Immediate versus delayed palliative thoracic radiotherapy in patients with unresectable locally advanced non-small cell lung cancer and minimal thoracic symptoms: Randomised controlled trial. BMJ 2002;325(7362):465-8.

[7]   Auchter RM, Scholtens D, Adak S, Wagner H, Cella DF, Mehta MP. Quality of life assessment in advanced non-small-cell lung cancer patients undergoing an accelerated radiotherapy regimen: Report of ECOG Study 4593. Int J Radiat Oncol Biol Phys 2001;50(5):1199-206.

SECTION SEVEN: ACKNOWLEDGMENTS

In: Advanced Cancer
Editors: N. Thavarajah, N. Pulenzas, B. Lechner et al.

ISBN: 978-1-62808-239-5

© 2013 Nova Science Publishers, Inc.

Chapter 42

About the editors

Natalie Pulenzas, BSc(C) is a clinical research assistant in the Rapid Response Radiotherapy Program at the Odette Cancer Centre, Sunnybrook Health Sciences Centre, Toronto, Canada and also an undergraduate student at the University of Waterloo. She was awarded an Applied Health Sciences Undergraduate Scholarship from the University of Waterloo in 2013 for academic excellence. E-mail: Natalie.Pulenzas@sunnybrook.ca

Breanne Lechner, BSc(C) is a clinical research assistant in the Rapid Response Radiotherapy Program at the Odette Cancer Centre, Sunnybrook Health Sciences Centre, Toronto, Canada and also an undergraduate student at the University of Waterloo. She was the recepient of the J. Frank Brookfield Scholarship from the University of Waterloo in 2012 for excellence in biology. E-mail: breanne.lechner@sunnybrook.ca

Nemica Thavarajah, BSc(C) is a clinical research assistant in the Rapid Response Radiotherapy Program at the Odette Cancer Centre, Sunnybrook Health Sciences Centre, Toronto, Canada and also an undergraduate student at the University of Waterloo. She was awarded the 2012 Marion J. Todd award and Co-op Student of the Year award from the University of Waterloo for high achievment in health related research during her co-operative work terms. E-mail: nemica.thavarajah@hotmail.com

Edward Chow, MBBS, MSc, PhD, FRCPC is professor of radiation oncology at the University of Toronto in Canada. He is the chair of the Rapid Response Radiotherapy Program and Bone Metastases Site Group at the Odette Cancer Centre, Sunnybrook Health Sciences Centre, Toronto, Canada and also a senior scientist at the Sunnybrook Research Institute. He has published in the area of palliative radiotherapy and end of life care issues. E-mail: Edward.Chow@sunnybrook.ca

Joav Merrick, MD, MMedSci, DMSc, is professor of pediatrics, child health and human development affiliated with Kentucky Children's Hospital, University of Kentucky, Lexington, United States and the Division of Pediatrics, Hadassah Hebrew University Medical Center, Mt Scopus Campus, Jerusalem, Israel, the medical director of the Health Services, Division for Intellectual and Developmental Disabilities, Ministry of Social Affairs and Social Services, Jerusalem, the founder and director of the National Institute of Child Health and Human Development in Israel. Numerous publications in the field of pediatrics, child health and human development, rehabilitation, intellectual disability, disability, health, welfare, abuse, advocacy, quality of life and prevention. Received the Peter Sabroe Child

Award for outstanding work on behalf of Danish Children in 1985 and the International LEGO-Prize ("The Children's Nobel Prize") for an extraordinary contribution towards improvement in child welfare and well-being in 1987. E-mail: jmerrick@zahav.net.il

Acknowledgments

The editors want to acknowledge Stacy Yuen BA, CMS, Sunnybrook Health Sciences and Odette Cancer Centre, Department of Radiation Oncology, Toronto, Canada, administrative assistant to Edward Chow for her dedication, effective work and handling of the logistic work around the creation of this book.

In: Advanced Cancer
Editors: N. Thavarajah, N. Pulenzas, B. Lechner et al.

ISBN: 978-1-62808-239-5
© 2013 Nova Science Publishers, Inc.

Chapter 43

About the Rapid Response Radiotherapy Program at the Odette Cancer Centre, Sunnybrook Health Sciences Centre, Toronto, Canada

The Odette Cancer Centre, the comprehensive cancer program of Sunnybrook Health Sciences Centre is a leading regional cancer centre in Toronto, Ontario, Canada. It is the sixth largest cancer centre in North America in terms of number of new cancer patients seen per year. The Department of Radiation Oncology at Sunnybrook is an academic unit fully affiliated with the University of Toronto. Palliative radiotherapy is one of the key research foci in the Department of Radiation Oncology. The Rapid Response Radiotherapy Program (RRRP) is a specialized clinic designed to provide timely palliative radiotherapy. The RRRP was developed in 1996, and approximately 500-600 patients are seen in one year. This program aims to improve the quality of life of palliative cancer patients, while decreasing wait time and allowing for same day treatment.

Contact:
Professor Edward Chow, MBBS, PhD, FRCPC, Department of Radiation Oncology, Odette Cancer Centre, Sunnybrook Health Sciences Centre, 2075 Bayview Avenue, Toronto, Ontario, Canada M4N 3M5. E-mail: Edward.Chow@sunnybrook.ca

In: Advanced Cancer   ISBN: 978-1-62808-239-5
Editors: N. Thavarajah, N. Pulenzas, B. Lechner et al.   © 2013 Nova Science Publishers, Inc.

Chapter 44

About the National Institute of Child Health and Human Development in Israel

The National Institute of Child Health and Human Development (NICHD) in Israel was established in 1998 as a virtual institute under the auspicies of the Medical Director, Ministry of Social Affairs and Social Services in order to function as the research arm for the Office of the Medical Director. In 1998 the National Council for Child Health and Pediatrics, Ministry of Health and in 1999 the Director General and Deputy Director General of the Ministry of Health endorsed the establishment of the NICHD. In 2011 the NICHD became affiliated with the Division of Pediatrics, Hadassah Hebrew University Medical Center, Mt Scopus Campus in Jerusalem.

Mission

The mission of a National Institute for Child Health and Human Development in Israel is to provide an academic focal point for the scholarly interdisciplinary study of child life, health, public health, welfare, disability, rehabilitation, intellectual disability and related aspects of human development. This mission includes research, teaching, clinical work, information and public service activities in the field of child health and human development.

Service and academic activities

Over the years many activities became focused in the south of Israel due to collaboration with various professionals at the Faculty of Health Sciences (FOHS) at the Ben Gurion University of the Negev (BGU). Since 2000 an affiliation with the Zusman Child Development Center at the Pediatric Division of Soroka University Medical Center has resulted in collaboration around the establishment of the Down Syndrome Clinic at that center. In 2002 a full course on "Disability" was established at the Recanati School for Allied Professions in the Community, FOHS, BGU and in 2005 collaboration was started with the Primary Care Unit of the faculty and disability became part of the master of public health course on "Children and society". In the academic year 2005-2006 a one semester course on "Aging with disability" was started as part of the master of science program in gerontology in our collaboration with the Center for Multidisciplinary Research in Aging. In 2010 collaborations with the Division of Pediatrics, Hadassah Hebrew University Medical Center, Jerusalem, Israel around the National Down Syndrome Center and teaching students and residents about intellectual and developmental disabilities as part of their training at this campus.

Research activities

The affiliated staff have over the years published work from projects and research activities in this national and international collaboration. In the year 2000 the International Journal of Adolescent Medicine and Health and in 2005 the International Journal on Disability and Human Development of De Gruyter Publishing House (Berlin and New York) were affiliated with the National Institute of Child Health and Human Development. From 2008 also the International Journal of Child Health and Human Development (Nova Science, New York), the International Journal of Child and Adolescent Health (Nova Science) and the Journal of Pain Management (Nova Science) affiliated and from 2009 the International Public Health Journal (Nova Science) and Journal of Alternative Medicine Research (Nova Science). All peer-reviewed international journals.

National collaborations

Nationally the NICHD works in collaboration with the Faculty of Health Sciences, Ben Gurion University of the Negev; Department of Physical Therapy, Sackler School of Medicine, Tel Aviv University; Autism Center, Assaf HaRofeh Medical Center; National Rett and PKU Centers at Chaim Sheba Medical Center, Tel HaShomer; Department of Physiotherapy, Haifa University; Department of Education, Bar Ilan University, Ramat Gan, Faculty of Social Sciences and Health Sciences; College of Judea and Samaria in Ariel and in 2011 affiliation with Center for Pediatric Chronic Diseases and National Center for Down Syndrome, Department of Pediatrics, Hadassah Hebrew University Medical Center, Mount Scopus Campus, Jerusalem.

International collaborations

Internationally with the Department of Disability and Human Development, College of Applied Health Sciences, University of Illinois at Chicago; Strong Center for Developmental Disabilities, Golisano Children's Hospital at Strong, University of Rochester School of Medicine and Dentistry, New York; Centre on Intellectual Disabilities, University of Albany, New York; Centre for Chronic Disease Prevention and Control, Health Canada, Ottawa; Chandler Medical Center and Children's Hospital, Kentucky Children's Hospital, Section of

Adolescent Medicine, University of Kentucky, Lexington; Chronic Disease Prevention and Control Research Center, Baylor College of Medicine, Houston, Texas; Division of Neuroscience, Department of Psychiatry, Columbia University, New York; Institute for the Study of Disadvantage and Disability, Atlanta; Center for Autism and Related Disorders, Department Psychiatry, Children's Hospital Boston, Boston; Department of Paediatrics, Child Health and Adolescent Medicine, Children's Hospital at Westmead, Westmead, Australia; International Centre for the Study of Occupational and Mental Health, Düsseldorf, Germany; Centre for Advanced Studies in Nursing, Department of General Practice and Primary Care, University of Aberdeen, Aberdeen, United Kingdom; Quality of Life Research Center, Copenhagen, Denmark; Nordic School of Public Health, Gottenburg, Sweden, Scandinavian Institute of Quality of Working Life, Oslo, Norway; The Department of Applied Social Sciences (APSS) of The Hong Kong Polytechnic University Hong Kong.

Targets

Our focus is on research, international collaborations, clinical work, teaching and policy in health, disability and human development and to establish the NICHD as a permanent institute at one of the residential care centers for persons with intellectual disability in Israel in order to conduct model research and together with the four university schools of public health/medicine in Israel establish a national master and doctoral program in disability and human development at the institute to secure the next generation of professionals working in this often non-prestigious/low-status field of work.

Contact:

Joav Merrick, MD, DMSc

Professor of Pediatrics, Child Health and Human Development

Medical Director, Health Services, Division for Intellectual and Developmental Disabilities, Ministry of Social Affairs and Social Services, POB 1260, IL-91012 Jerusalem, Israel.

E-mail: jmerrick@zahav.net.il

In: Advanced Cancer
ISBN: 978-1-62808-239-5
Editors: N. Thavarajah, N. Pulenzas, B. Lechner et al.   © 2013 Nova Science Publishers, Inc.

Chapter 45

About the book series "Health and Human Development"

Health and human development is a book series with publications from a multidisciplinary group of researchers, practitioners and clinicians for an international professional forum interested in the broad spectrum of health and human development. Books already published:

- Merrick J, Omar HA, eds. Adolescent behavior research. International perspectives. New York: Nova Science, 2007.
- Kratky KW. Complementary medicine systems: Comparison and integration. New York: Nova Science, 2008.
- Schofield P, Merrick J, eds. Pain in children and youth. New York: Nova Science, 2009.
- Greydanus DE, Patel DR, Pratt HD, Calles Jr JL, eds. Behavioral pediatrics, 3 ed. New York: Nova Science, 2009.
- Ventegodt S, Merrick J, eds. Meaningful work: Research in quality of working life. New York: Nova Science, 2009.
- Omar HA, Greydanus DE, Patel DR, Merrick J, eds. Obesity and adolescence. A public health concern. New York: Nova Science, 2009.
- Lieberman A, Merrick J, eds. Poverty and children. A public health concern. New York: Nova Science, 2009.
- Goodbread J. Living on the edge. The mythical, spiritual and philosophical roots of social marginality. New York: Nova Science, 2009.
- Bennett DL, Towns S, Elliot E, Merrick J, eds. Challenges in adolescent health: An Australian perspective. New York: Nova Science, 2009.
- Schofield P, Merrick J, eds. Children and pain. New York: Nova Science, 2009.
- Sher L, Kandel I, Merrick J, eds. Alcohol-related cognitive disorders: Research and clinical perspectives. New York: Nova Science, 2009.
- Anyanwu EC. Advances in environmental health effects of toxigenic mold and mycotoxins. New York: Nova Science, 2009.

- Bell E, Merrick J, eds. Rural child health. International aspects. New York: Nova Science, 2009.
- Dubowitz H, Merrick J, eds. International aspects of child abuse and neglect. New York: Nova Science, 2010.
- Shahtahmasebi S, Berridge D. Conceptualizing behavior: A practical guide to data analysis. New York: Nova Science, 2010.
- Wernik U. Chance action and therapy. The playful way of changing. New York: Nova Science, 2010.
- Omar HA, Greydanus DE, Patel DR, Merrick J, eds. Adolescence and chronic illness. A public health concern. New York: Nova Science, 2010.
- Patel DR, Greydanus DE, Omar HA, Merrick J, eds. Adolescence and sports. New York: Nova Science, 2010.
- Shek DTL, Ma HK, Merrick J, eds. Positive youth development: Evaluation and future directions in a Chinese context. New York: Nova Science, 2010.
- Shek DTL, Ma HK, Merrick J, eds. Positive youth development: Implementation of a youth program in a Chinese context. New York: Nova Science, 2010.
- Omar HA, Greydanus DE, Tsitsika AK, Patel DR, Merrick J, eds. Pediatric and adolescent sexuality and gynecology: Principles for the primary care clinician. New York: Nova Science, 2010.
- Chow E, Merrick J, eds. Advanced cancer. Pain and quality of life. New York: Nova Science, 2010.
- Latzer Y, Merrick, J, Stein D, eds. Understanding eating disorders. Integrating culture, psychology and biology. New York: Nova Science, 2010.
- Sahgal A, Chow E, Merrick J, eds. Bone and brain metastases: Advances in research and treatment. New York: Nova Science, 2010.
- Postolache TT, Merrick J, eds. Environment, mood disorders and suicide. New York: Nova Science, 2010.
- Maharajh HD, Merrick J, eds. Social and cultural psychiatry experience from the Caribbean Region. New York: Nova Science, 2010.
- Mirsky J. Narratives and meanings of migration. New York: Nova Science, 2010.
- Harvey PW. Self-management and the health care consumer. New York: Nova Science, 2011.
- Ventegodt S, Merrick J. Sexology from a holistic point of view. New York: Nova Science, 2011.
- Ventegodt S, Merrick J. Principles of holistic psychiatry: A textbook on holistic medicine for mental disorders. New York: Nova Science, 2011.
- Greydanus DE, Calles Jr JL, Patel DR, Nazeer A, Merrick J, eds. Clinical aspects of psychopharmacology in childhood and adolescence. New York: Nova Science, 2011.
- Bell E, Seidel BM, Merrick J, eds. Climate change and rural child health. New York: Nova Science, 2011.
- Bell E, Zimitat C, Merrick J, eds. Rural medical education: Practical strategies. New York: Nova Science, 2011.
- Latzer Y, Tzischinsky. The dance of sleeping and eating among adolescents: Normal and pathological perspectives. New York: Nova Science, 2011.

- Deshmukh VD. The astonishing brain and holistic consciousness: Neuroscience and Vedanta perspectives. New York: Nova Science, 2011.
- Bell E, Westert GP, Merrick J, eds. Translational research for primary healthcare. New York: Nova Science, 2011.
- Shek DTL, Sun RCF, Merrick J, eds. Drug abuse in Hong Kong: Development and evaluation of a prevention program. New York: Nova Science, 2011.
- Ventegodt S, Hermansen TD, Merrick J. Human Development: Biology from a holistic point of view. New York: Nova Science, 2011.
- Ventegodt S, Merrick J. Our search for meaning in life. New York: Nova Science, 2011.
- Caron RM, Merrick J, eds. Building community capacity: Minority and immigrant populations. New York: Nova Science, 2012.
- Klein H, Merrick J, eds. Human immunodeficiency virus (HIV) research: Social science aspects. New York: Nova Science, 2012.
- Lutzker JR, Merrick J, eds. Applied public health: Examining multifaceted Social or ecological problems and child maltreatment. New York: Nova Science, 2012.
- Chemtob D, Merrick J, eds. AIDS and tuberculosis: Public health aspects. New York: Nova Science, 2012.
- Ventegodt S, Merrick J. Textbook on evidence-based holistic mind-body medicine: Basic principles of healing in traditional Hippocratic medicine. New York: Nova Science, 2012.
- Ventegodt S, Merrick J. Textbook on evidence-based holistic mind-body medicine: Holistic practice of traditional Hippocratic medicine. New York: Nova Science, 2012.
- Ventegodt S, Merrick J. Textbook on evidence-based holistic mind-body medicine: Healing the mind in traditional Hippocratic medicine. New York: Nova Science, 2012.
- Ventegodt S, Merrick J. Textbook on evidence-based holistic mind-body medicine: Sexology and traditional Hippocratic medicine. New York: Nova Science, 2012.
- Ventegodt S, Merrick J. Textbook on evidence-based holistic mind-body medicine: Research, philosophy, economy and politics of traditional Hippocratic medicine. New York: Nova Science, 2012.
- Caron RM, Merrick J, eds. Building community capacity: Skills and principles. New York: Nova Science, 2012.
- Lemal M, Merrick J, eds. Health risk communication. New York: Nova Science, 2012.
- Ventegodt S, Merrick J. Textbook on evidence-based holistic mind-body medicine: Basic philosophy and ethics of traditional Hippocratic medicine. New York: Nova Science, 2013.
- Caron RM, Merrick J, eds. Building community capacity: Case examples from around the world. New York: Nova Science, 2013.
- Steele RE. Managed care in a public setting. New York: Nova Science, 2013.
- Srabstein JC, Merrick J, eds. Bullying: A public health concern. New York: Nova Science, 2013.

Contact:
Professor Joav Merrick, MD, MMedSci, DMSc
Medical Director, Health Services
Division for Intellectual and Developmental Disabailities
Ministry of Social Affairs and Social Services
POBox 1260, IL-91012 Jerusalem, Israel
E-mail: jmerrick@zahav.net.il

SECTION EIGHT: INDEX

Index

E

F

N

O

S

T